Cholangiocarcinoma

Editor Jae Bock Chung

The Korean Society of Pancreatobiliary Diseases

KOON JA PUBLISHING INC.

KOONJA PUBLISHING INC.
3F Dongwon B/D 112-1,
Inui-dong Jongno-gu,
Seoul, Korea 110-717

Cholangiocarcinoma
Editor Jae Bock Chung

For permission to use material from this text or product, contact us by
Tel (822) 762-9194
Fax (822) 764-0209
admin@koonja.co.kr
www.Koonja.co.kr

Printed in The Republic of Korea.
ISBN 978-89-6278-036-9

Foreword

Publishing an expert book about cholangiocarcinoma is meaningful for doctors who study pancreatobiliary field and treat patients with pancreatobiliary diseases.

Among many digestive tract diseases, incidence rate of cholangiocarcinoma in Asian countries including the South Korea is especially higher than western countries. Various new treatments of cholangiocarcinoma have developed in the South Korea. And internationally released papers are also outstanding in the South Korea. So, we think that it is meaningful and our responsibility to publish an expert book about cholangiocarcinoma in English.

Korean Society of Pancreatobiliary Diseases is publishing English version of 'Cholangiocarcinoma' by help of authoritative professors for two years under the leadership of former president Jae Bock Chung, M.D..

With authors' ample experiences, we organized wide range of up-to-date medical information about cholangiocarcinoma in detail.

We sincerely hope that this book will be helpful to people not only in the field of education and research but doctors, so that they can give practical help to patients with cholangiocarcinoma.

Finally, I would like to thank to authors of this book and board members of the Korean Society of Pancreatobiliary Diseases for their sustained efforts.

Sun-Joo Kim, M.D.
President
Korean Society of Pancreatobiliary Diseases

Preface

Cholangiocarcinoma is a relatively rare neoplasm of the bile ducts which is increasing in incidence. Approximately 3~10% of resected bile duct cancers have been reported to be early cancers in the literature. The development of endoscopic techniques (ERCP, EUS and PTCS) and cross sectional imagings (MRI, MDCT and PET-CT) has markedly improved diagnostic accuracy and staging of cholangiocarcinoma. But, unfortunately, the majority of patients present with unresectable disease at the time of diagnosis.

This book attempts to review all medical and surgical aspects of cholangiocarcinoma in a systematic manner. The anatomy and development of the biliary duct, classification, etiology and risk factors, epidemiology, histopathology, pathogenesis, diagnostic modalities, preoperative assessment for resectability, surgical and nonsurgical treatment including palliative treatments of cholangiocarcinoma are described. Special types of cholangiocarcinoma, such as mucin-producing cholangiocarcinoma, biliary papillomatosis, and Klatskin tumor are also included.

The goals of this book are to provide those who are studying cholangiocarcinoma with a chance of complete understanding; to present to the practicing physician the principles for the management of cholangiocarcinoma; and to give a stimulation to the student, resident, or fellow to continue to search for knowledge of cholangiocarcinoma.

I am deeply grateful to all authors for their painstaking writing and contributions to prepare a concise and informative book. The publisher have also made a significant contribution to this book and have turned out an impressive volume with illustration of the highest quality.

Seoul December 2008

J. B. Chung

Editorial Boards

Contributors

Ho Soon Choi, M.D., Ph.D.

Professor
Department of Internal Medicine
Hanyang University Medical Center
Seoul, Korea

Dong Hee Koh, M.D.

Department of Internal Medicine
Hanyang University Medical Center
Seoul, Korea

Yong-Tae Kim, M.D., Ph.D.

Professor
Division of Gastroenterology Department of Internal medicine Seoul National University College of Medicine
Seoul National University Hospital
Seoul, Korea

Ho Gak Kim, M.D.

Professor
Department of Internal Medicine,
Catholic University of Daegu School of Medicine,
Daegu, Korea

Jimin Han, M.D.

Department of Internal Medicine,
Catholic University of Daegu School of Medicine,
Daegu, Korea

Chang Duck Kim, M.D., Ph.D.

Professor
Department of Internal Medicine,
Korea University Anam Hospital
Seoul, Korea

So-Young Jin, M.D.

Professor
Department of Pathology
Soonchunhyang University Hospital
Seoul, Korea

Seungmin Bang, M.D.

Assistant professor
Department of Internal Medicine,
Yonsei University College of Medicine
Seoul, Korea

Kyung Sik Kim, M.D., Ph.D.

Associate Professor
Deparmennt of Surgery
Pancreatobiliary Cancer Special Clinic, Severance Hospital
Yonsei University College of Medicine
Seoul, Korea

Sae Byeol Choi, M.D.

Deparmennt of Surgery
Pancreatobiliary Cancer Special Clinic, Severance Hospital
Yonsei University College of Medicine
Seoul, Korea

Yong Bum Yoon, M.D., Ph.D.

Professor
Division of Gastroenterology Department of Internal medicine Seoul National University College of Medicine
Seoul National University Hospital
Seoul, Korea

Myeong-Jin Kim, M.D., Ph.D.

Professor
Department of Radiology
Yonsei University College of Medicine
Seoul, Korea

Yong Eun Chung, M.D.

Department of Radiology
Yonsei University College of Medicine
Seoul, Korea

Chan Sup Shim, M.D., Ph.D.

Professor
Institute for Digestive Research,
Department of Internal Medicine,
College of Medicine, Soon Chun Hyang University
Seoul, Korea

Dong Wan Seo, M.D.

Division of Gastroenterology
Department of Internal Medicine
Asan Medical Center
University of Ulsan College of Medicine
Seoul, Korea

Young Deok Cho, M.D.

Institute for Digestive Research,
Department of Internal Medicine,
College of Medicine, Soon Chun Hyang University
Seoul, Korea

Jae Bock Chung, M.D., Ph.D.

Professor
Department of Internal Medicine
Yonsei University College of Medicine
Seoul, Korea

Chang Mo Moon, M.D.

Department of Internal Medicine
Yonsei University College of Medicine
Seoul, Korea

Sun Whe Kim, M.D.

Professor
Department of Surgery,
Seoul National University College of Medicine
Seoul, Korea

Hee Jung Wang, M.D,

Professor
Department of Surgery, Ajou University School of Medicine
Suwon, Korea

Myung Wook Kim, M.D.

Professor
Department of Surgery, Ajou University School of Medicine
Suwon, Korea

Seungwoo Park, M.D., Ph.D.

Associate professor
Department of Internal Medicine,
Yonsei University College of Medicine
Seoul, Korea

Jinsil Seong, M.D., Ph.D.

Professor
Department of Radiation Oncology
Yonsei Cancer Center, Yonsei University College of Medicine
Seoul, Korea

Woong Sub Koom, M.D.

Department of Radiation Oncology
Yonsei Cancer Center, Yonsei University of Medicine College
Seoul, Korea

Young Koog Cheon, M.D.

Associate Professor
Institute for Digestive Research,
Department of Internal Medicine,
College of Medicine, Soon Chun Hyang University
Seoul, Korea

Jin Hong Kim, M.D., Ph.D.

Professor
Department of Gastroenterology, Ajou University School of Medicine
Suwon, Korea

Sung Koo Lee, M.D., Ph.D.

Professor
Division of Gastroenterology,
Department of Internal Medicine
Asan Medical center University of Ulsan College of Medicine
Seoul, Korea

DongKi Lee, M.D., Ph.D.

Professor
Department of Internal Medicine,
Youngdong Severance Hospital,
Yonsei University College of Medicine
Seoul, Korea

Myung-Hwan Kim, M.D

Professor
Division of Gastroenterology,
Department of Internal Medicine
Asan Medical center University of Ulsan College of Medicine
Seoul, Korea

Jae Myung Cha, M.D.

Division of Gastroenterology,
Department of Internal Medicine
Asan Medical center University of Ulsan College of Medicine

Contents

I. Anatomy and Development of the Biliary Tract

I Anatomy and Development of the Biliary Tract

Dong Hee Koh, M.D., Ho Soon Choi, M.D., Ph.D.

I

Anatomy and Development of the Biliary Tract

1. Development of the Liver and Biliary Tract

The liver primodium is formed in the third week of gestation as an outgrowth (known as the hepatic diverticulum or liver bud) of the endodermal epithelium at caudal part of the forgut (Fig. 1).[1] Before the hepatic diverticulum become recognizable, cardiac mesoderm induce the foregut endoderm to become a precursor of the hepatic epithelium by fibroblast growth factor signaling (FGF-1, FGF-2 and FGF-8) and joined with bone morphogenetic protein signaling (BMP-2, BMP-4 and BMP-7) from the septum transversum.[2,3] The hepatic diverticulum grows into the mesenchyme of septum transversum between the pericardial cavity and stalk of yolk sac (Fig. 1).[1] The transcription factors hepatocyte nuclear factor 3β (HNF3β) and GATA-4 are necessary for the development of the ventral foregut endoderm and hepatic gene expression.[2]

This outgrowth of the hepatic diverticulum consists of rapidly proliferating cells that penetrate the septum transversum. The homeodomain transcription factor Hex, which is expressed in the anterior endoderm and the hepatic diverticulum, are necessary for migration of hepatic progenitor cells into the septum transversum and undergoing liver morphogenesis.[5] Another homeodomain transcrtional factor HIx is expressed in visceral mesenchyme and required for hepatic progenitor cells proliferation.[5]

This diverticulum has a caudal and a cranial portion. The larger cranial part of the hepatic diverticulum is the primordium of the liver (Fig. 1). The proliferating

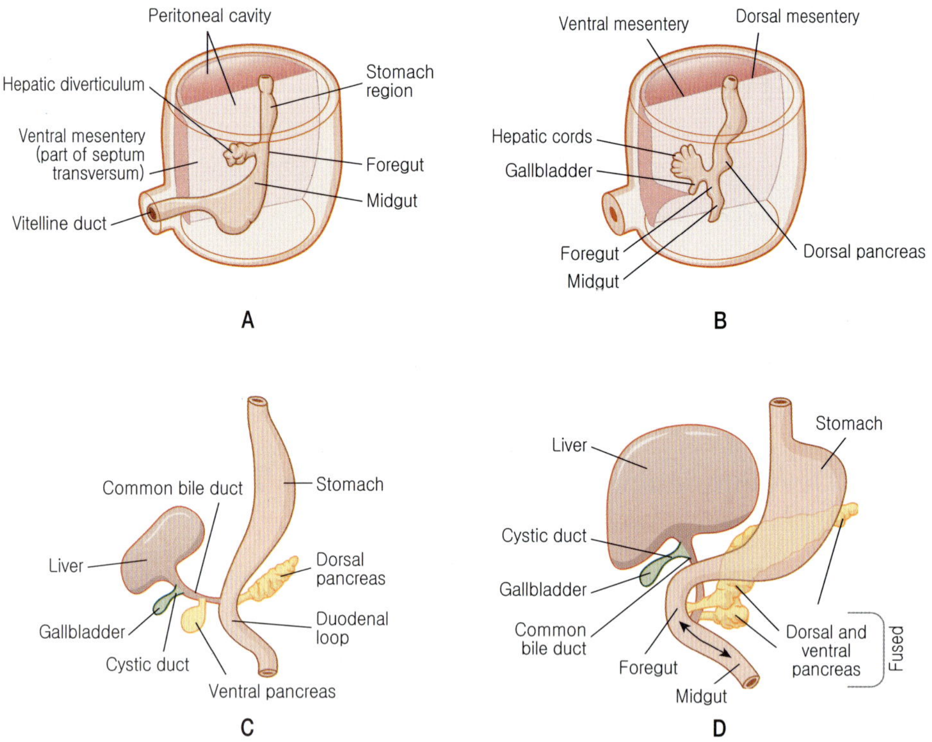

Fig. 1 Stages in the embryologic development of the liver, gallbladder, extrahepatic bile ducts, pancreas, and duodenum. A, 4 weeks; B and C, 5 weeks; D, 6 weeks. *(From Moore KL: The Developing Human. Philadelphia, WB Saunders, 1973.)*

endodermal cells give rise to interlacing cords of hepatic cells of liver parenchyma and to the epithelial lining of the intrahepatic bile duct. The fibrous and hematopoietic tissue and Kupffer cells of the liver are derived from mesenchyme in the septum transversum. The epithelial liver cords intermingle with the vitelline and umbilical veins, which form hepatic sinusoids. HNF4α in hepatocytes are necessary for develop the sinusoidal architecture.[6] The transcrtion factors Hes1, HNF6 and HNF1β, are necessary for gallbladder and bile duct development.[5,7,8]

The liver grows rapidly in size and comes to occupy the greater part of the abdominal cavity from the fifth to tenth weeks. The main hepatic bud and its right and left terminal branches become canalized to form the common hepatic duct and the right and left hepatic ducts. Initially, the right and left lobes are about the same size, but the right lobe soon becomes larger. The important role of fetal liver is hematopoesis. It begins during the sixth week, making the liver a bright red appearance. In the 10th week of gestation, the weight of the liver is approximately 10% of the total body weight, which is due to developing hepatic sinusoids and active hematopoiesis. During the last 2 months of intrauterine life, this activity gradually subsides and the weight of the liver is only 5% of the total body weight.[4,9]

The small caudal portion of hepatic diverticulum forms the gallbladder, and the stalk connecting the cystic duct. The transcription factor foxf1 participates in mesenchymal epithelial cell inductive signaling of gallbladder.[5] The stalk connecting the hepatic and the cystic ducts to the duodenum narrows and becomes the common bile duct. Due to growing and rotation of the duodenum, the entrance of the bile duct gradually shifts from the initial ventral aspect of the duodenum to the dorsal aspect of the duodenum (Fig. 1). At approximately the 12th week of gestation, the hepatocytes begin to produce bile, draining down the newly formed bile duct system and being stored in the gallbladder. The bile released the duodenum through the bile duct after the thirteenth week gives the meconium (intestinal content) a dark green color.[10]

Many minor variations in the shape of the bile duct and gallbladder occur, but these defects are of no clinical importance. One of the most serious malformations of biliary tract is biliary atresia. This occurs in 1:10,000 to 15,000 live birth.[9] Failure of the bile ducts to canalize during development cause atresia. Biliary atresia can any level from the tiny bile canaliculi to the major bile ducts. Jaundice appears soon after birth. Clay-colored stools and very dark colored urine are present. Surgical correction of the atresia should be attempted when possible. If the atresia cannot be corrected, the child may die of liver failure.

Agenesis of gallbladder without extrahepatic biliary atresia is very rare. It arises either because the outgrowth of cells from the hepatic bud fails to develop, resulting in the absence of both gallbladder and cystic duct, or as a result of lack of vacuolation of the epithelium leaving an atretic gallbladder, although the cystic duct may have been present.[11]

Another anomalies of gallbladder are duplication, partial subdivision, diverticulum and malposition of the gallbladder.

2. Anatomy of the Biliary Tract and Gallbladder

The biliary system is comprised of intrahepatic bile ducts, extrahepatic bile ducts, and the gallbladder. Extrahepatic bile duct is classified as perihilar or distal bile duct, and intrahepatic bile ducts are classified as either intrahepatic large or small bile ducts. Intrahepatic large bile ducts roughly correspond to ducts from the first to the fourth branches of the right and left hepatic ducts. Intrahepatic small bile ducts are further classified as septal bile ducts, interlobular bile ducts, or bile ductules according to their size and location. Microscopically, the wall of bile duct constitute with mucosa lined by cholangiocyte, fibromuscular layer consisted of intermixed dense fibrous tissue and muscle fibers, subserosa, and serosa, but muscularis mucosa, submucosa, and muscle layer are very scant or absent.

Bile is transported in the biliary ductal system. The length of the biliary ductal system in humans is about 2 kilometers. A layer of epithelial cells lines this extensive network. In general, cholangiocytes is defined as the epithelial cells that line the intrahepatic bile ducts. The extrahepatic ductal epithelial cells and gallbladder epithelial cells share many features of cholangiocytes.

The primary cell target of biliary disorders is the biliary epithelium. Cholangiocytes have many functions, not limited to bile production. Cholangiocytes are involved in transport processes that regulate the volume and composition of bile. Cholangiocytes undergo proliferation and cell death under a variety of conditions. Cholangiocytes have functional and morphological heterogenecity-not all cholangiocytes are the same functionally and morphologically. The immunobiology of the cholangiocyte is important, particulary to the understanding of biliary disease. Secretion of different pro-inflammatory mediators, cytokines, and chemokines indicates a major role of cholangiocytes in the inflammatory reaction. Furthermore, paracrine secretion of growth factors and peptides mediates an extensive cross-talk with other liver cells, including hepatocytes, stellate cells, and endothelial and inflammatory cells.

1) Intrahepatic bile duct

The right and left livers are drained by the right and the left hepatic ducts, whereas the caudate lobe is drained by several ducts joining both the right and left hepatic ducts (Fig. 2). The intrahepatic bile ducts are terminal branches of the main right and left hepatic ductal branches which invaginate Glisson's capsule at the hilum along with the corresponding portal vein and hepatic artery branches forming the portal triads. In the intrahepatic portal triad, the bile ducts are usually situated above the portal vein, whereas hepatic arterial branches are located inferiorly to the veins.[12]

The left hepatic ducts drains segment II, III, and IV, which constitute the left liver. The duct draining segment III run slightly behind the left horn of the umbilical recess and join with the ducts from segment II, IVb and IVa to form the main left duct at the point where the left branch of the portal vein turns forward and caudally. The left hepatic duct courses transversely beneath the left liver at the base of segment IV to join the right hepatic duct. In its transverse portion, the left hepatic duct drains one to three small branches from segmental IV (Fig. 3).

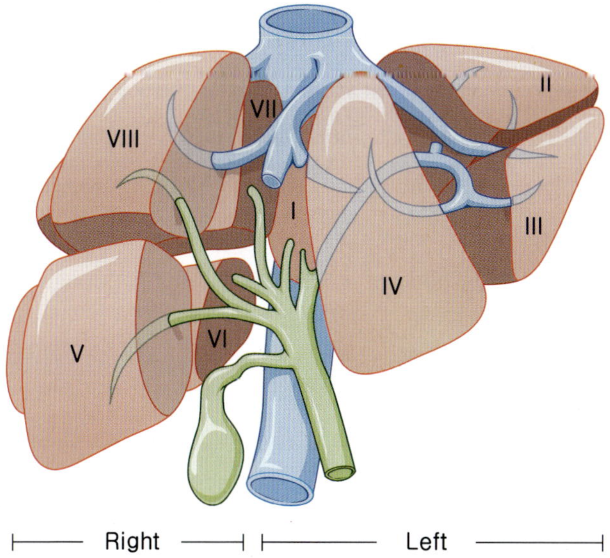

Fig. 2 Biliary drainage of the two functional hemilivers. The liver segment according to Couinaud's nomenclature.

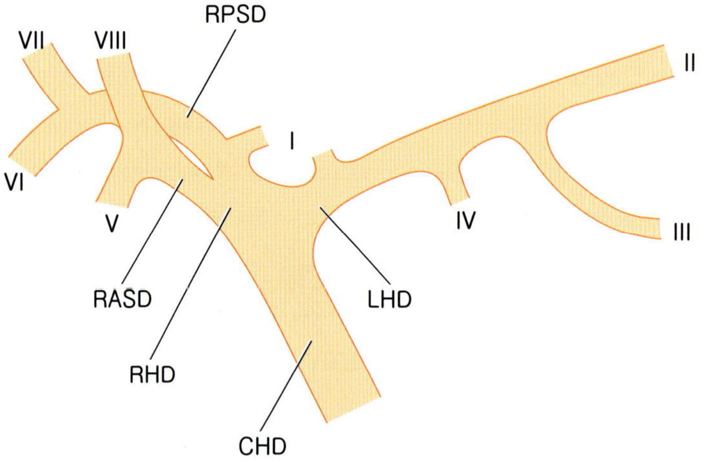

Fig. 3 Standard intrahepatic ductal anatomy.
CHD, common hepatic duct; LHD, left hepatic duct; RHD, right hepatic duct; RASD, right anterior sectoral duct; RPSD, right posterior sectoral duct.

The right hepatic duct drains segment V, VI, VII and VIII and is formed by the joining of the anterior sectoral duct (draining segments V and VIII) and posterior sectoral duct (draining segments VI and VII). The posterior sectoral duct runs in a horizontal and posterior direction and runs to join the anterior sectoral duct as it descends vertically. The junction of these two sectoral ducts usually occurs above the right branch of the portal vein. The short right hepatic duct joined the longer left hepatic duct in front of the right portal vein to form the common hepatic duct (Fig. 3).

The caudate lobe (segment I) has its own biliary drainage, which is usually through both right and left hepatic ducts, but in up to 15% of cases drainage is through the left hepatic ductal system only and in 5% it is through the right hepatic ductal system only.[13]

2) Extraheptic bile duct

The right and left hepatic ducts may join deep in the porta hepatis and form common hepatic duct, which is usually 3 cm long.[14] From the porta hepatis, the common hepatic duct runs along the right side of the hepatoduodenal ligament and lies on the right side of the hepatic artery in front of the portal vein.[15] The common hepatic duct constitutes the left border of triangle of Calot with the cystic duct and the inferior surface of the right lobe of the liver.[16] The common hepatic duct is joined by cystic duct to form the common bile duct (Fig. 4).

The walls of cystic, common hepatic and common bile duct constitute mucosa, submucosa, and muscularis. The mucosa of the bile ducts is lined by a single layer of columnar epithelium and contains numerous mucous-secreting glands.

The common bile duct is normally 0.5 to 1.5 cm in diameter and 7 cm long. Using ultrasound, the diameter is 2 to 7 mm, with diameter greater than 7 mm being regarded as abnormal. Using endoscopic cholangiography, the duct diameter is usually less than 11 mm, although it may be more without obstruction in postcholecystecomy state, old age or periampullary diverticulum.[17] The common bile

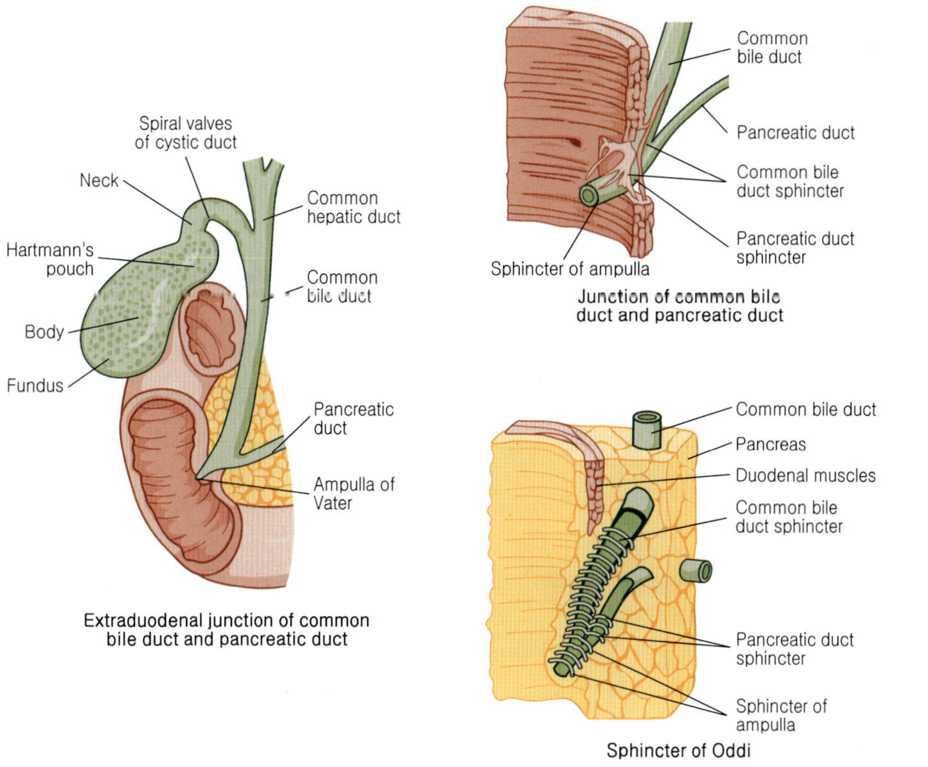

Fig. 4 Schematic representation of the gallbladder, the extrahepatic biliary tract, and the choledochoduodenal junction
(From Lindner HH: Clinical Anatomy. East Norwalk, CT, Appleton & Lange, 1989.)

duct course is divided according correlation of duodenum and pancreas. In the supraduodenal part of its course, It descends between layers of the lesser omentum and lies anterior to the portal vein and to the right of the hepatic artery.[18] In the retroduodenal part of its course, It is situated the first part of the duodenum to the right of the gastroduodenal artery. In the pancreatic part of its course, it lies in a groove or tunnel on the back of the head of the pancreas and enters the left of the posteromedial wall of the descending duodenum.

In the head of the pancreas, the common bile duct is joined by main pancreatic duct to form ampulla of Vater. The ampulla opens into the lumen of duodenum by means of a small papilla, the major duodenal papilla (Fig. 4). Fusion the two lumen usually occurs in the submucosal layer of the duodenum to form a common channel varying in length between 5 mm and 15 mm.[19] Occasionally, the common channel is longer than 15 mm, which is called anomalous union of pancreaticobiliary duct (AUPBD).[20] It often occur in association with choledochal cysts and results in a long common channel and free reflux of pancreatic secretions into the biliary tract. This reflux of pancreatic juice into the biliary tract results in increased biliary pressures and inflammatory changes in the biliary epithelium and may be related to the formation of choledochal cysts.

The junction of the terminal common bile duct, pancreatic duct, and duodenum at the papilla assumes one of three configurations (Fig. 5). In approximately 70% of subjects, the ducts join before entering the duodenum to open into papilla and have a Y-shape configuration. In approximately 20% of subjects, the common channel is

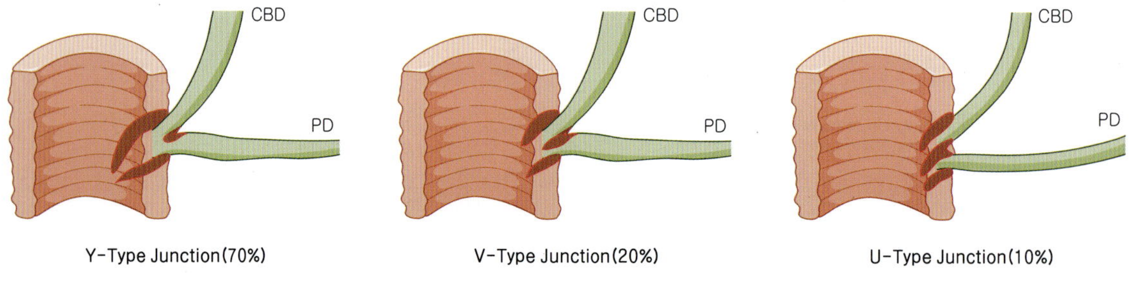

Fig. 5 Variation in the union of common bile duct and pancreatic duct.

almost nonexistent, and two ducts have a common V-shape opening on the papilla. In approximately 10% of subjects, the common bile duct and pancreatic duct have open separately on the tip of the papilla and have a U-shape configulation.[18]

In the duodenal wall, the bile duct and pancreatic ducts are surrounded by thickening of both longitudinal and circular muscle fibers derived from the intestine known as the sphincter of Oddi (Fig. 4). It regulates bile flow and prevents reflux of duodenal contents into the biliary tree. The longitudinal and circular muscles of the duodenum swing around the ducts to create potential weaknesses in duodenal wall. This is predisposing factor to duodenal diverticula.[21] All three sphincters are apparently independent of the muscle coat of the duodenum. The sphincter choledochus is a circular muscle surrounding the intramural portion of the common bile dcut before junction with pancreatic duct and serves to regulate bile flow and the filling of the gallbladder; the pancreatic sphincter, which is present to variable degrees and surrounds the intraduodenal pancreatic duct; and the sphincter ampulla, consisted of longitudinal muscle, serves to prevent duodenal reflux.[22]

The arterial blood supply to the supra-duodenal bile duct is generally by two main vessels which run beside the bile duct. These are supplied predominantly by the retro-duodenal artery from below, and the right hepatic artery from above, although many other vessels contribute. This pattern of arterial supply would explain why vascular damage results in bile duct stricturing.[23]

3) Gallbladder and cystic duct

The gallbladder is a storage reservoir which bile is concentrated and excretion to duodenum for the solubilization of dietary lipid. It lies on the undersurface of the right lobe of the liver within the cystic fossa and seperated from the liver by cystic plate that is an extension of the hilar plate.[12] The gallbladder varies in size but is usually about 7 cm long and 3 cm wide and has a capacity of 30 to 50 mL.[24] The gallbladder is composed of a fundus, body and neck (Fig. 4). The fundus usually projects beyond the inferior margin of the liver and is in the contact with the anterior abdominal wall just below the ninth costal cartilage. The body extends into a narrow neck which continues into the cystic duct. Hartmann's pouch is pouch like dilatation close to the neck of the gallbladder. This is common site for gallstone to lodge. Extensive inflammation in Hartman's pouch can lead to obstruction of adjacent common hepatic duct (Mirizzi's syndrome).[24] The gallbladder wall consist of a mucosa, lamina propria, tunica muscularis, and serosa. The peritoneum completely surrounds the fundus of the gallbladder and binds the body and neck to the visceral surface of the liver.

The cystic duct is usually 4 cm long and joins the common hepatic duct in its supraduodenal segment by angle. The course and union of cystic duct are variable such as anterior, posterior, spiral, or parallel (Fig. 6). The mucous membrane of gallbladder neck and cystic duct is arranged in spiral folds known as the valves of Heister, which regulate the filling and emptying of the gallbladder.

The source of blood supply of gallbladder is cystic artery, which usually arise from the right hepatic artery. The venous drainage is into cystic vein and thence into portal vein and, occasionally, directly into the hepatic sinusoids.[26]

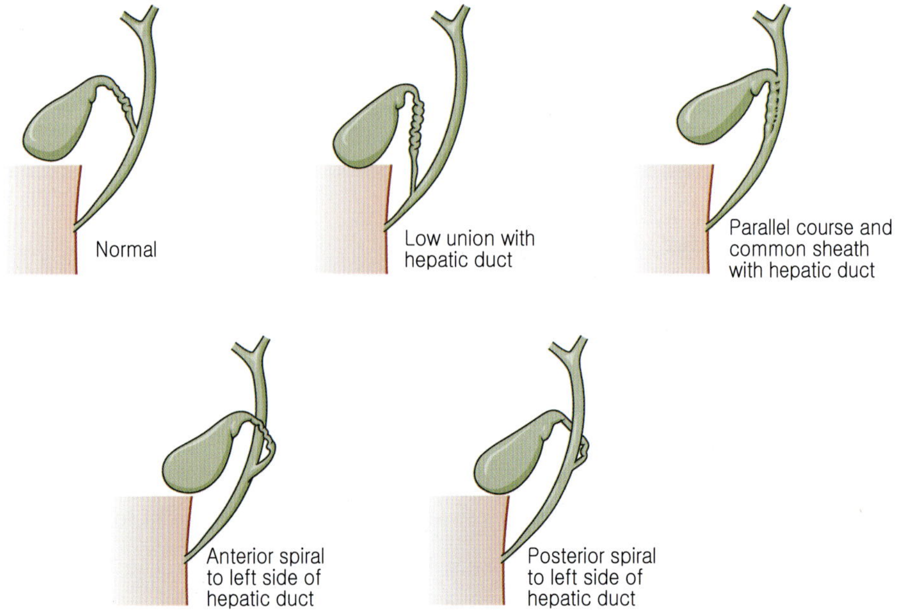

Fig. 6 Variation in cystic duct insertion.

Reference

1. Severn CB. A Morphological study of the development of the human liver. I. Development of the hepatic diverticulum. Am J Anat 1971;131:133-158.
2. Zaret KS. Liver specification and early morphogenesis. Mech Dev 2000;92:83-88.
3. Carlson BM. Human embryology and developmental biology. 3rd Ed. Philadelphia: Mosby, 2004.
4. Sadler TW. Langman's Medical Embryology. 6th Ed. Baltimore: Wiliams & Wilkins, 1990.
5. Costa RH, Kalinichenko VV, Holterman AX, Wang X. Transcription factors in liver development, differentiation, and regeneration. Hepatology 2003;38:1331-1347.
6. Parviz F, Matullo C, Garrison WD, et al. Hepatocyte nuclear factor 4alpha controls the development of a hepatic epithelium and liver morphogenesis. Nat Genet 2003;34:292-296.
7. Sumazaki R, Shiojiri N, Isoyama S, et al. Conversion of biliary system to pancreatic tissue in Hes1-deficient mice. Nat Genet 2004;36:83-87.
8. Clotman F, Lannoy VJ, Reber M, et al. The onecut transcription factor HNF6 is required for normal development of the biliary tract. Development 2002;129:1819-1828.
9. Moore KL, Persaud TVN. The developing human. 6th Ed. Philadelphia, WB Saunders, 1998.
10. Beath SV:Hepatic function and physiology in the newborn. Semin Neonatol 2003;8: 337-346.
11. Lamah M, Karanjia ND, Dickson GH. Anatomical variations of the extrahepatic biliary tree: Review of the world literature. Clin Anat 2001;14:167-172.
12. Blumgart LH. Surgery of the liver, Biliary tract, and Panceras. 4th ed. Philadelphia, Saunders Elsevier, 2007.
13. Healey Jr JE, Schroy PC. Anatomy of the biliary ducts within the human liver: Analysis of the prevailing pattern of branchings and the major variations of the biliary ducts. Arch Surg 1953;66:599-616.
14. Dowdy GS Jr, Waldron GW, Brown WG. Surgical anatomy of the pancreato-biliary ductal system. Arch Surg 1962;84:229-246.
15. Townsend CM, Beauchamp RD, Evers BM, Mattox KL. Sabiston textbook of surgery, 17th Ed. Philadelphia, Saunders Elsevier, 2004.
16. Wood M. Presidential address: Eponyms in biliary tract surgery. AM J Surg 1979;138: 746-754.
17. Sherlock SD, Dooley J. Diseases of the liver and biliary system. 11th ed. Malden, MA: Blackwell Science, 2002.
18. Adkins RB, Chapman WC, Reddy VS. Embryology, anatomy, and surgical applications of the extrahepatic biliary system. Surg Clin North Am 2000;80:363-379.

19. Wiedmeyer DA, Stewart ET, Dodds WJ, et al. Choledochal cyst: finding on cholangiopancreatography with emphasis on ectasia of the common channel. AJR Am J Roentgenol 1989;153:969-972.

20. Kim MH, Yoo BM, Seo DW et al. Choledochal cyst and anomalus union of pancreaticobiliary duct in adult. Korean J Gastrointest Endosc 1996;16:41-48.

21. Rosse C, Gaddum-Rosse P. Hollinshead's textbook of anatomy. 5th Ed. Philadelphia: Lippincott-Raven publisher, 1997.

22. Boyden EA. The anatomy of the choledochoduodenal junction in man. Surg Gynecol Obstet 1957;104:641-652.

23. Northover JM, Terblanche J. A new look at the arterial supply of the bile duct in man and its surgical implications. Br J surg 1979;66:379-384.

24. Frierson Jr HF. The gross anatomy and histology of the gallbladder, extrahepatic bile ducts, Vaterian system, and minor papilla. Am J Surg Pathol 1989;13:146.

25. Feldman M, Friedman LS, Brandt LJ. Sleisenger & Fordtran's Gastrointestinal and liver disease, 8th Ed. Philadelphia, WB Saunders, 2006.

26. Lee CM, Stewart L, Way LW. Postcholecystectomy abdominal bile collections. Arch Surg 2000;135:538-544.

II · Classification of Cholangicarcinoma

II · I Anatomic Location

Yong Tae Kim, M.D., Ph.D.

II · II Gross Morphology

Yong Tae Kim, M.D., Ph.D.

II·I
Anatomic Location

Cholangiocarcinoma is classified into extrahepatic and intrahepatic types. Intrahepatic cholangiocarcinoma originates at the second branch or the proximal branch of the bile duct. Extrahepatic cholangiocarcinoma is defined as that which originates at the first branch, lobular branch of the bile duct or at the common bile duct (Fig. 1).[1]

The extrahepatic cholangiocarcinoma is further divided into hilar, middle, and distal tumors according to its location in the biliary tree (Fig. 1). The hilar cholangiocarcinoma is also named as Klatskin tumor and occupies approximately 60%

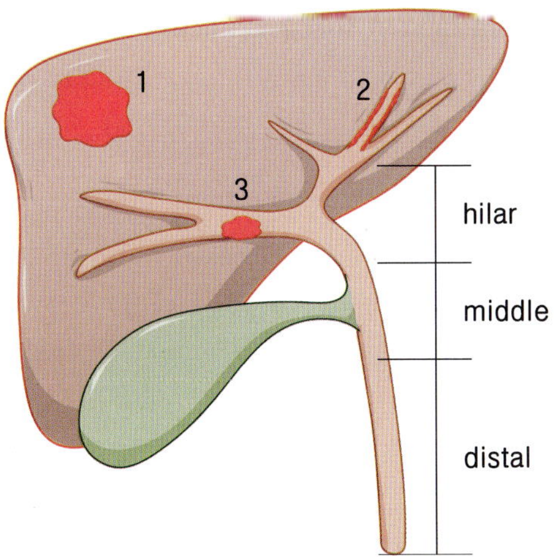

Fig. 1 Anatomic and morphologic classification of intrahepatic and extrahepatic cholangiocarcinoma.
1, mass-forming type; 2, periductal-infiltrative type; 3, Intraductal-growing type.

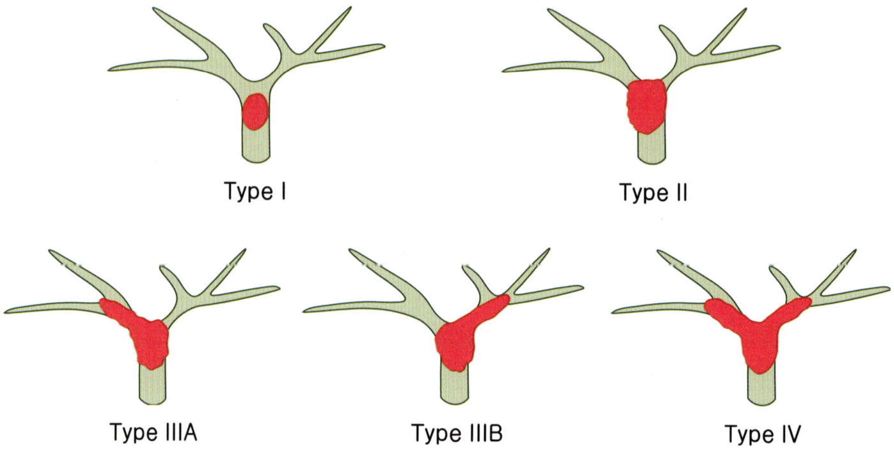

Fig. 2 Bismuth classification of hilar cholangiocarcinoma.

of all extrahepatic cholangiocarcinoma. Hilar cholangiocarcinoma are commonly classified according to Bismuth type with respect to the level of ductal obstruction (Fig. 2).[2] In Bismuth type I, tumor involves only the proximal common hepatic duct with communication between left and right hepatic ducts. Bismuth type II tumor involves the bifurcation and separately obstruct the left and right hepatic ducts but do not extend into the right or the left segmental hepatic ducts. Bismuth type IIIA or IIIB tumors involve either the right or left secondary intrahepatic ducts, respectively with the contralateral secondary intrahepatic duct intact. Bismuth type IV lesion involves both secondary right and left hepatic ducts. Bismuth type IV lesion is usually considered as unresectable. However, some tumors with type IV obstruction can be resected due to the individual variation of biliary anatomy.

II·II
Gross Morphology

Extrahepatic cholangiocarcinoma presents as sclerosing, nodular, or papillary types. The sclerosing type is the most frequent and infiltrates into surrounding bile ducts or periductal tissue. This results in annular thickening of the bile ducts. The papillary type can spread along the whole bile ducts and is termed papillomatosis at that stage. The prognosis is best in papillary type and worst in sclerosing type.

The intrahepatic cholangiocarcinoma are classified into the following three growth types: mass-forming, periductal-infiltrating, and intraductal-growing types.[3] Compared with other classifications, this classification is considered to be more reasonable because it represents the gross morphology, radiologic feature, tumor growth pattern, tumor biology, and patient's prognosis.

1) Mass-forming type

Mass forming type is the most frequent form of intrahepatic cholangiocarcinoma. Mass is formed at the proximal bile ducts irrespective of location of the major bile ducts and grossly looks like hepatocellular carcinoma. The size of tumor is enlarged as the tumor is growing. This type cholangiocarcinoma is usually large, firm and whitish gray because of fibrous stroma. The margin is well circumscribed or lobulated. It is not surrounded by capsule and is usually accompanied by daughter nodules around the main mass because tumor frequently metastasis to adjacent liver via portal veins.

2) Periductal-infiltrative type

Periductal-infiltrative cholangiocarcinoma is located in the major bile ducts and grows and infiltrates alongside the bile ducts and the portal veins. Therefore, it is elongated and branchlike. Most of hilar cholangiocarcinoma belong to this type of cholangiocarcinoma. It tends to spread far away from the original site and can form a mass when it grows. Bile ducts are usually obstructed or markedly narrowed. Lymphatic invasion is more frequent than intrahepatic metastasis. This periductal-infiltrative type of cholangiocarcinoma tends to be associated with hepatolithiasis.

3) Intraductal-growing type

Intraductal-growing choalngiocarcinoma is rare and the tumor protrudes into the lumen. It forms a polypoid nodule inside the bile ducts without infiltrating into the liver parenchyma and rarely forms a mass. The tumors are usually small and sessile or polypoid. Biliary papillomatosis is characterized by multiple papillary adenomas spreading superficially along the mucosal surface of biliary tree. Biliary papillomatosis is rare and is a borderline or low grade malignant neoplasm with a high malignant potential. The metastatic potential of intraductal-growing choalngiocarcinoma is very low and the prognosis is usually very good.[4]

Reference

1. Liver Cancer Study Group of Japan. Intrahepatic cholangiocarcinoma, macroscopic typing. In: Okamoto E ed. Classification of primary liver cancer. Tokyo: Kanehara, 1997:6-7.
2. Bismuth H, Castaing D, Traynor O. Resection or palliation: priority of surgery in the treatment of hilar cancer. World J Surg 1988;12:39-47.
3. Yamasaki S. Intrahepatic cholangiocarcinoma: macroscopic type and stage classification. J Hepatobiliary Pancreat Surg 2003;10:288-291.
4. Suh KS, Roh HR, Koh YT, Lee KU, Park YH, Kim SW. Clinicopathologic features of the intraductal growth type of peripheral cholangiocarcinoma. Hepatology 2000;31:12-17.

III • Etiology and Risk Factors

III Etiology and Risk Factors

Jimin Han, M.D., Ho Gak Kim, M.D.

III
Etiology and Risk Factors

Introduction

Recognized risk factors for cholangiocarcinoma include (1) hepatolithiasis, (2) hepatobiliary parasitic infestations, (3) primary sclerosing cholangitis, (4) congenital anomalies with ectatic ducts, such as choledochal cyst, Caroli disease and anomalous union of pancreaticobiliary duct, (5) primary sclerosing cholangitis, and (6) others which include biliary papillary neoplasm, chronic liver disease and occupational exposure to possible biliary tract carcinogens (Table 1). Unfortunately, only a few cases of cholangiocarcinoma are associated with specific risk factors.[1]

Table 1. Risk factors for cholangiocarcinoma

Established risk factors	Probable risk factors
Hepatolithiasis	*Clonorchis sinensis* infection
Opisthorchis viverrini infection	Hepatitis B virus infection
Primary sclerosing cholangitis	Environmental or occupational toxin exposure-dioxin, polyvinyl chloride
Choledochal cysts	Biliary tract-enteric drainage procedures
Anomalous union of pancreaticobiliary junction	Diabetes
Thorotrast® exposure	HIV infection
Biliary papillary neoplasm	
Liver cirrhosis	
Hepatitis C virus infection	

1. Hepatolithiasis

Stone disease affecting only the intrahepatic bile ducts is rare in the West, but endemic in Taiwan, China, South Korea, and Japan. Many studies showed a clear association exists between hepatolithiasis and cholangiocarcinoma.[2-7] In Taiwan, 50 to 70 percent of patients undergoing resection for cholangiocarcinoma have associated hepatolithiasis.[4,5] In Japan, the incidence of cholangiocarcinoma associated with hepatolithiasis is 6 to 18 percent.[6]

The etiology of hepatolithiasis is not clearly known, but various conditions such as congenital ductal abnormalities, diet, and chronic inflammation from bacterial or parasitic infections have been implicated.[8] In hepatolithiasis, the calculi are usually composed of calcium bilirubinate (brown pigment stone) rather than cholesterol,[8] and the stones are thought to cause bile stasis, predisposing to recurrent bacterial infections and chronic inflammation.[8]

It is often difficult to diagnose cholangiocarcinoma arising as a complication of hepatolithiasis (Fig. 1). However, presence of cholangiocarcinoma should be suspected in a patients over the age of 40 with a long history of hepatolithiasis, weight loss, elevated serum alkaline phosphatase, serum CEA level above 4.2 ng/mL, and

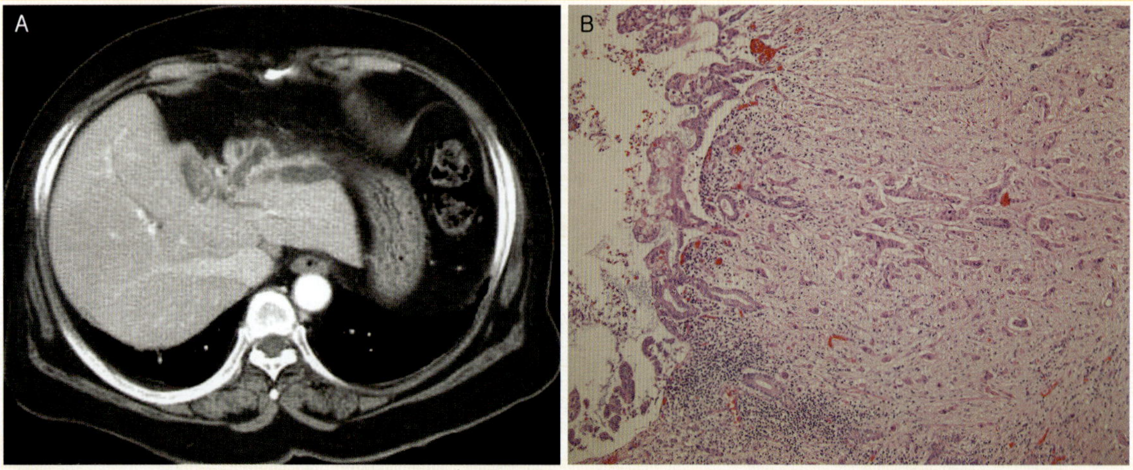

Fig. 1 CT finding and post-operative microscopic finding of in the patient with cholangiocarcinoma arising from hepatolithiasis

A: Abdominal CT scan shows multiple stones and dilated bile duct in atrophied left lobe of liver. B: Adenocarcinoma was notified after resection of left lobe of liver (H & E stain, ×200).

hepatolithiasis in either the right or both lobes of the liver.[9]

2. Liver Flukes: Opisthorchiasis, Clonorchiasis

The liver fluke infestations may be complicated by cholangiocarcinoma of the intrahepatic bile ducts. Cholangiocarcinoma usually arise in the heavily parasitized bile ducts near the hilum. In Asia, infestation with liver flukes of the genera Clonorchis and Opisthorchis is associated with intrahepatic cholangiocarcinoma.[10-12] Although the association between *Clonorchis sinensis* and cholangiocarcinoma remains only probable, the role of *Opisthorchis viverrini* as an etiologic factor in cholangiocarcinoma has been clearly established.[11]

Humans contact liver flukes by consuming raw or undercooked fish. Adult worms inhabit and lay eggs in the biliary system. Liver flukes induce a chronic inflammatory state in the biliary system, presumably leading to malignant transformation of the bile duct epithelium. Carcinogens that are produced by bacteria in the fish and other foods, smoking and alcohol might also act as cofactors.[13,14]

Opisthorchis viverrini infestation is prevalent in Thailand, Laos and western Malaysia.[15] Through the production of carcinogens and free radicals, the parasites induce DNA changes, mutations and stimulate proliferation of intrahepatic bile duct epithelium.[16]

Clonorchis sinensis infestation is prevalent in China, Hong Kong, South Korea, and Vietnam. An association between *Clonorchis sinensis* and cholangiocarcinoma is supported by epidemiological data. Hou estimated that 15% of primary liver cancers in Hong Kong were cholangiocarcinoma associated with *Clonorchis sinensis*.[17-19] In certain areas of Korea with an extremely high prevalence of clonorchiasis, fluke infection increased the relative risk of cholangiocarcinoma six times.[20] A hamster animal model has been developed which showed that development of cholangiocarcinoma in Clonorchis-infected hamsters was related to simultaneous administration of the carcinogen demethylnitrosamine, suggesting that Clonorchis infection alone is insufficient for development of cholangiocarcinoma.[21]

In 1994, the International Agency for Research (IARC) on Cancer Working Group evaluated three previous case-control studies in Hong Kong and Korea.[22] According to these studies and another recent study,[12] the relative risk of clonorchiasis for cholangiocarcinoma ranges from 2.7% to 6.5%. The IARC concluded that *Clonorchis sinensis* is a presumed carcinogen for cholangio-carcinoma.[22]

3. Primary Sclerosing Cholangitis

Primary sclerosing cholangitis (PSC) is an inflammatory disorder of the biliary tree that leads to fibrosis and stricturing of the intrahepatic bile ducts and/or extrahepatic bile ducts. PSC is the most common known risk factor for cholangiocarcinoma in the Western countries.[13]

According to several studies of patients with PSC, the annual incidence of cholangiocarcinoma in patients with PSC has been estimated to be between 0.6 and 1.5 percent per year, with a lifetime risk of 10 to 15 percent.[23-28] However, the incidence is much higher in one study.[29] In a group of 70 patients with PSC, 15 patients died of liver failure during follow-up for a mean of 30 months. Five of 12 patients (40%) who underwent an autopsy had cholangiocarcinoma; cholangiocarcinoma was found in 7% of the total group.[29]

Cholangiocarcinoma in patients with PSC is characterized by development in at a significantly younger age (between the ages of 30 and 50) than in patients without this condition. Early diagnosis of cholangiocarcinoma is also more difficult because of the diffusely abnormal biliary system.[30] In addition, about 30% of cholangiocarcinoma are diagnosed in patients with ulcerative colitis and PSC.[31] Patients with PSC and ulcerative colitis who also have colorectal dysplasia/carcinoma are at greater risk of cholangiocarcionoma than those without colorectal malignancy.[31]

However, cholangiocarcinoma is not necessarily a late complication of PSC. In one case control study, 30% of patients have been diagnosed with cholangiocarcinoma within one year of the first evidence of underlying liver disease based on abnormal liver function tests.[32] Similar to this finding, over one-third of cholangiocarcinoma are diagnosed within two years of the initial diagnosis of PSC, and the risk seems to be unrelated to the duration of inflammatory bowel disease.[26,29,33]

The reason why patients with PSC develop cholangiocarcinoma is not well understood. Smoking and alcohol consumption have been implicated as risk factors.[26,34] However, the authors could not test for a dose-response relationship between alcohol consumption and cholangiocarcinoma due to inadequate data, and they could not confirm the link between smoking and cholangiocarcinoma in PSC.[23]

In patients with PSC, the development of cholangiocarcinoma is heralded by rapid clinical deterioration with jaundice, body weight loss, abdominal discomfort and elevated CA 19-9 and CEA.[29,35] Tumors are often detected at an advanced stage making curative resection impossible.[29,35] Screening strategies are often used to diagnose the malignancy at an early and treatable stage. Many clinicians suggest an interval physical examination, transabdominal ultrasound, and serum levels of CA 19-9; these tests are often recommended annually in patients without cirrhosis and semi-annually in those with cirrhosis.[27] An alternative approach may involve annual or semi-annual CA 19-9, ultrasound, and endoscopic retrograde cholangio-pancreatography (ERCP) with brush cytology/biopsy in those without cellular atypia on initial ERCP.[27] However, the efficacy of tumor markers as screening tests for cholangiocarcinoma in patients with PSC has not been established. In one three-year prospective study of 75 patients with PSC without clinical signs of cholangiocarcinoma, serum levels of CEA, CA19-9, CA-50 and CA-242 were not useful in diagnosing bile duct cancer because of low specificity,[36] On the other hand, a more recent study of 208 patients found a sensitivity, specificity, positive and negative predictive value of 78, 98, 56 and 99 percent, respectively, using an absolute CA 19-9 level of 129 U/ml.[35]

4. Choledochal Cyst

Choledochal cysts are congenital cystic dilatations of the bile ducts, while Caroli disease is a variant of choledochal cyst disease that is characterized by multiple cystic dilations of the intrahepatic bile ducts.[37] It is well established that 10~30% of adults

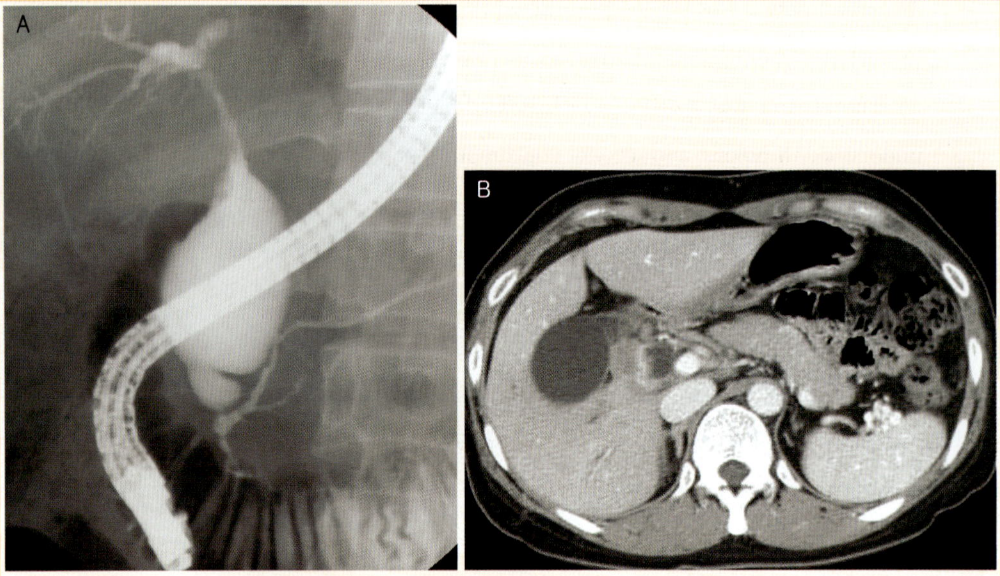

Fig. 2 Cholangiogram and CT findings of common hepatic duct cancer in the patient with choledochal cyst and anomalous union of pancreaticobiliary duct.

A: On endoscopic retrograde cholangiography, there shows large protruding mass at right wall of common hepatic duct and common bile duct. B: On contrast enhancing CT, there shows thickened enhancing mucosa at right wall of dilated common hepatic duct level.

with choledochal cysts develop cholangiocarcinoma and harbor approximately 15 percent lifetime risk of malignant change (Fig. 2).[13,38,39]

The mechanism underlying carcinogenesis in patients with choledochal cysts is unclear yet. Development of cholangiocarcinoma have been related to biliary stasis, chronic inflammation from reflux of pancreatic juice, or abnormalities in bile salt transporter proteins that result in unstable bile content, or deconjugation of carcinogens that were previously conjugated in the liver.[13] The cancer may arise either in the cyst wall itself,[40] or in remnant tissue or undilated parts of the extrahepatic or intrahepatic bile duct.[41]

Cholangiocarcinoma is the most common malignancy in patients with choledochal cysts. Compared to the general population, these patients have a 20-30 fold higher risk of developing cholangiocarcinoma and about 120 times greater incidence of cholangiocarcinoma and the risk remains high even after surgical treatment.[41,42] And the incidence of cholangiocarcinoma increases with age (0.7% in the first decade to more than 14% after 20 years of age),[43] and the mean age at which malignancy develops in choledochal cysts is 32 years, which is about two decades earlier than in the general population. Cholangiocarcinoma have been reported even in children with choledochal cysts,[40,44] which makes the early diagnosis and treatment very important. All types of choledochal cysts develop cholangiocarcinoma, but type I and type IV cysts are associated with a higher incidence even after cyst excision.[41,45] The poor prognosis is the same as that for patients in the general population with cholangiocarcinoma.

Complete excision of choledochal cysts is recommended as soon as possible, preferably before puberty, in order to decrease malignant transformation. All patients with choledochal cysts require lifelong follow-up even after surgical excision. The following patients should be subjected to more intense long term surveillance: those with type I and IV cysts, those with an anomalous union of pancreaticobiliary duct[45-49] and those with incompletely excised cyst parts, as in the instance of intrahepatic dilatation of type IV cysts.[41]

5. Anomalous Union of Pancreaticobiliary Duct (AUPBD)

AUPBD is defined as a congenital anomaly in which a junction of the pancreatic and biliary duct is detected radiologically and/or anatomically outside the duodenal wall.[50] The presence of an AUPBD combined with choledochal cyst has been known to increase the risk for gallbladder and bile duct cancer.[45-49]

Since pancreatic duct and bile duct unite outside the sphincter of Oddi, both pancreaticobiliary and biliopancreatic refluxes may occur. However, intraductal pressure in the pancreatic duct is generally higher than that in the bile duct. Resultant pancreaticobiliary reflux causes pancreatic enzyme activation and recurrent inflammation. The reflux seems very likely to play a crucial role in carcinogenesis in patients with AUPBD, but the precise mechanism has not been elucidated.

In patients with both choledochal cyst and AUPBD, reflux of pancreatic enzymes, bile stasis, and an increased intraductal concentration of bile acids contribute to the proliferative activity of bile acids.[44,51,52] Premalignant alterations in the epithelial wall of the cyst increase with age,[53] which is in accordance with the age-related increased in cancer incidence.[43] Both dilated and undilated non-cancerous parts of the bile duct in patients with an AUPBD exhibit K-ras and p53 mutations, reflecting the high risk of malignant change in the biliary epithelium.[54,55]

Many hypotheses that have been proposed for carcinogenesis in patients with only AUPBD are not different from the above findings. One in vitro study showed that pancreatic juice incubated with bile contained mutagens that was a complex of low-molecular-weight, stable substances that included amino acids and peptides.[56] Mutations of the p53 and K-ras genes have been found in both cancerous and noncancerous biliary epithelia of patients with AUPBD.[54]

6. Other Risk Factors

1) Toxic exposure

There is a clear association exists between exposure to the radiologic contrast agent Thorotrast® (a radiology contrast agent banned in the 1960s for its carcinogenic properties) and cholangiocarcinoma; malignancy usually develops 30 to 35 years after exposure.[57] An increased incidence of cholangiocarcinoma has been less strongly associated with several occupations, including the automobile, rubber, chemical, and wood-finishing industries. Studies on the association between smoking and alcohol intake and risk of cholangiocarcinoma have been conflicting.[26,34]

2) Biliary papillary neoplasm

Intraductal papillary mucin producing neoplasm of the bile duct is a rare disease entity characterized by multiple adenomatous polyps in the bile ducts, closely resembling intraductal papillary mucinous tumor of the pancreas.[58,59] This type tumor secretes large amount of mucin into the bile duct lumen, leading to intermittent obstruction and thus resulting in bile duct dilatation and repeated episodes of abdominal pain, jaundice, and acute cholangitis.[58,59] Microscopic examination of the tumor often shows a wide range of histologic findings, such as hyperplasia, adenoma, carcinoma in situ, and invasive carcinomas. This finding suggests that the pathogenesis of this tumor is in the hyperplasic-adenoma-carcinoma sequence.[58] Biliary papillomatosis should be considered a premalignant condition since 83-89 percent of these lesions undergo malignant transformation.[58-60]

3) Chronic liver disease

Hepatitis B virus (HBV) and hepatitis C virus (HCV) as well as liver cirrhosis regardless of etiology, have been scrutinized as risk factors for intrahepatic cholangiocarcinoma.[7,12,13,61,62]

Several reports have noted a higher than expected rate of HCV-related cirrhosis in patients with cholangiocarcinoma, although the risk is much lower than for hepatocellular carcicnoma.[3,13,61,63-67] A prospective case-control study from Japan reported the risk of developing cholangiocarcinoma in patients with HCV-related cirrhosis was 3.5% at 10 years.[61] The role of HCV in the pathogenesis of cholangiocarcinoma is unclear. An association between HBV and cholangiocarcinoma has also been suggested although the data are much less compelling than for HCV.[7,12]

Similar to hepatocellular carcinoma, chronic liver disease of nonviral etiology also appears to be associated with cholangiocarcinoma.[7,12,41,62-64] In a case-control study, risk factors that were significantly more prevalent among patients with intrahepatic cholangiocarcinoma included nonspecific cirrhosis (adjusted OR 27.2) and alcoholic liver disease (adjusted OR 7.4).[64] A Danish cohort study that followed 11,605 persons with cirrhosis from any cause for an average of approximately six years found a significant 10-fold risk for intrahepatic cholangiocarcinoma among these patients compared to the general population.[62]

Conclusion

In conclusion, common features among known risk factors for cholangiocarcinoma are chronic biliary inflammation and cholestasis. Both of these events resulting from hepatolithiasis, liver flukes, PSC, congenital cystic disease of the bile duct and environmental exposures contribute to malignant transformation of bile duct epithelium. Early detection and elimination of these risk factors may lead to curative treatment of cholangiocarcinoma. Unfortunately, a specific risk factor cannot be identified for the majority of patients.

Reference

1. Chapman RW. Risk factors for biliary tract carcinogenesis. Ann Oncol 1999;10 Suppl 4:308-311.
2. Chijiiwa K, Yamashita H, Yoshida J, Kuroki S, Tanaka M. Current management and long-term prognosis of hepatolithiasis. Arch Surg 1995;130:194-197.
3. Okuda K, Nakanuma Y, Miyazaki M. Cholangiocarcinoma: Recent progress. part 1: Epidemiology and etiology. J Gastroenterol Hepatol 2002;17:1049-1055.
4. Chen MF. Peripheral cholangiocarcinoma (cholangiocellular carcinoma): Clinical features, diagnosis and treatment. J Gastroenterol Hepatol 1999;14:1144-1149.
5. Su CH, Shyr YM, Lui WY, P'Eng FK. Hepatolithiasis associated with cholangiocarcinoma. Br J Surg 1997;84:969-973.
6. Okuda K, Kubo Y, Okazaki N, Arishima T, Hashimoto M. Clinical aspects of intrahepatic bile duct carcinoma including hilar carcinoma: A study of 57 autopsy-proven cases. Cancer 1977;39:232-246.
7. Donato F, Gelatti U, Tagger A, et al. Intrahepatic cholangiocarcinoma and hepatitis C and B virus infection, alcohol intake, and hepatolithiasis: A case-control study in italy. Cancer Causes Control 2001;12:959-964.
8. Kim MH, Sekijima J, Park HZ, Lee SP. Structure and composition of primary intrahepatic stones in korean patients. Dig Dis Sci 1995;40:2143-2151.
9. Kim YT, Byun JS, Kim J, et al. Factors predicting concurrent cholangiocarcinomas associated with hepatolithiasis. Hepatogastroenterology 2003;50:8-12.
10. Watanapa P. Cholangiocarcinoma in patients with opisthorchiasis. Br J Surg 1996;83:1062-1064.
11. Watanapa P, Watanapa WB. Liver fluke-associated cholangiocarcinoma. Br J Surg 2002;89:962-970.
12. Shin HR, Lee CU, Park HJ, et al. Hepatitis B and C virus, clonorchis sinensis for the risk of liver cancer: A case-control study in Pusan, Korea. Int J Epidemiol 1996;25:933-940.
13. Khan SA, Thomas HC, Davidson BR, Taylor-Robinson SD. Cholangiocarcinoma. Lancet 2005;366:1303-1314.

14. Honjo S, Srivatanakul P, Sriplung H, et al. Genetic and environmental determinants of risk for cholangiocarcinoma via opisthorchis viverrini in a densely infested area in Nakhon Phanom, Northeast Thailand. Int J Cancer 2005;117:854-860.

15. Kurathong S, Lerdverasirikul P, Wongpaitoon V, et al. Opisthorchis viverrini infection and cholangiocarcinoma. A prospective, case-controlled study. Gastroenterology 1985;89:151-156.

16. Parkin DM, Ohshima H, Srivatanakul P, Vatanasapt V. Cholangiocarcinoma: Epidemiology, mechanisms of carcinogenesis and prevention. Cancer Epidemiol Biomarkers Prev 1993;2:537-544.

17. Hou PC. The pathology of clonorchis sinensis infestation of the liver. J Pathol Bacteriol 1955;70:53-64.

18. Hou PC. The relationship between primary carcinoma of the liver and infestation with clonorchis sinensis. J Pathol Bacteriol 1956;72:239-246.

19. Hou PC. Primary carcinoma of bile duct of the liver of the cat (felis catus) infested with clonorchis sinensis. J Pathol Bacteriol 1964;87:239-244.

20. Chung CS, Lee SK. An epidemiological study of primary liver carcinomas in Pusan areas with special reference to clonorchiasis. Korean J Pathol 1976;10:33-64.

21. Lee JH, Yang HM, Bak UB, Rim HJ. Promoting role of clonorchis sinensis infection on induction of cholangiocarcinoma during two-step carcinogenesis. Korean J Parasitol 1994;32:13-18.

22. Infection with liver flukes (opisthorchis viverrini, opisthorchis felineus and clonorchis sinensis). IARC Monogr Eval Carcinog Risks Hum 1994;61:121-175.

23. Bergquist A, Ekbom A, Olsson R, et al. Hepatic and extrahepatic malignancies in primary sclerosing cholangitis. J Hepatol 2002;36:321-327.

24. Lee YM, Kaplan MM. Primary sclerosing cholangitis. N Engl J Med 1995;332:924-933.

25. Wiesner RH. Current concepts in primary sclerosing cholangitis. Mayo Clin Proc 1994; 69: 969-982.

26. Bergquist A, Glaumann H, Persson B, Broome U. Risk factors and clinical presentation of hepatobiliary carcinoma in patients with primary sclerosing cholangitis: A case-control study. Hepatology 1998;27:311-316.

27. de Groen PC. Cholangiocarcinoma in primary sclerosing cholangitis: Who is at risk and how do we screen? Hepatology 2000;31:247-248.

28. Burak K, Angulo P, Pasha TM, Egan K, Petz J, Lindor KD. Incidence and risk factors for cholangiocarcinoma in primary sclerosing cholangitis. Am J Gastroenterol 2004;99:523-526.

29. Rosen CB, Nagorney DM, Wiesner RH, Coffey RJ, Jr, LaRusso NF. Cholangiocarcinoma complicating primary sclerosing cholangitis. Ann Surg 1991;213:21-25.

30. LaRusso NF, Wiesner RH, Ludwig J, MacCarty RL. Current concepts. primary sclerosing cholangitis. N Engl J Med 1984;310:899-903.

31. Broome U, Lofberg R, Veress B, Eriksson LS. Primary sclerosing cholangitis and ulcerative colitis: Evidence for increased neoplastic potential. Hepatology 1995;22:1404-1408.

32. Leidenius M, Hockersted K, Broome U, et al. Hepatobiliary carcinoma in primary sclerosing cholangitis: A case control study. J Hepatol 2001;34:792-798.

33. Broome U, Olsson R, Loof L, et al. Natural history and prognostic factors in 305 Swedish patients with primary sclerosing cholangitis. Gut 1996;38:610-615.

34. Chalasani N, Baluyut A, Ismail A, et al. Cholangiocarcinoma in patients with primary sclerosing cholangitis: A multicenter case-control study. Hepatology 2000;31:7-11.

35. Levy C, Lymp J, Angulo P, Gores GJ, Larusso N, Lindor KD. The value of serum CA 19-9 in predicting cholangiocarcinomas in patients with primary sclerosing cholangitis. Dig Dis Sci 2005;50:1734-1740.

36. Hultcrantz R, Olsson R, Danielsson A, et al. A 3-year prospective study on serum tumor markers used for detecting cholangiocarcinoma in patients with primary sclerosing cholangitis. J Hepatol 1999;30:669-673.

37. Dayton MT, Longmire WP,Jr, Tompkins RK. Caroli's disease: A premalignant condition? Am J Surg 1983;145:41-48.

38. Scott J, Shousha S, Thomas HC, Sherlock S. Bile duct carcinoma: A late complication of congenital hepatic fibrosis. case report and review of literature. Am J Gastroenterol 1980; 73:113-119.

39. Lipsett PA, Pitt HA, Colombani PM, Boitnott JK, Cameron JL. Choledochal cyst disease. A changing pattern of presentation. Ann Surg 1994;220:644-652.

40. Todani T, Watanabe Y, Narusue M, Tabuchi K, Okajima K. Congenital bile duct cysts: Classification, operative procedures, and review of thirty-seven cases including cancer arising from choledochal cyst. Am J Surg 1977;134:263-269.

41. Kobayashi S, Asano T, Yamasaki M, Kenmochi T, Nakagohri T, Ochiai T. Risk of bile duct carcinogenesis after excision of extrahepatic bile ducts in pancreaticobiliary maljunction. Surgery 1999;126:939-944.

42. Watanabe Y, Toki A, Todani T. Bile duct cancer developed after cyst excision for choledochal cyst. J Hepatobiliary Pancreat Surg 1999;6:207-212.

43. Voyles CR, Smadja C, Shands WC, Blumgart LH. Carcinoma in choledochal cysts. age-related incidence. Arch Surg 1983;118:986-988.

44. Imazu M, Iwai N, Tokiwa K, Shimotake T, Kimura O, Ono S. Factors of biliary carcinogenesis in choledochal cysts. Eur J Pediatr Surg 2001;11:24-27.

45. Ishibashi T, Kasahara K, Yasuda Y, Nagai H, Makino S, Kanazawa K. Malignant change in the biliary tract after excision of choledochal cyst. Br J Surg 1997;84:1687-1691.

46. Sugiyama M, Atomi Y, Kuroda A. Pancreatic disorders associated with anomalous pancreaticobiliary junction. Surgery 1999;126:492-497.

47. Song HK, Kim MH, Myung SJ, et al. Choledochal cyst associated the with anomalous union of pancreaticobiliary duct (AUPBD) has a more grave clinical course than choledochal cyst alone. Korean J Intern Med 1999;14:1-8.

48. Tashiro S, Imaizumi T, Ohkawa H, et al. Pancreaticobiliary maljunction: Retrospective and nationwide survey in Japan. J Hepatobiliary Pancreat Surg 2003;10:345-351.

49. Matsumoto Y, Fujii H, Itakura J, et al. Pancreaticobiliary maljunction: Pathophysiological and clinical aspects and the impact on biliary carcinogenesis. Langenbecks Arch Surg 2003;388:122-131.

50. The Japanese Study Group on Pancreaticobiliary Maljunction (JSPBM). The Committee of JSPBM for Diagnostic Criteria. Diagnostic criteria of pancreaticobiliary maljunction. J Hepatobiliary Pancreat Surg 1994;1:219-221.

51. Wu GS, Zou SQ, Luo XW, Wu JH, Liu ZR. Proliferative activity of bile from congenital choledochal cyst Patients. World J Gastroenterol 2003;9:184-187.

52. Reveille RM, Van Stiegmann G, Everson GT. Increased secondary bile acids in a choledochal cyst. possible role in biliary metaplasia and carcinoma. Gastroenterology 1990;99:525-527.

53. Komi N, Tamura T, Tsuge S, Miyoshi Y, Udaka H, Takehara H. Relation of patient age to premalignant alterations in choledochal cyst epithelium: Histochemical and immunohistochemical studies. J Pediatr Surg 1986;21:430-433.

54. Matsubara T, Sakurai Y, Zhi LZ, Miura H, Ochiai M, Funabiki T. K-ras and p53 gene mutations in noncancerous biliary lesions of patients with pancreaticobiliary maljunction. J Hepatobiliary Pancreat Surg 2002;9:312-321.

55. Nagai M, Watanabe M, Iwase T, Yamao K, Isaji S. Clinical and genetic analysis of noncancerous and cancerous biliary epithelium in patients with pancreaticobiliary maljunction. World J Surg 2002;26:91-98.

56. Mizuno M, Kato T, Koyama K. An analysis of mutagens in the contents of the biliary tract in pancreaticobiliary maljunction. Surg Today 1996;26:597-602.

57. Sahani D, Prasad SR, Tannabe KK, Hahn PF, Mueller PR, Saini S. Thorotrast-induced cholangiocarcinoma: Case report. Abdom Imaging 2003;28:72-74.

58. Kim HJ, Kim MH, Lee SK, et al. Mucin-hypersecreting bile duct tumor characterized by a striking homology with an intraductal papillary mucinous tumor (IPMT) of the pancreas. Endoscopy 2000;32:389-393.

59. Lee SS, Kim MH, Lee SK, et al. Clinicopathologic review of 58 patients with biliary papillomatosis. Cancer 2004;100:783-793.

60. Taguchi J, Yasunaga M, Kojiro M, Arita T, Nakayama T, Simokobe T. Intrahepatic and extrahepatic biliary papillomatosis. Arch Pathol Lab Med 1993;117:944-947.

61. Kobayashi M, Ikeda K, Saitoh S, et al. Incidence of primary cholangiocellular carcinoma of the liver in Japanese patients with hepatitis C virus-related cirrhosis. Cancer 2000;88: 2471-2477.

62. Sorensen HT, Friis S, Olsen JH, et al. Risk of liver and other types of cancer in patients with cirrhosis: A nationwide cohort study in Denmark. Hepatology 1998;28:921-925.

63. Shaib YH, Davila JA, McGlynn K, El-Serag HB. Rising incidence of intrahepatic cholangiocarcinoma in the united states: A true increase? J Hepatol 2004;40:472-477.

64. Shaib YH, El-Serag HB, Davila JA, Morgan R, McGlynn KA. Risk factors of intrahepatic cholangiocarcinoma in the United States: A case-control study. Gastroenterology 2005;128:620-626.

65. Tomimatsu M, Ishiguro N, Taniai M, et al. Hepatitis C virus antibody in patients with primary liver cancer (hepatocellular carcinoma, cholangiocarcinoma, and combined hepatocellular-cholangiocarcinoma) in Japan. Cancer 1993;72:683-688.

66. Yamamoto S, Kubo S, Hai S, et al. Hepatitis C virus infection as a likely etiology of intrahepatic cholangiocarcinoma. Cancer Sci 2004;95:592-595.

67. Liu XF, Zou SQ, Qiu FZ. Pathogenesis of cholangiocarcinoma in the porta hepatis and infection of hepatitis virus. Hepatobiliary Pancreat Dis Int 2003;2:285-289.

IV. Epidemiology of Cholangiocarcinoma

IV Epidemiology of Cholangiocarcinoma

Chang Duck Kim, M.D., Ph.D.

IV
Epidemiology of Cholangiocarcinoma

Cholangiocarcinoma (CC) is a malignant tumor arising from biliary epithelial cells or cholangiocytes. Although rare and comprising only 10~15% of hepatobiliary tumors, its incidence has been rising worldwide.[1,2] This tendency of increase is estimated by some authors as a result of increased recognition of the intrahepatic type of CC, or a real increase of cases because of major tertiary referral care with an interest in this disease.[2] CC is commonly subdivided into two distinct types, intrahepatic cholangiocarcinoma (ICC) and extrahepatic cholangiocarcinoma (ECC), or ductal cholangiocarcinoma. This classification seems to conform to the site of tumor-originating cells, with discrete epidemiological, clinical, and therapeutic differences.[1] However, overlap in features causes some confusion due to incorrect classification. For instance, ICC is sometimes grouped as a primary liver tumor with hepatocellular carcinomas (HCC) in some studies because of intrahepatic mass formation. Klatskin tumor has traditionally been classified as ECC, based on the origination from the bifurcation of right and left hepatic ducts. In practice, however, many studies have classified Klatskin tumors as an ICC, probably erroneously influencing the correct epidemiology of CC. Conversely, gallbladder (GB) carcinomas are commonly reported collectively with primary ECC, and this may influence the epidemiologic and pathogenetic associations.[3] From data collected worldwide, ICC has been increasing in incidence and mortality rates. In contrast, incidence and mortality rates of ECC are decreasing.

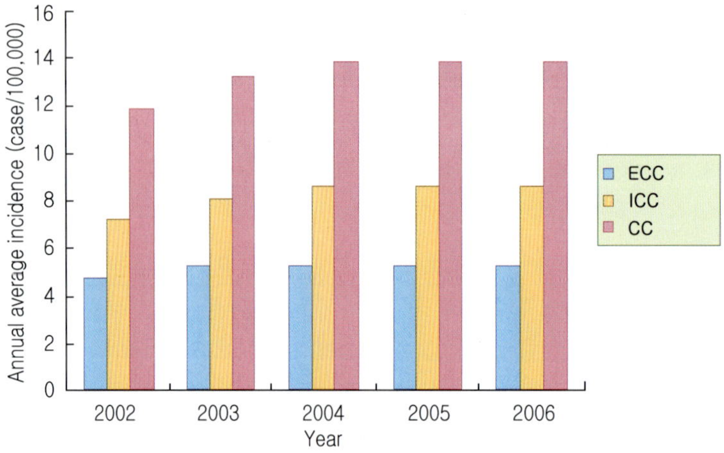

Fig. 1 Annual average incidence rates of ICC, ECC, and CC including ICC and ECC from 2002 to 2006 in Korea.
(CC: cholangiocarcinoma, ICC: intrahepatic cholangiocarcinoma, ECC: extrahepatic cholangiocarcinoma)

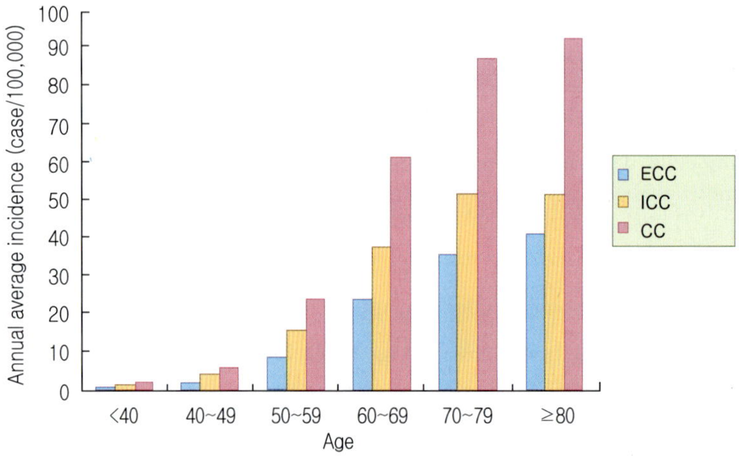

Fig. 2 Annual average incidence rates of ICC, ECC, and CC including ICC and ECC from 2002 to 2006 in Korea.
Annual average incidence rates of ICC, ECC, and CC including ICC and ECC according to the age in Korea. (CC: cholangiocarcinoma, ICC: intrahepatic cholangiocarcinoma, ECC: extrahepatic cholangiocarcinoma)

Unfortunately, nationwide survey of CC in Korea is not yet available. The prevalence of cholangiocarcinoma of Korea in 1999 was 1.5%, comprising about 5%

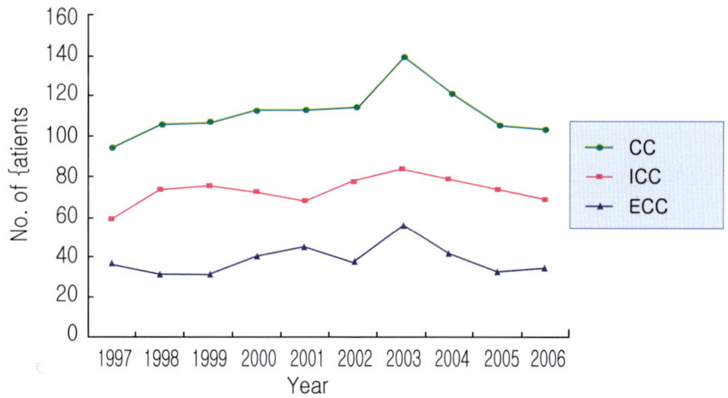

Fig. 3 Temporal trends in the incidence of ICC, ECC, and CC including ICC and ECC in patients who were admitted to Korea University Medical Center from 1997 to 2006.
(CC: cholangiocarcinoma, ICC: intrahepatic cholangiocarcinoma, ECC: extrahepatic cholangiocarcinoma)

of whole gastrointestinal malignancies. Annual Report of the Korea Central Cancer Registry (KCCR) collects nationwide biliary cancer cases as a whole, instead of subdividing it into ICC, ECC, or GB cancer. The age-standardized incidence rate of biliary cancer was 8.2 per 100,000 population in male and 5.7 per 100,000 in female on 2002. According to the collected data from Korea's Health Insurance Review and Assessment Service (HIRA), the annual average incidence rate per 100,000 population of CC including ICC and ECC were 11.8 on year 2002, 13.2 on 2003, 13.8 on 2004, 13.7 on 2005 and 13.7 on 2006, respectively, showing no obvious change of incidence for the recent 5 years (Fig. 1). Incidence rates of CC according to patients' age are less than 1 per 100,000 until 30s, but rapidly rise on their 5th decades: incidence rates are 5.4 per 100,000 on 40s, 23.4 on 50s, 60.3 on 60s, 86.3 on 70s, and 92.0 on 80s (Fig. 2). On the analysis of 1108 cases of CC admitted to Korea University Medical Center from 1997 to 2006, there was no distinct change of annual cases during last decade (Fig. 3).

In this chapter, we will observe the epidemiologic characteristics of CC, commenting ICC and ECC separately. We will also briefly review the recent epidemiological characteristics of CC in Korea.

1. Intrahepatic Cholangiocarcinoma

1) Incidence

According to the report published in 2002 by International Agency of Research on Cancer (IARC), incidence of ICC differs among nations of the world in an wide-ranging variation (Fig. 4).[1] ICC incidence rates are as high as 96 per 100,000 population in men and 38 per 100,000 in women in the Northeast Thailand. In contrast, Australia has the lowest incidence rates of 0.2 and 0.1 per 100,000 among men and women, respectively. Difference of ICC incidence exists even within the same nation, related to variation in prevalence of risk factors on a specific region of a certain country. In Thailand, the northeast zone (e.g., Khon Kaen) is an endemic area of liver fluke infestation: this characteristics associate with a higher incidence of ICC in this region.[4]

ICC incidence is rising as a whole, and there are reports describing increasing ICCs in several regions of the world. In the United States, the age-adjusted incidence

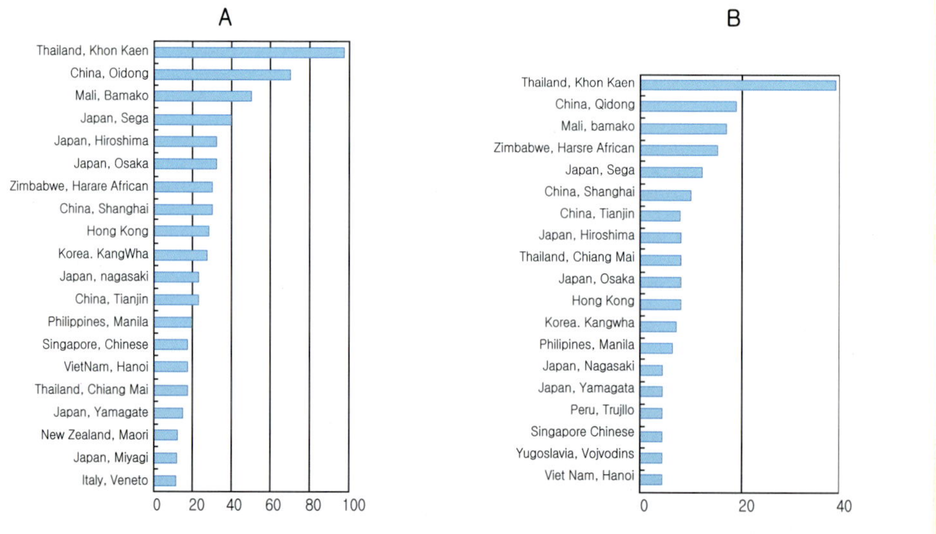

Fig. 4 The age-adjusted incidence rates of ICC in men (left) and women (right) in 20 different geographic regions (modified from Shaib et al.[1])

rates of ICC increased from 0.32 per 100,000 in 1975 to 1979, to 0.85 per 100,000 in 1995 to 1999.[1] A Japanese study revealed a slight increase of ICC frequency from 0.31% in 1976 to 1977, to 0.58% in 1996 to 1997 after collecting autopsied cases.[5] A study from Crete also reported an increased ICC incidence from 0.998 per 100,000 in 1992 to 1994, to 3.327 per 100,000 in 1998 to 2000.[6] In Korea, data collected by HIRA from 2002 to 2006 showed an annual average incidence rate of 7.2 per 100,000 on 2002, 8.0 on 2003, 8.6 on 2004, 8.5 on 2005, and 8.6 on 2006, respectively (Fig. 1). We suppose that the high incidence of ICC in Korea is related with liver fluke infestation.

Globally, male predominance is distinct (although less than that of the HCC), and ICC incidence is higher among men in various areas in the world. Male-female ratio for ICC is about 1.5 in the United States,[7] and 3.3 in France.[1] In Korea, the male-female ratio is 1.3.

ICC rarely occurs before the age of 40. Internationally, the average age of presentation is approximately 50 years. However, there has been a shift toward an older age at diagnosis, being discovered in ages more than 65 years old. The reasons of shift are supposed to be a change of risk factors.[1] As an example of evidence supporting this estimation, chronic conditions such as cirrhosis of any cause seems to overcome the "traditional" risk factors such as primary sclerosing cholangitis (PSC) or choledocal cyst, which are diagnosed at a younger age. Referring to the data from HIRA, annual average incidence rates according to age groups in Korea were low on 30s of less than 1 case per 100,000, but rose sharply of 3.37 on 40s, 20.7 on 50s, 53.6 on 60s, 75.8 on 70s, and 83.2 on 80s of age (Fig. 2). This trend of rise of incidence along the increase of age is similar to different areas of the world.

2) Mortality and survival

In general, mortality rates of ICC are increasing. By analyzing the data from the World Health Organization (WHO) database, Khan et al described a trend of increasing ICC mortality.[8] From 1979 to 1997, the United States, Japan, Australia, the United Kingdom, France, and Italy all showed an increase of mortality rate, with an age-standardized rate ranging from 130 % to 600%. The increase of ICC mortality is

Table 1. Reported Survivals after Surgical Resection of Intrahepatic Cholangiocarcinoma

	Publication year	No. of Patient	No. of Resection (RR/CR)	Median Survival	Cumulative Survival Rate (%)		
					1-year	3-year	5-year
Roayaie et al.[18]	1998	26	16 (61.5/42.3%)	42.9	86.0%	64.0%	21.0%
Kim et al.[19]	1999	28	25 (89.3/53.6%)	17.0	50.8%	32.3%	22.1%
Weber et al.[20]	2001	53	33 (62.3/37.7%)	37.4	83.0%	55.0%	31.0%
Jan et al.[21]	2005	373	187(50.1/36.2%)	13.0	25.3%	17.9%	10.2%
Song et al.[10]	2007	318	292(91.8/68.9%)	-	68.3%	39.3%	29.0%

(RR: resection rate; CR: curative resection rate)

likely a result of the increasing incidence of ICC, indicating poor survival with this malignancy.[1] Actually, the mortality rate of ICC is greater than that of HCC.[7] On estimating the reason of mortality rate increase, there may be an artefactual trend originating from the improvement in diagnosis and diagnostic techniques, or from misclassification of disease coding. However, an alternative explanation is a real increase in the incidence. This may be due to the vast surface area of the intrahepatic bile duct that enables larger exposure to potential carcinogens; natural substances or xenobiotic chemical residues in the environment are excreted and concentrated in the bile juice.[8]

Survival of patients of ICC is still correspondingly low. According to the report which studied the registries of ICCs of the Surveillance Epidemiology and End Results (SEER), the overall observed and relative survival rates of ICC remained unacceptably low. This study revealed that the 1-year relative survival rate (1-YSR) increased, but 5-year survival rate (5-YSR) did not show any significant change in the United States.[1,9] From 1975 to 1979 and from 1995 to 1999, 1-YSR was 16.4% and 27.6%, respectively. On the contrary, the 5-YSR of the both time period were less than 5%, showing no discernible improvement in survival. The improved short-term but not long-term survival, as the authors analyzed, can be attributed to improved palliative treatments such as stenting and drainage, or improved general supportive medical care. Some researchers, however, hold a pessimistic view, emphasizing that this unchanging trend of 5-YSR persisted over the past 20 years despite diagnoses at less advanced stages, introduction of novel therapeutic measures, or better surgical manipulations.[7] The poor survival of ICC may be explained by several factors, such as few etiological risk factors, late presentation, and frequently aggressive tumor biology.[10]

Regrettably, the exact survival rate or mortality rates of ICC in Korea are not available to date. The KCCR of Ministry of Health and Welfare issued a report about incidence and survival of various types of cancer from 1993 to 2002. Of these, "malignant neoplasm of liver and intrahepatic bile ducts" (coded C22 of the ICD-10) which includes the ICC showed a 5-YSR of 13.3%, while "malignant neoplasm of other and unspecified parts of biliary tract" (coded C24) that includes ECC showed a 5-YSR of 19.3%.

In the meantime, some researchers showed a relatively better survival after surgical treatment of ICC. In a Korean report of analyzing the clinical outcome and prognostic factors of patients with hilar cholangiocarcinoma, 3-year overall survival and disease-free survival rates were 41.2% and 52.5%, respectively, after curative resection.[11] In this study, the mean survival period of subjects who had curative resection was 49 months, in contrast to 17 months who had bypass surgery. The 1-, 2-, 3-, and 5-YSR after curative resection were 71.0%, 50.3%, 41.2%, and 32.9%, respectively. Another Korean publication, reporting analysis of survival and factors affecting the survival after surgical resection of peripheral CC, showed that the 1-, 3-, 5-, and 10-YSR of R0 resection were 74.9%, 46.9%, 36.9%, and 15.2%, respectively.[10] Table 1 shows a number of reports relevant to survival after surgical resection of ICC.

2. Extrahepatic Cholangiocarcinoma

1) Incidence and prevalence

Fewer data are available and collected concerning ECC. In general, the incidence rate of ECC is decreasing. Incidence rates of ECC range from 0.53 per 100,000 population (the United Kingdom) to 1.14 per 100,000 (Canada) according to a survey from Strom et al.[12] After analysis of incidence rates of ECC using the SEER registry, some authors concluded that incidence of ECC has an evidence of declining over time.[1] According to this report, the age-adjusted incidence decreased from 1.08 per 100,000 in 1979 to 0.82 per 100,000 in 1998 in the United States. The annual average incidence of ECC in Korea were 4.7 per 100,000 on 2002, 5.2 on 2003, 5.2 on 2004, 5.2 on 2005, and 5.1 on 2006, respectively, with an average of 5.1 per 100,000 based on data collected by HIRA (Fig. 1).

Demographic features of ECC are a little different to that of ICC, in terms of race, gender, and age.[13] In the United States, the incidence rates were slightly lower in blacks (0.8 per 100,000) than in whites (1.0 per 100,000). The age-adjusted incidence of ECC was 1.2 per 100,000 for men and 0.8 per 100,000 for women as reported by SEER registry between 1973 and 1987. Meanwhile, of all patients with ECC, 48% were female, and 65% were older than 65 years of age, and most were within the 70 to 74 year age group.[13] In a Korean report of studying prognostic factors after major resection for 154 cases of distal ECC, male patients comprised of 66.9%, whereas female patients 33.1%.[14] According to the HIRA data, Korean patients in their 40s were diagnosed of ECC on an annual average rate of 1.7 per 100,000 populations, 8.2 on 50s, 23.1 on 60s, 35.2 on 70s, and 41.0 on their 80s (Fig. 2). Therefore, ECC cases increased rapidly in patients on 6th decades, comprising more than 97% of total cases.

2) Mortality and survival

A report studying age-standardized mortality rates from 1978 to 1998 were gained from the World Health Organization mortality database.[8] This study revealed a downward trend in deaths from ECC and GB cancers. However, there were some exceptions from Italy and Japan, with a mortality rate of men as 1.43 to 2.10 and 4.30 to 5.87, respectively. Another study published on the same year, which also utilized the WHO database, showed a similar result of global tendency of decreasing estimated annual percent change in age-adjusted mortality rates.[15]

In the United States, 5-YSR of ECC revealed to slightly increase after population-based studies.[13] From 1973 to 1987, 5-YSR of ECC patients was 11.7% in 1973 to 1977, whereas it increased to 15.1% in 1983 to 1987. In Korea, Joo et al reported that the overall 1, 2, 3, and 5-YSR in clinical study on 193 cases of ECC were 49.9%, 32.2%, 23.4% and 17.8%, respectively.[16] However, in 85 patients without curative surgery, 1-, 2-, 3-, and 5-YSR were 24.0%, 12.5%, 7.1%, and 3.0%, respectively. On the other hand, in the 108 patients with curative surgery, the 1-, 2-, 3-, and 5- YSR was 70.0%, 48.0%, 37.1%, and 27.2%, respectively. Also, a single center survey collecting data of 34 ECC cases that underwent segmental resections revealed 2- and 4-YSR of 64% and 22%, respectively.[17] Recently, Kim et al reported that after major resection for distal ECC, 3- and 5-YSR were 48.0% and 32.8%, respectively, with a mean 47.2 months (range 39.1 ~ 55.3 months).[14]

Reference

1. Shaib Y, El-Serag HB. The epidemiology of cholangiocarcinoma. Semin Liver Dis 2004;24:115-125.
2. Gores GJ. Cholangiocarcinoma: current concepts and insights. Hepatology 2003;37: 961-969.
3. Ben-Menachem T. Risk factors for cholangiocarcinoma. Eur J Gastroenterol Hepatol 2007;19:615-617.
4. Parkin DM, Ohshima H, Srivatanakul P, Vatanasapt V. Cholangiocarcinoma: epidemiology, mechanisms of carcinogenesis and prevention. Cancer Epidemiol Biomarkers Prev 1993;2:537-544.
5. Okuda K, Nakanuma Y, Miyazaki M. Cholangiocarcinoma: recent progress. Part 1: epidemiology and etiology. J Gastroenterol Hepatol 2002;17:1049-1055.
6. Mouzas IA, Dimoulios P, Vlachonikolis IG, Skordilis P, Zoras O, Kouroumalis E. Increasing incidence of cholangiocarcinoma in Crete 1992-2000. Anticancer Res 2002;22:3637-3641.
7. Lazaridis KN, Gores GJ. Cholangiocarcinoma. Gastroenterology 2005;128:1655-1667.
8. Khan SA, Taylor-Robinson SD, Toledano MB, Beck A, Elliott P, Thomas HC. Changing international trends in mortality rates for liver, biliary and pancreatic tumours. J Hepatol 2002;37:806-813.
9. Shaib YH, Davila JA, McGlynn K, El-Serag HB. Rising incidence of intrahepatic cholangiocarcinoma in the United States: a true increase? J Hepatol 2004;40:472-477.
10. Song GW, Lee SG, Lee YJ, et al. Analysis of survival and factors affecting the survival after surgical resection of peripheral cholangiocarcinoma: 318 cases in single institute. Korean J Hepatol 2007;13:208-221.

11. Kim SJ, Lee CY, Kim DG. Analysis of the clinical outcome and prognostic factors of patients with hilar cholangiocarcinoma. J Korean Surg Soc 2007;73:156-164.

12. Strom BL, Hibberd PL, Soper KA, Stolley PD, Nelson WL. International variations in epidemiology of cancers of the extrahepatic biliary tract. Cancer Res 1985;45:5165-5168.

13. Carriaga MT, Henson DE. Liver, gallbladder, extrahepatic bile ducts, and pancreas. Cancer 1995;75:171-190.

14. Kim JW, Jo S, Moon HJ, et al. Prognostic factors after major resection for distal extrahepatic cholangiocarcinoma. Korean J Gastroenterol 2006;47:144-152.

15. Patel T. Worldwide trends in mortality from biliary tract malignancies. BMC Cancer 2002;2:10.

16. Joo YH, Myung SJ, Kim MH, et al. Clinical study on 193 cases of extrahepatic bile duct carcinoma and Its prognostic factors. Korean J Gastroenterol 1999;33:114-123.

17. Kim JH, Kim YI. Segmental resection for extrahepatic bile duct cancer (excluding GB cancer). J Korean Surg Soc 2001;61:593-599.

18. Roayaie S, Guarrera JV, Ye MQ, et al. Aggressive surgical treatment of intrahepatic cholangiocarcinoma: predictors of outcomes. J Am Coll Surg 1998;187:365-372.

19. Kim H, Yun S, Jung K, Kwun W, Choi J. Intrahepatic cholangiocarcinoma in Korea. J Hepatobiliary Pancreat Surg 1999;6:142-148.

20. Weber SM, Jarnagin WR, Klimstra D, DeMatteo RP, Fong Y, Blumgart LH. Intrahepatic cholangiocarcinoma: resectability, recurrence pattern, and outcomes. J Am Coll Surg 2001;193:384-391.

21. Jan YY, Yeh CN, Yeh TS, Hwang TL, Chen MF. Clinicopathological factors predicting long-term overall survival after hepatectomy for peripheral cholangiocarcinoma. World J Surg 2005;29:894-898.

V. Pathology of Cholangiocarcinoma

V Pathology of Cholangiocarcinoma

So-Young Jin, M.D.

V

Pathology of Cholangiocarcinoma

Cholangiocarcinoma is an adenocarcinoma arising from a bile duct. It can be classified into intrahepatic or peripheral cholangiocarcinoma, hilar cholangiocarcinoma, and extrahepatic cholangiocarcinoma according to the anatomic sites. This type of classification make easy to understand the clinical presentation of each type. However, the pathologic findings are similar regardless of the origin of the sites. The Korean Liver Cancer Study Group suggested the macroscopic classification of cholangiocarcinoma into 4 types; mass forming type, periductal infiltrating type, intraductal growth type, and mixed type.[1]

1. Intrahepatic Cholangiocarcinoma

1) Gross

Intrahepatic cholangiocarcinoma is a malignant tumor of cells resembling those of bile ducts. It can arise from any portion of intrahepatic bile ducts from the large bile ducts to small ducts. The mass is mostly gray to gray-white, firm, and solid nodules, usually coalescent, resulting in bosselated margin (Fig. 1). Central necrosis or scarring are common and occasionally mucin can be identifiable on cut section. The surrounding liver is usually non-cirrhotic. In cases associated with hepatolithiasis, the neoplastic process tends to grow and spread along the dilated intrahepatic ducts. The dependent liver lobe or segments containing stones are atrophic.

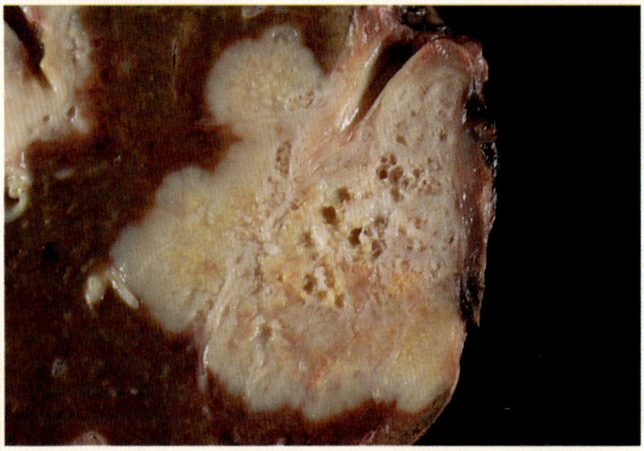

Fig. 1 Cut surface of the peripheral cholangiocarcinoma

A gray-white firm gritty nodular mass with lobulated margin is seen on non-cirrhotic liver.

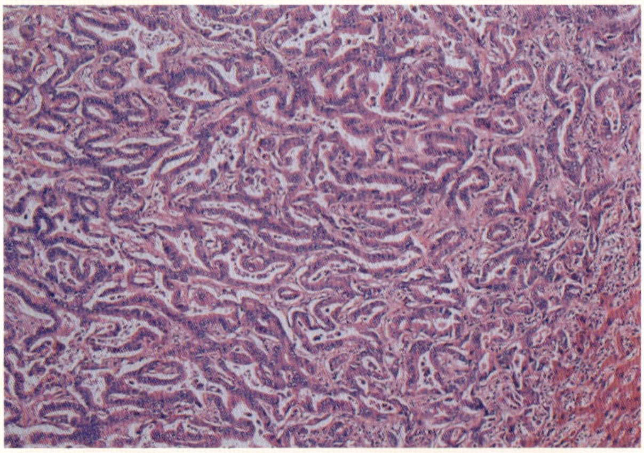

Fig. 2 Microscopic findings of cholangiocarcinoma

Well formed tubulo-papillary glandular structures are seen on desmoplastic stroma (H-E, ×100).

2) Micro

Most intrahepatic cholangiocarcinomas are adenocarcinoma. Proliferation of tubular and and/or papillary structures with variable differentiation is seen without fibrous capsule. Abundant desmoplastic stromal reaction is common (Fig. 2). Tumor cells are cuboidal or columnar in shape and their nuclei are small with less prominent nucleoli. Most cells have abundant pale eosinophilic or vacuolated cytoplasm. More dense proliferation of glands are seen in the peripheral portions, otherwise, glandular cells are more hypocellular or acellular and the stroma is sclerotic or hyalinized in the central portions of the tumor. Carcinoma arising from the large intrahepatic bile ducts shows intraductal micropapillary carcinoma and in situ like spread along the biliary lumen. Neoplastic glands can grow along the sinusoids and spread into portal tracts and bile ducts. Vascular invasion is frequent. When the tumor infiltrate into the peribiliary glands of the intrahepatic large ducts, particularly in cases of well differentiated type, it may be difficult to distinguish neoplastic glands from reactive proliferating glands due to bland looking appearance. Entrapped normal bile ducts can be seen in the periphery of the mass.

Mucin can be demonstrated by mucicarmine, diastase-PAS, and alcian blue stains and immunohistochemical mucin markers of MUC1 and MUC2. Bile production by tumor cells themselves is not found. Another immunohistochemical markers include cytokeratin 7, cytokeratin 19, carcinoembryonic antigen, and epithelial membrane antigen. Reduced membranous expression and aberrant nuclear expression of β-catenin, higher COX-2 expression, and p53 protein overexpression can be seen. MUC2 expression is relatively frequent in well differentiated cholangiocarcinoma, suggesting a somewhat more favorable prognosis.

The most common genetic abnormalities in intrahepatic cholangiocarcinoma are mutations of the RAS and TP53 genes. The incidence of KRAS mutation is variable and in a study using Korean cases of 40 surgically resected intrahepatic cholangiocarcinomas, it was reported as 22.5%.[2] The gross morphology may be related to the mutation pattern. In a Japanese group, KRAS gene alterations were prevalent in the periductal and spicular forming infiltrating subtype and TP53 mutations were predominant in the mass forming type.[3]

Other types include adenosquamous and squamous carcinoma, cholangiolocellular carcinoma, mucinous carcinoma, signet-ring cell carcinoma, pseudosarcomatous cholangiocarcinoma, lymphoepithelioma-like carcinoma, clear cell variant of cholangiocarcinoma, and mucoepidermoid carcinoma.

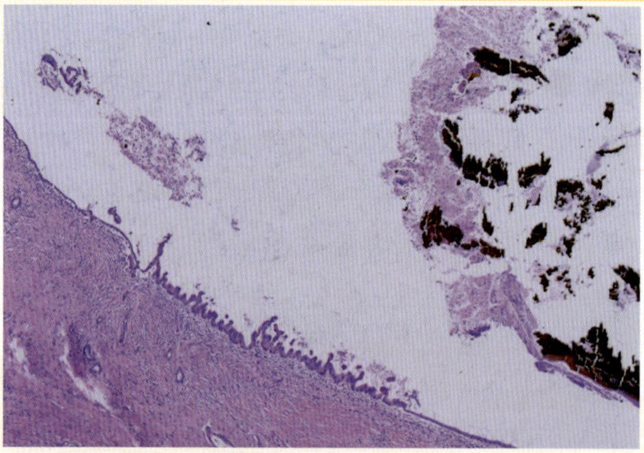

Fig. 3 Biliary intraepithelial neoplasia lesion in hepatolithiasis

An area of transformation from normal flat epithelium to micropapillary BilIN lesion is noted in a markedly distended intrahepatic bile duct filled with stone (H-E, ×40).

2. Biliary Intraepithelial Neoplasia (BilIN)

Intrahepatic cholangiocarcinoma, especially arising in hepatolithiasis show varying spectrum of atypical biliary epithelial change (Fig. 3). The concept of premalignant or non-invasive neoplastic lesions of bile duct was proposed using the liver of patients with hepatolithiasis. An international interobserver agreement study and proposal for diagnostic criteria of biliary intraepithelial neoplasia was published in 2007. They divided noninvasive dysplastic lesions of biliary epithelium excluding intraductal papillary neoplasm into three histological grades; BilIN-1, BilIN-2, and BilIN-3(including carcinoma in situ).[4]

3. Mucin Hypersecreting Papillary Cholangiocarcinoma

Biliary papillomatosis consists of dilated intrahepatic and extrahepatic bile ducts filled with papillary or villous excrescences. The latter consists of delicate fibrovascular stalk covered with a columnar or glandular epithelium. The affected bile ducts are variably dilated and contain papillary or villous growths of columnar epithelial cells supported by delicate fibrovascular stalk. The epithelial cells may be biliary, foveolar, or colonic in appearance. Mucin production is commonly seen. There may be varying degrees of

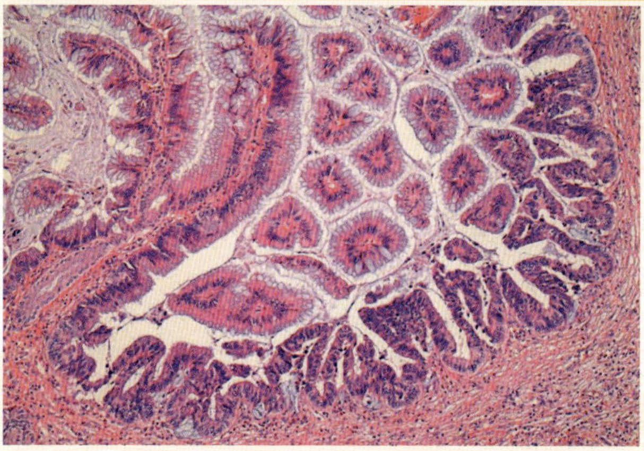

Fig. 4 Intraductal papillary cholangiocarcinoma arising in biliary papillomatosis

A spectrum of benign to high grade dysplasia upto carcinoma in situ in the intraductal papillary mass can be observed (H-E, ×100).

dysplasia, carcinoma in situ, and even invasive adenocarcinoma (Fig. 4). Even though after the malignant transformation, they have prominent intraductal papillary proliferation and abundant mucin hypersecretion, resulting in dilation of intrahepatic bile ducts. The immunohistochemistry disclose positive starning for MUC2, CDX2, and CK20, commonly.[5] These findings suggest a biliary counterpart of pancreatic papillary mucinous neoplasm.[6]

4. Differential Diagnosis

1) Hepatocellular Carcinoma

Hepatocellular cords are lined by sinusoids and bile canaliculi are not seen. Immunohistochemical hepatocytic markers such as hepatocyte antigen and albumin are not found in cholangiocarcinoma. Otherwise, cytokeratin 7 and 19 seen in cholangiocarcinoma are not expressed in hepatocellular carcinoma.

2) Combined Hepatocellular and Cholangiocarcinoma

This tumor have both elements of hepatocellular and cholagiocarcinoma.

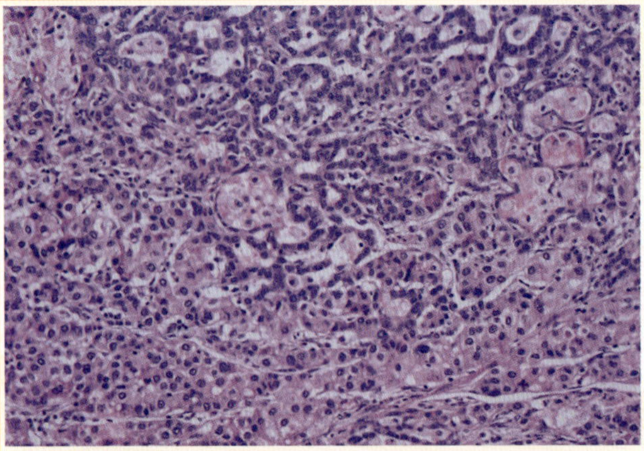

Fig. 5 Intermediate carcinoma subtype of combined hepatocellular-cholangiocarcinoma

Mixed proliferation of cholangiocyte, hepatocyte, and small poorly differentiated progenitor cells are intermingled (H-E, ×200).

Unequivocal elements can be seen either in the same mass with transitional area or separately in the same liver("collision tumor"). Currently it is regarded as a subtype of hepatocellular carcinoma by WHO classification. However, some groups suggested the close relation of combined hepatocellular and cholangiocarcinoma to cholangiocarcinoma rather than to hepatocellular carcinoma.[7] Some tumors are poorly differentiated with intermediate or hepatic progenitor cell phenotype (Fig. 5), represented by positive expression for CD117. These group of tumors were called as "intermediate carcinoma".[8]

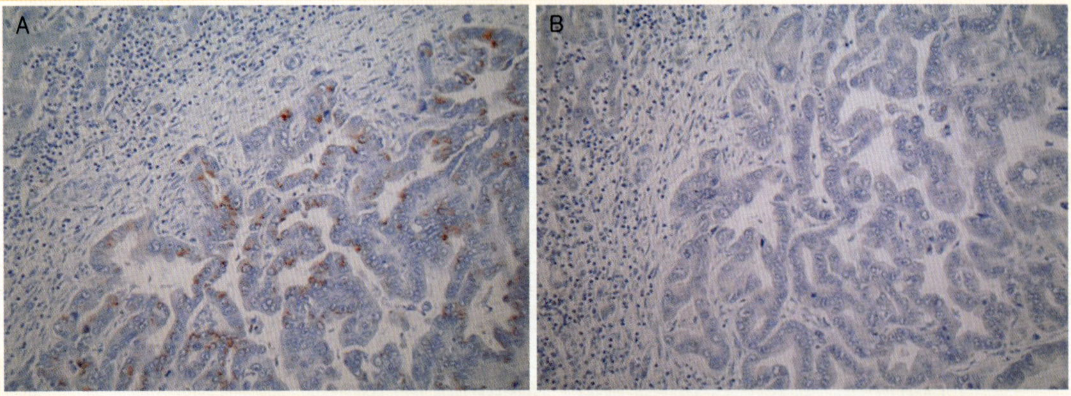

Fig. 6 CK7/CK20 profile of cholangiocarcinoma

Tumor cells are positive for CK7(A) and negative for CK20(B) (Immunohistochemistry, ×200).

3) Metastatic carcinoma

Most frequent origin of metastatic carcinoma is colon, in which cytokeratin 7/20 profile is useful for the differentiation of origin sites. CK7(-)/CK20(+) expression is universal in metastatic colon cancers; whereas CK7(+)/CK20(-) is usual in cholangiocarcinomas (Fig. 6).

4) Sclerosing cholangitis

Marked cytologic atypia, random diffuse infiltration of the duct wall, and perineural invasion favor the possibility of periductal spread of cholangio-carcinoma, rather than sclerosing cholangitis.

5) Epithelioid hemangioendothelioma

It can mimick neoplastic epithelial glandular structures on desmoplastic stroma. However, it lacks mucin production and express the endothelial cell markers.

5. Klatskin's Tumor (Hilar Cholangiocarcinoma and Extrahepatic Cholangiocarcinoma)

1) Gross

An half of carcinoma of extrahepatic bile ducts occurs in the upper third or hilar area. Cholangiocarcinoma arising from the right and left main hepatic ducts at or near their junction is named as Klatskin's tumor (Fig. 7). Tumors occurring at the bifurcation of the common hepatic duct make a problem such as obstruction or biliary stricture, resulting in obstructive jaundice even in their small size, and sometimes death attributed to liver failure or sepsis rather than to massive invasion of the liver or widespread metastases. Extrahepatic cholangiocarcinoma is presented by a small firm gray-white and poorly demarcated intramural nodule or relatively flat plaque-like induration. Fibrous collar encircling and constricting the one or both hepatic ducts is not uncommon. Some may have a papillary or polypoid shape with endoluminal growth. The mucosa may be granular, friable, or necrotic in appearance. For the proper pathologic evaluation, anatomic orientation of resected extrahepatic bile duct specimens should be provided by the surgeon.

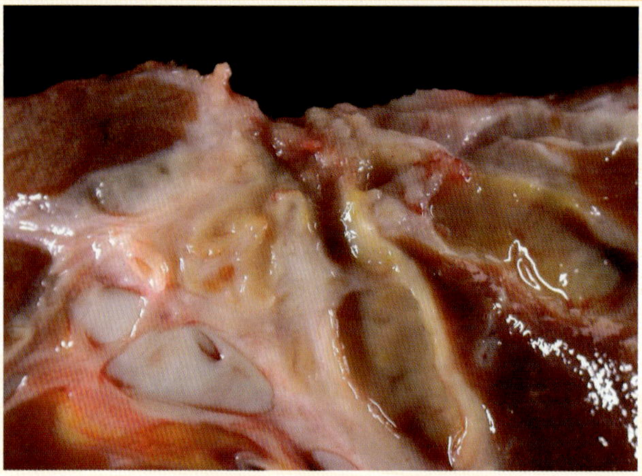

Fig. 7 Cut surface of hilar cholangiocarcinoma

Flat plaque-like nodular mass is noted at the bifurcation of main hepatic ducts with spread to the branch ducts.

2) Micro

Adenocarcinomas are usually well to moderately well differentiated with stromal desmoplasia (Fig. 8). Well-differentiated adenocarcinomas lined by cells with minimal atypia, basal nuclei, inconspicuous nucleoli, and a low N/C ratio may have a deceptively bland appearance. It frequently invades vertically beyond the confines of the duct wall because there are no formal anatomic barriers. And it

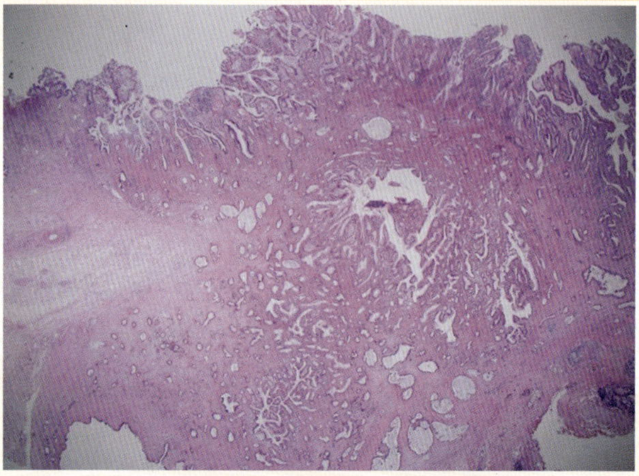

Fig. 8 Microscopic finding of extrahepatic cholangiocarcinoma

Whole layer of bile duct wall is involved by well differentiated adenocarcinoma (H-E, ×12.5).

also spreads laterally both in the proximal and the distal directions. It is very difficult to make a decision of reactive atypia and dysplasia/carcinoma of the surface epitheliums and to differentiate between atypical intramural glands and invading neoplastic glands, particularly at the time of frozen section of surgical resection margins. The presence of perineural or intraneural invasion is very helpful in the diagnosis of adenocarcinoma. Absence of true stratification of the epithelium, gradual transition between atypical areas and epithelial regions, that are more clearly reactive in appearance, and the presence of prominent neutrophilic inflammation and/or ulceration favor the benign reactive atypia.

6. Cytology of the Biliary Tract

Direct sampling of biliary secretions and endobiliary brushing are used to sample the biliary system lesions, when stricture or obstruction of the biliary tree. Recently liquid based cytology technique can be applied to the biliary tract brushing cytology. The overall sensitivity is not high (about 60%) due to limitation of information for the origin sites and degeneration or dryness of tumor cells. Repeated cytology can decrease the false negative rates.

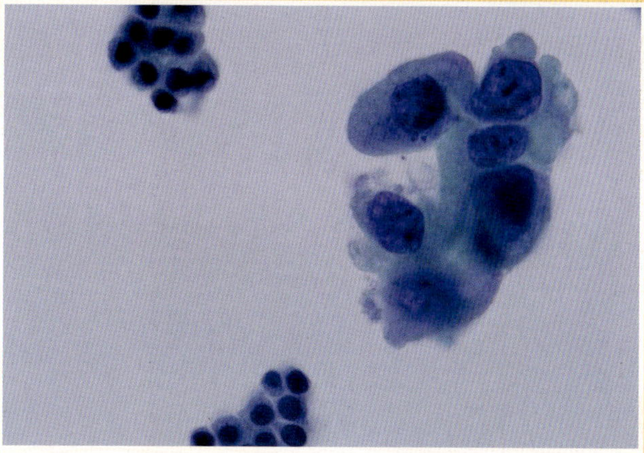

Fig. 9 Liquid based cytology preparation of bile duct brushing cytology

A cluster of overlapping large atypical cells is seen with two clusters of normal reactive cells. Tumor cells have large irregular nuclei with one or more prominent nucleoli and abundant pale cytoplasm (Papanicolaou, ×1,000).

Low grade dysplasia is characterized by sheets and clusters of cells that show nuclear crowding and overlapping. Nuclear membranes are smooth, and the nucleus-to-cytoplasm ratio is moderate. High grade dysplasia is characterized by more pronounced nuclear crowding and overlapping, irregular nuclear membrane, and increased N/C ratio. Adenocarcinoma shows highly cellular smear with a greater number of single cells. The chromatin is usually coarse, and nucleoli are usually distinct, however, the N/C ratio does not appear increased due to abundant cytoplasm (Fig. 9). The differential diagnosis between a reactive process and an adenocarcinoma may be extremely difficult. Japanese group suggested features highly associated with malignancy; loss of a honeycomb arrangement, an increase in the size of nuclei, loss of polarity, a bloody background, the presence of flat nuclei, and a "cell-in-cell" arrangement.[9]

7. Biliary Cystadenocarcinoma

Biliary cystadenocarcinoma is a continuum of biliary cystic neoplasm. It is usually multilocular cystic tumor filled with mucoid fluid. A large papillary mass or solid areas of grey-white mural nodule are found in the cyst wall (Fig. 10). Although it is a malignant tumor, well circumscription makes feasible to complete removal and prognosis is good. The cyst wall of benign cystadenoma have a single layer of columnar mucinous epithelium and underlying ovarian type stroma. Varying degree of cytologic atypia of mucinous epithelium, mitosis, and invasion of the underlying stroma are observed in cystadenocarcinoma.

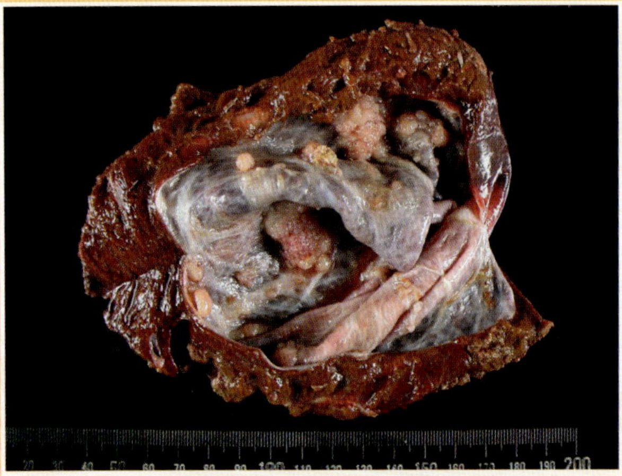

Fig. 10 Macroscopic finding of biliary cystadenocarcinoma

A huge unilocular cystic mass demonstrate multiple varying sized papillary mural nodules.

Reference

1. The Korean Liver Cancer Study Group. The general rules for the study of primary liver cancer. 3rd ed. Seoul: Jin, 2007.
2. Kang YK, Kim WH, Lee HW, Lee HK, Kim YI. Mutation of p53 and K-ras, and loss of heterozygosity of APC in intrahepatic cholangiocarcinoma. Lab Invest 1999;79:477-483.
3. Ohashi K, Nakajima Y, Kanehiro H, et al. Ki-ras mutations and p53 protein expressions in intrahepatic cholangiocarcinomas: relation to gross tumor morphology. Gastroenterology 1995;109:1612-1617.
4. Zen Y, Adsay NV, Bardadin K, et al. Biliary intraepithelial neoplasia: an international interobserver agreement study and proposal for diagnostic criteria. Mod Pathol 2007;20:701-709.
5. Zen Y, Fujii T, Itatsu K, et al. Biliary papillary tumors share pathological features with intraductal papillary mucinous neoplasm of the pancreas. Hepatology 2006;44:1333-1343.
6. Kloppel G, Kosmahl M. Is the intraductal papillary mucinous neoplasia of the biliary tract a counterpart of pancreatic papillary mucinous neoplasm? J Hepatol 2006;44:249-250.
7. Cazals-Hatem D, Rebouissou S, Bioulac-Sage P, et al. Clinical and molecular analysis of combine hepatocellular-cholangiocarcinomas. J Hepatol 2004;41:292-298.
8. Kim H, Park C, Han KH, et al. Primary liver carcinoma of intermediate (hepatocyte-cholangiocyte) phenotype. J Hepatol 2002;40:298-304.
9. Rabinovitz M, Zajko AB, Hassanein T, et al. Diagnostic value of brush cytology in the diagnosis of bile duct carcinoma: A study in 65 patients with bile duct strictures. Hepatology 1990;2:747-752.
10. Nakajima T, Tajima Y, Sugano I, et al. Multivariate statistical analysis of bile cytology. Acta Cytol 1994;38:51-55.

VI. Pathogenesis of Cholangiocarcinoma

VI Pathogenesis of Cholangiocarcinoma

Seungmin Bang, M.D.

VI
Pathogenesis of Cholangiocarcinoma

Introduction

Cholangiocarcinomas are rare cancers developing from the epithelial or blast-like cells lining the bile ducts. A variety of known predisposing factors and experimental

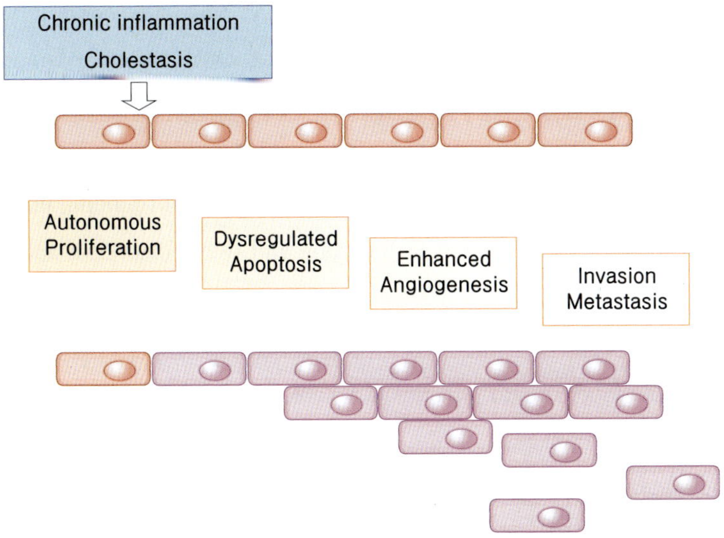

Fig. 1 Molecular multi-step carcinogenesis of cholangiocarcinomas.
Cholangiocarcinoma cells express altered molecular mechanisms that allow enhanced cell proliferation, deregulation of the apoptotic process, high capacity of tissue invasion, metastasize and angiogenesis. In this process, various molecular and genomic alterations are developed.

models of biliary carcinogenesis have elucidated the complex events of biliary tumorigenesis.[1] Cholangiocarcinogenesis is a multi-step process constituted by several hallmarks: enhanced susceptibility to proliferation stimuli and escape from inhibitory growth stimuli, dysregulation from the apoptotic process, and the development of a rich vessel network with the capacity for invasiveness and metastasis. Chronic inflammatory processes, generation of active oxygen radicals, altered cellular detoxification mechanisms, activation of oncogenes, functional loss of tumor-suppressor genes have been identified as important contributors in this process (Fig. 1).[2-6] And recent researches suggest 'liver progenitor cells' has a key role in the development of cholagniocarcinomas.[7,8] In this chapter, the known mechanisms involved in the multi-step carcinogenesis of biliary epithelium are summarized with mainly focusing the molecular aspects.

1. Enhanced Proliferation Signaling and Dysregulation of Apoptosis

The previously described etiologic factors, including liver fluke infestation, primary sclerosing cholantitis, and intrahepatic bile duct stones, create an environment of chronic inflammation predisposing biliary epithelium to malignant transformation.[1] Chronic inflammation and cholestasis have been linked to carcinogenesis in cholangiocarcinoma. In other words, the noxious environment surrounding inflamed cholangiocytes can cause autonomous proliferation and dysregulation of apoptosis mechanisms in cholangiocarcinogenesis.

Chronic inflammation results in the expression of multiple cytokines and chemokines by cholangiocytes and inflammatory cells. This milieu caused by chronic inflammation can lead a fundamental step-autonomous proliferating signaling.[9,10] The growth of malignant cholangiocytes is favored and constantly enhanced by the mitogenic factors locally produced by the tumor cells and by the constitutive activation of cellular receptors or various components of the intracellular signaling pathway. In the liver, hepatocytes, sinusoidal endothelial cells, hepatic stellate cells and Kupffer cells secrete cytokines, which are abundant in the course of chronic inflammation.

And, cholangiocytes produce and release cytokines such as interleukin-6 (IL-6), transforming growth factor-β (TGF-β), IL-8, tumor necrosis factor-α (TNF-α) and platelet-derived growth factor (PDGF) B chain.[11,12] These molecules play an important function in the development of cholangiocarcinomas. Although it is not clear how the cholangiocyte gets the abnormal functions by these cytokines initially, an explanation can be that cholangiocyte intracellular signaling in response to cytokine stimuli is altered during the course of malignancy. This altered mechanism could elicit the development and growth of biliary tract cancers.

One of the key cytokines in cholangiocarcinoma carcinogenesis is interleukin-6 (IL-6). IL-6 secretion is proven to be increased during the course of chronic inflammation and the neoplastic processes of biliary ducts and results in sustained proliferation by an autocrine/paracrine mechanism (Fig. 2).[11,13] Specifically, IL-6 increases the activation state of p44/p42 and p38 mitogen activated phosphorylation kinase (MAPK) pathways, which in turn, decreases the expression of p21.[14,15]

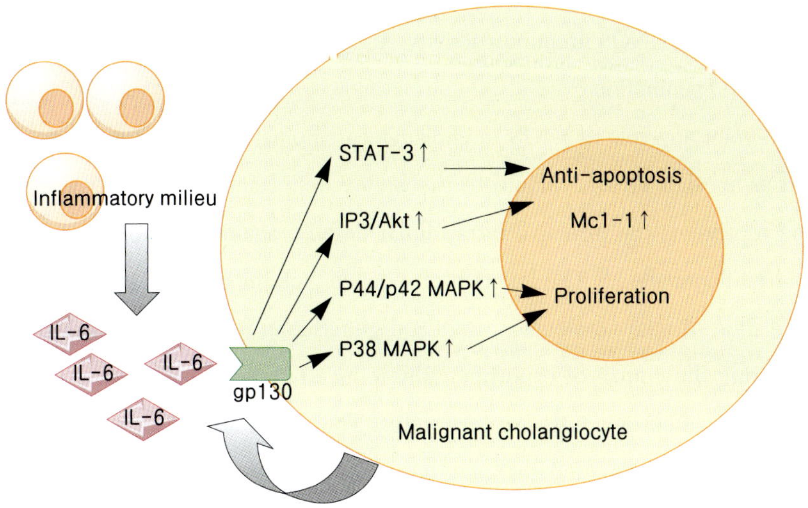

Fig. 2 Mechanisms of autocirne and paracrine action of IL-6 on malignant cholangiocyte.

IL-6, through an activation of STAT-3, upregulates Mcl-1 transcription. IL-6 also stimulates p38 and p44/p42 mitogen activated protein kinases in cholangiocarcinoma cells thus sustain their malignant growth.

However, it is the most interesting that IL-6-induced carcinogenicity has been shown to depend on the up-regulation of myeloid cell leukemia-1 (Mcl-1), a key anti-apoptotic B-cell lymphoma/leukemia 2 (Bcl-2) family member protein.[16] This effect is dependent upon IL-6 induced constitutive activation of STAT3 in malignant cholangiocytes, which regulates Mcl-1 transcription.[17] Cellular Mcl-1 protein levels are further enhanced by bile acid-induced epidermal-derived growth factor receptor (EGFR) activation. Furhtermore, IL-6 mediates escape from senescence by the induction of telomerase.[18]

Further damage is mediated by cytokine induction of inducible nitric oxide synthase (iNOS) in inflammatory cells and cholangiocytes. Increased iNOS expression has been observed in cholangiocytes in primary sclerosing cholangitis and cholangiocarcinoma, and elevated serum nitrate concentrations have been identified in patients with liver fluke infection.[19] Increased expression of iNOS results in increased generation of nitric oxide (NO), which inhibits DNA repair proteins and pro-apoptosis enzymes such as caspase-9.[10] Promotion of cancer development induced by iNOS and NO has also lead to the up-regulation of Notch-1, which is an important signaling pathway in bile duct and pancreas development.[20,21] Notch-1 was found overexpressed in cholangiocytes in PSC as well as in cholangiocarcinoma cells and it co-localizes with iNOS immunoreactivity. And, Notch-1 expression was actually dependent on NO generation.[20]

With the emerging role of iNOS in cholangiocarcinoma, reduced glutathione is considered as another factors related to the biliary neoplasms. Basically, reduced glutathione represents the principal intracellular defense against oxidative stress in the course of inflammation.[22] The function of reduced glutathione is to participate in the detoxification of many molecules. Reduced glutathione levels are decreased in bile juice during the course of experimentally induced cholestasis and also in the biliary epithelium of chronic inflammatory status. Thus, such alterations of reduced glutathione levels in cholangiocytes may dysregulate apoptosis and lead to DNA damage.[23] However, the role of reduced glutathione in the cholangiocarcinogenesis needs to be fully elucidated.

The molecular link between chronic inflammation and cholangiocarcinoma is further intensified by the potential roles of cyclooxygenase-2 (COX-2). In a murine model of biliary adenocarcinoma, developed upon overexpression of erythroblastic leukemia viral oncogene homolog 2 (ErbB-2), upregulation of COX-2 was initially observed. And overexpression of COX-2 enhanced cell growth in rat cholangiocarcinoma cells.[24,25] During the chronic inflammatory processes and cholestasis, 'oxysterols'- the oxidative derivatives of cholesterol-are produced and they are able to modulate gene expression of COX-2.[26,27] Actually, it is proven that increased COX-2 expression occurs in human cholangiocarcinoma cells with exposure to oxysterols.[26]

Recently, several another genes get spotlight in the aspect of malignant transformation of cholangiocytes. ErbB-2 and Met are proto-oncogenes that are very important for invasiveness and metastases of many types of malignancies. Interestingly, Met expression is increased in early phases of cholangiocarcinoma genesis, whereas ErbB-2 is thought to play a substantial role in the development and progression of cholangiocarcinomas.[28] And both ErbB-2 and Met can facilitate COX-2 formation.[2] And additional molecular alterations have been reported including TGF-β, Smad4, and PTEN gene.[29-31]

In the development of malignant tumors, dysregulation of apoptosis is inevitable mechanisms. A decrease or impairment of apoptotic mechanisms leads to the survival of mutated cholangiocytes, which lead to malignant transformation with multi-step events of various genetic mutations. Until now, Bcl-2, K-ras mutation and/or dysresgulation of p53 have been associated with dysregulation of apoptosis in cholangiocarcinomas.

Bcl-2 represents a superfamily of anti-apoptotic proteins. Bcl-2, the prototype of this family, is expressed by only small bile ductules.[32] The anti-apoptotic activity of Bcl-2 is exerted by preventing caspase 3 activation. Bcl-2 has shown to be overexpressed in cholangiocarcinoma cells, which possess a significantly increased apoptotic threshold compared to normal cholangiocytes.[33]

Point mutations of the K-ras oncogene noted in a wide variety of human tumors are also found in cholangiocarcinomas. Such mutations have been detected in codon 12, 13, and 61.[34] Interestingly, the expression of K-ras varies in accordance to the growth pattern of the neoplastic lesions. Indeed, K-ras gene alterations are frequent in the periductal-spreading type tumor but absent in the mass-forming type tumor, suggesting that such a mutation is important in cholangiocarcinoma arising near the hepatic hilum rather than peripheral cholangiocarcinomas.

The mutation of p53 gene in intrahepatic cholangiocarcinomas has been reported in relatively high incidence ranging 20~80%.[3] Interestingly, these mutations are more frequent in the mass-forming type tumors, thus suggesting that p53 mutation is related to the development of intrahepatic cholangiocarcinoma arising from the peripheral small bile ductules.[3,34,35]

Several other factors, including NO, COX-2 and Notch-1 are implicated in the dysregulation of apoptosis. Besides inducing malignant transformation of biliary cells, NO is also able to promote cholangiocyte immortalization by inhibiting apoptosis, which can occur through an event that occurs through the nitrosylation of caspase 9.[36] Notch-1 leads the cholangiocarcinoma cells to escape from apoptosis by attenuation of tumor necrosis factor-related apoptosis-inducing ligand (TRAIL)-mediated apoptosis. COX-2 also can prevent apoptosis of cholangiocarcinma cells with neutralizing the Fas-induced apoptosis.[20,37]

Finally, cellular senescence leads to a growth arrest due to telomere shortening. However, the over-expression of the enzyme telomerase maintains chromosomal length, thus conserving cell replication in malignant cells. The expression of human telomerase was detected in intrahepatic cholangiocarcinoma cells, and precancerous dysplatic cells, whereas its expression was not detected in non-dysplastic biliary epithelial cells and normal livers, thus suggesting that malignant cholangiocytes acquire telomerase activity at the dysplastic cell status thus triggering the carcinogenesis.[38]

2. Enhanced Angiogenesis, Invasiveness and Metastasis

Cholangiocarcinoma cells lead to development of a rich neovascular network for sustainig the metabolic needs and ensuring an adequate support of oxygen and nutrients to the malignant cells. High levels of the vascular endothelial growth factor (VEGF) play an important role in maintaining biliary tumor vascularization. Furthermore, VEGF expression is stimulated by β-catenin and TGF-β that are more expressed by the surrounding stromal cells and, to a lesser extent, by the malignant cells. Thus it suggests an autocrine/paracrine mechanism which stimulates the production of VEGF necessary for tumor growth.[39,40]

The high capacity of invasion and metastasis are two important features of cholangiocarcinomas. In this aspect, matrix metalloproteinases (MMPs) are considered as a key mediators. Cholangiocarcinoma expressed a large amount of MMP and a positive correlation between degree of MMP expression and clinical invasiveness exists. Human aspartyl (asparaginyl) b-hydroxylase and proteins related to the connective tissue growth factors are also overexpressed in cholangiocarcinomas, the levels of which correlate with the increase in malignant cholangiocyte motility and invasiveness.[41,42]

The expression of cell adhesion molecules (CAMs), which are considered as playing a critical role in invasion and metastasis, has been extensively evaluated in cholangiocarcinoma.[43] Indeed, membranous expression of E-cadherin, α-catenin, and β-catenin is reduced in a majority of biliary tract cancers. Especially, β-catenin down-regulation is associated with c-erbB2 down-regulation. Furthermore, MUC1 and Met have been demonstrated to interact with β-catenin, an interaction capable of increasing the invasive and metastatic properties of cholangiocarcinoma.[44]

Conclusion

The difficulty to overcome cholangiocarcinomas is due to the fact that cholangiocarcinoma is usually diagnosed in advanced stage. Unfortunately, at this stage any therapeutic modalities are no longer curative but assume a role of palliation. Moreover, chemotherapy and radiation therapy offer inadequate clinical outcomes. With this dismal situation, studies must be focused on the investigation of the molecular mechanisms involved in the development and progression of biliary malignancies. Recently, many studies have demonstrated that during the course of cholestasis and chronic inflammation, a multitude of factors released in the environment chronically stimulate the proliferation of cholangiocytes compounded by an accumulation of genetic damage leading to malignant transformation. These progresses in elucidating the molecular carcinogenetic mechanisms of cholangiocarcinomas can offer the possibility of developing new and more accurate tools for an earlier diagnosis and a potent therapy for cholangiocarcinoma.

Reference

1. Khan SA, Thomas HC, Davidson BR, Taylor-Robinson SD. Cholangiocarcinoma. Lancet 2005;366:1303-1314.
2. Sirica AE. Cholangiocarcinoma: molecular targeting strategies for chemoprevention and therapy. Hepatology 2005;41:5-15.
3. Berthiaume EP, Wands J. The molecular pathogenesis of cholangiocarcinoma. Semin Liver Dis 2004;24:127-137.
4. Sirica AE, Lai GH, Zhang Z. Biliary cancer growth factor pathways, cyclooxygenase-2 and potential therapeutic strategies. J. Gastroenterol Hepatol 2001;16:363-372.
5. Fava G, Marzioni M, Benedetti A, Glaser S, DeMorrow S, Francis H, et al. Molecular pathology of biliary tract cancers. Cancer Lett 2007;250:155-167.
6. Gores SJ. Cholangiocarcinoma: current concepts and insights. Hepatology 2003;37: 961-969.
7. Kim H, Park C, Han KH, Choi J, Kim YB, Kim JK, et al. Primary liver carcinoma of intermediate (hepatocytecholangiocyte) phenotype. J Hepatol 2004;40:298-304.
8. Libbrecht L, Roskams T. Hepatic progenitor cells in human liver diseases. Semin Cell Dev Biol 2002;13:389-396.
9. Lazaridis KN, Gores GJ. Cholangiocarcinoma. Gastroenterology 2005;128:1655-1667.
10. Jaiswal M, LaRusso NF, Burgart LJ, Gores GJ. Inflammatory cytokines induce DNA damage and inhibit DNA repair in cholangiocarcinoma cells by a nitric oxide dependent mechanism. Cancer Res 2000;60:184-190.
11. Yasoshima M, Kono N, Sugawara H, Katayanagi K, Harada K, Nakanuma Y. Increased expression of interleukin-6 and tumor necrosis factor-alpha in pathologic biliary epithelial cells: in situ and culture study. Lab Invest 1998;78:89-100.
12. Grappone C, Pinzani M, Parola M, Pellegrini G, Caligiuri A, DeFranco R, et al. Expression of platelet-derived growth factor in newly formed cholangiocytes during experimental biliary fibrosis in rats. J Hepatol 1999;31:100-109.
13. Okada K, Shimizu Y, Nambu S, Higuchi K, Watanabe A. Interleukin-6 functions as an autocrine growth factor in a cholangiocarcinoma cell line. J Gastroenterol Hepatol 1994;9:462-467.

14. Park J, Tadlock L, Gores GJ, Patel T. Inhibition of interleukin 6-mediated mitogen-activated protein kinase activation attenuates growth of a cholangiocarcinoma cell line. Hepatology 1999;30:1128-1133.

15. Tadlock L, Patel T. Involvement of p38 mitogen-activated protein kinase signaling in transformed growth of a cholangiocarcinoma cell line. Hepatology 2001;33:43-51.

16. Yoon JH, Werneburg NW, Higuchi H, Canbay AE, Kaufmann SH, Akgul C, et al. Bile acids inhibit Mcl-1 protein turnover via an epidermal growth factor receptor/Raf-1-dependent mechanism. Cancer Res 2002;62:6500-6505.

17. Isomoto H, Kobayashi S, Werneburg NW, Bronk SF, Guicciardi ME, Frank DA, et al. Interleukin 6 upregulates myeloid cell leukemia-1 expression through a STAT3 pathway in cholangiocarcinoma cells. Hepatology 2005;42:1329-1338.

18. Yamagiwa Y, Meng F, Patel T. Interleukin-6 decreases senescence and increases telomerase activity in malignant human cholangiocytes. Life Sci 2006;78:2494-2502.

19. Spirli C, Fabris L, Duner E, Fiorotto R, Ballardini G, Roskams T, et al. Cytokine-stimulated nitric oxide production inhibits adenylyl cyclase and cAMP-dependent secretion in cholangiocytes. Gastroenterology 2003;124:737-753.

20. Ishimura N, Bronk SF, Gores GJ. Inducible nitric oxide synthase up-regulates Notch-1 in mouse cholangiocytes: implications for carcinogenesis. Gastroenterology 2005;128:1354-1368.

21. Louis AA, Van Eyken P, Haber BA, Hicks C, Weinmaster G, Taub R, et al. Hepatic jagged1 expression studies. Hepatology 1999;30:1269-1275.

22. Celli A, Que FG, Gores GJ, LaRusso NF. Glutathione depletion is associated with decreased Bcl-2 expression and increased apoptosis in cholangiocytes. Am J Physiol Gastrointest Liver Physiol 1998;275:G749-G757.

23. Okuda K, Nakanuma Y, Miyazaki M. Cholangiocarcinoma: recent progress. Part 2: molecular pathology and treatment. J Gastroenterol Hepatol 2002;17:1056-1063.

24. Kiguchi K, Carbajal S, Chan K, Beltran L, Ruffino L, Shen J, et al. Constitutive expression of ErbB-2 in gallbladder epithelium results in development of adenocarcinoma. Cancer Res 2001; 61:6971-6976.

25. Zhang Z, Lai GH, Sirica AE. Celecoxib-induced apoptosis in rat cholangiocarcinoma cells mediated by Akt inactivation and Bax translocation. Hepatology 2004;39:1028-1037.

26. Yoon JH, Canbay AE, Werneburg NW, Lee SP, Gores GJ. Oxysterols induce cyclooxygenase-2 expression in cholangiocytes: implications for biliary tract carcinogenesis, Hepatology 2004;39:732-738.

27. Haigh WG, Lee SP. Identification of oxysterols in human bile and pigment gallstones, Gastroenterology 2001;121:118-123.

28. Aishima SI, Taguchi KI, Sugimachi K, Shimada M, Tsuneyoshi M. c-erbB-2 and c-Met expression relates to cholangiocarcinogenesis and progression of intrahepatic cholangiocarcinoma. Histopathology 2002;40:269-278.

29. Yazumi S, Ko K, Watanabe N, Shinohara H, Yoshikawa K, Chiba T, et al. Disrupted transforming growth factor-beta signaling and deregulated growth in human biliary tract cancer cells. Int J Cancer 2000;86:782-789.

30. Hahn SA, Bartsch D, Schroers A, Galehdari H, Becker M, Ramaswamy A, et al. Mutations of the DPC4/Smad4 gene in biliary tract carcinoma. Cancer Res 1998;58:1124-1126.

31. Xu X, Kobayashi S, Qiao W, Li C, Xiao C, Radaeva S, et al. Induction of intrahepatic cholangiocellular carcinoma by liver-specific disruption of Smad4 and Pten in mice. J Clin Invest 2006;116:1843-1852.

32. Skopelitou A, Hadjiyannakis M, Alexopoulou V, Krikoni O, Kamina S, Agnantis N. Topographical immunohistochemical expression of bcl-2 protein in human liver lesions. Anticancer Res 1996;16:975-978.

33. Harnois DM, Que FG, Celli A, LaRusso NF, Gores GJ. Bcl-2 is overexpressed and alters the threshold for apoptosis in a cholangiocarcinoma cell line. Hepatology 1997;26:884-890.

34. Ohashi K, Nakajima Y, Kanehiro H, Tsutsumi M, Taki J, Aomatsu Y, et al. Ki-ras mutations and p53 protein expressions in intrahepatic cholangiocarcinomas: relation to gross tumor morphology. Gastroenterology 1995;109:1612-1617.

35. Furubo S, Harada K, Shimonishi T, Katayanagi K, Tsui W, Nakanuma Y. Protein expression and genetic alterations of p53 and ras in intrahepatic cholangiocarcinoma. Histopathology 1999;35:230-240.

36. Torok NJ, Higuchi H, Bronk S, Gores GJ. Nitric oxide inhibits apoptosis downstream of cytochrome c release by nitrosylating caspase 9. Cancer Res 2002;62:1648-1653.

37. Nzeako UC, Guicciardi ME, Yoon JH, Bronk SF, Gores GJ. COX-2 inhibits Fas-mediated apoptosis in cholangiocarcinoma cells. Hepatology 2002;35:552-559.

38. Ozaki S, Harada K, Sanzen T, Watanabe K, Tsui W, Nakanuma Y. In situ nucleic acid detection of human telomerase in intrahepatic cholangiocarcinoma and its preneoplastic lesion. Hepatology 1999;30:914-919.

39. Easwaran V, Lee SH, Inge L, Guo L, Goldbeck C, Garrett E, et al. beta-Catenin regulates vascular endothelial growth factor expression in colon cancer. Cancer Res 2002;63: 3145-3153.

40. Benckert C, Jonas S, Cramer T, Von Marschall Z, Schafer G, Peters M, et al. Transforming growth factor beta 1 stimulates vascular endothelial growth factor gene transcription in human cholangiocellular carcinoma cells. Cancer Res 2003;63:1083-1092.

41. Terada T, Okada Y, Nakanuma Y. Expression of immunoreactive matrix metalloproteinases and tissue inhibitors of matrix metalloproteinases in human normal livers and primary liver tumors. Hepatology 1996;23:1341-1344.

42. Maeda T, Sepe P, Lahousse S, Tamaki S, Enjoji M, Wands JR, et al. Antisense oligodeoxynucleotides directed against aspartyl (asparaginyl) beta-hydroxylase suppress migration of cholangiocarcinoma cells. J Hepatol 2003;38:615-622.

43. Ashida K, Terada T, Kitamura Y, Kaibara N. Expression of E-cadherin, alpha-catenin, beta-catenin, and CD44 (standard and variant isoforms) in human cholangiocarcinoma: an immunohistochemical study. Hepatology 1998;27:974-982.

44. Schroeder JA, Adriance MC, Thompson MC, Camenisch TD, Gendler SJ. MUC1 alters beta-catenin-dependent tumor formation and promotes cellular invasion. Oncogene 2003;22:1324-1332.

VII. Staging of Cholangiocarcinoma

VII Staging of Cholangiocarcinoma

Sae Byeol Choi, M.D., Kyung Sik Kim, M.D., Ph.D.

VII
Staging of Cholangiocarcinoma

Introduction

Staging describes the severity of an individual's cancer based on the extent of the original (primary) tumor and spread in the body. Its importances are following:

- Staging helps a doctor to plan a treatment for patients .
- The stage can be used to estimate a person's prognosis (likely outcome or course of the disease).
- Knowing the stage helps in identifying clinical trials (research studies) that may be suitable for a particular patient.
- Staging helps researchers and health care providers to exchange information about patients and also gives them a common language for evaluating the results of clinical trials and comparing the results of different trials.

The clinical staging which includes patient's functional status generally depends on imaging procedures. These procedures demonstrate the size of the primary tumor and the presence of the hematogenous metastasis and lymph nodes involvements. On the other hand the pathological staging is mainly assessed from the surgically resected specimen.

Cholangiocarcinoma is a malignant neoplasm that arises from biliary epithelium. Anatomical classifications of this tumor are divided by two main tumor location; intrahepatic or extrahepatic. Extrahepatic cholangiocarcinomas are often subclassified into those involving hepatic duct bifurcation (perihilar or hilar lesion), and distal lesions. After hepatic resection that includes bile duct, the hilar bile duct cancer and intrahepatic cholangiocarcinoma involving the hepatic hilus appear to have different prognoses.[2] But it is very difficult to distinguish between the two by tumor location. The staging systems reflect the prognostic factors that significantly affect the survival of the patients. For the different pathophysiology of intrahepatic and extrahepatic tumors, there is no unified single staging system for all cholangiocarcinomas. There fore several modifications and alternatives have been proposed to improve the prognostic predictions for each cancer stage.

In this chapter, we describe the current staging systems available for cholangiocarcinoma according to intrahepatic (peripheral) and extrahepatic cholangiocarcinomas. The extrahepatic cholangiocarcinomas include hilar cholangiocarcinoma and distal bile duct cancer. As the techniques for liver resection and the supportive treatments for extensive surgery are beling developed, the active surgical approaches for hilar cholangiocarcinoma are strongly recommended.[3-5] First of all, it should be determined whether the tumor will be resectable based on preoperative tumor staging. Therefore the staging systems specific for hilar cholangiocarcinoma will also be described.

1. Intrahepatic (peripheral) Cholangiocarcinoma

The most common classification systems for primary cancers of the liver are the TNM International Union against Cancer (UICC)/American Joint Committee on Cancer (AJCC) classification[6-9] and the TNM classification of the Liver Cancer Study Group of Japan (LCSGJ).[10,11] Primary cancers of the liver are mostly composed of hepatocellular carcinoma (HCC) and intrahepatic cholangiocarcinoma (ICC). Intrahepatic cholangiocarcinomas (ICC) define tumors that originate at the second branch (segmental branch) or the proximal branch of the bile duct.[12] They account for approximately 10% of all cholangiocarcinomas and 5% of primary liver malignancies.[13-17] They are distinct from hepatocellular carcinomas (HCC) with regard to their etiology and biologic behavior.

Although the oncologic characteristics are different between the two cancers, the classification of the TNM staging for ICC is similar to that for HCC. The difference between HCC and ICC is that serous membrane invasion is a positive prognostic factor for ICC, but not for HCC. Vascular invasion is a positive prognostic factor in both HCC and ICC; however, the modes of vascular invasion of HCC and ICC are different. HCC forms a tumor thrombus in vascular structures, whereas ICC infiltrates into the walls of vessels.[18]

Several clinicopathological factors with significant influence on survival have been reported. Vascular invasion,[19-21] perineural invasion,[22,23] lymph node metastasis,[20-22,24,25] intrahepatic metastasis,[21,24] microscopic presence of tumor on resection margin,[19,21,22,26] multiple tumors,[19,25,26] tumor size,[21] and R0 resection[22,23,25] are found to be significant prognostic factors for survival in various studies.

1) AJCC TNM classification

Before the unification of UICC and AJCC staging system in 2002,[7,9] there were two main TNM classifications for primary liver carcinomas: UICC and AJCC. After the revision of the UICC system in 1997,[6] the T category of the UICC became the same as that of the AJCC.[8] The T category of the TNM classification of the AJCC 6th edition has been newly changed to reflect the tumor size, number, presence of vascular invasion, and invasion to adjacent organs (Table 1).

The N category is divided according to the presence of regional lymph node metastasis. The definition of regional lymph nodes in UICC/AJCC still was different in the 5th edition. In UICC 5th edition, the regional lymph nodes are limited to the hilar nodes (i.e. in the hepatoduodenal ligament).[6] In the AJCC 5th edition, the regional lymph nodes are the hilar, hepatic, and periportal lymph nodes, along with the hepatic artery, portal vein, and IVC.[8] Due to the different criteria for regional lymph nodes, the TNM stages of the cases according to the AJCC are not the same as those according to the UICC. Nozaki et al. reported that the status of the lymph nodes defined as "regional" according to the AJCC (5th edition) staging system more accurately predict prognosis than the status of those defined by the UICC (5th edition) staging system.[27]

Table 1. AJCC TNM staging system for ICC (6th edition)

TNM	
Tx	Primary tumor cannot be assessed
T0	No evidence of primary tumor
T1	Solitary tumor without vascular invasion
T2	Solitary tumor with vascular invasion or multiple tumors ≤5 cm
T3	Multiple tumors >5 cm or tumor involving a major branch of the portal or hepatic vein
T4	Tumor with direct invasion of adjacent organs other than gall bladder or with perforation of visceral peritoneum
Nx	Regional lymph nodes cannot be assessed
N0	No metastasis to lymph node
N1	Regional lymph node metastasis
Mx	Distant metastasis cannot be assessed
M0	No distant metastasis
M1	Distant metastasis
Stage I	T1N0M0
Stage II	T2N0M0
Stage IIIA	T3N0M0
Stage IIIB	T4N0M0
Stage IIIC	AnyTN1M0
Stage IV	AnyTAnyNM1

In the AJCC 6th edition, the regional lymph nodes are the hilar, hepatoduodenal ligament lymph nodes, and caval lymph nodes. The most prominent ones are the hepatic artery and portal vein lymph nodes. Histologic examination of a regional lymphadenectomy specimen ordinarily includes a minimum of three lymph nodes.[9]

The prognostic significance of the number and the extent of lymph node metastasis are controversial and not well characterized. Nozaki et al. reported that patients with only regional lymph node metastasis showed no difference in survival rate compared with those with distant lymph node metastasis.[27] Although the number of lymph node metastases did not affect survival (single vs. multiple lymph node metastasis, $p=0.26$),[28] the presence of lymph node metastasis is a poor prognostic factor for survival. In contrast, some authors have reported that the survival rates in patients with three or more positive nodes were significantly lower than in those with fewer than three ($p < 0.001$).[25]

The M category comprises cases with distant metastasis or non-regional lymph node metastasis. Nodal involvement beyond these lymph nodes is considered distant metastasis (M1). Invasion into the inferior phrenic lymph nodes should also be considered as M1 in the AJCC classification.[9] The stage grouping is shown in Table 1.

In one study, univariate analysis of prognostic factors on survival following surgical resection in 292 ICC patients showed that AJCC staging system is the one of significant factors for prognosis. The long-term survival of stage I/II patients is better than that of stage III/IV patients (Stage I vs. II, $p = 0.10$; Stage II vs. III, $p = 0.04$; Stage III vs. IV, $p = 0.06$). The 1-, 3-, 5-, and 10-year overall survival rates of these 292 patients were 68.3%, 39.0%, 29.0%, and 13.7%, respectively.[28]

In summary, the staging system proposed by AJCC has been formulated for HCC. It is the main limitation of AJCC classification in that two diseases with completely different biological behaviors as previously stated. Revision of ICC in the AJCC staging system is required to take into account the biological characteristics of ICC.

2) TNM classification of the Liver Cancer Study Group of Japan (LCSGJ)

In 1992, the Liver Cancer Study Group of Japan (LCSGJ) organized a committee to establish a macroscopic type classification and TNM staging system for ICC by using 245 collected resected ICC specimens from the leading institutes of hepatic surgery in Japan. ICCs were classified into one of three basic types:[10] (1) mass-forming type, (2) periductal-infiltrating type, and (3) intraductal growth type (Fig. 1).

The mass-forming type forms a definite round-shaped mass, located in the liver parenchyma without invasion of a major branch of the portal triad. The periductal infiltrating type is characterized by a tumor that extends mainly longitudinally along the bile duct. The tumor mass itself is often not detected upon imaging studies. The intraductal growth type showes a mass proliferating toward the lumen of the bile duct in a papillary pattern or like a tumor thrombus. This type of ICC is usually detected in a thick bile duct. 'Unclassified' is added as a fourth category. When the tumor has more than one component of the three basic types, the predominant type is described first and the following less dominant component, connected by a '+', is described

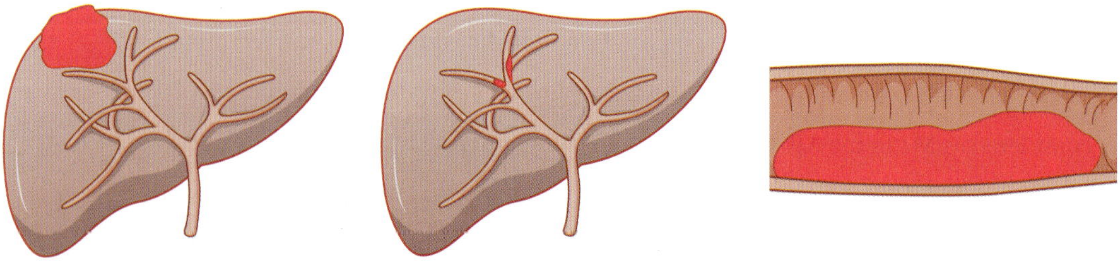

Fig. 1 Three macroscopic types of ICC.
A: mass-forming type; B: periductal infiltrating type; C: intraductal growth type

respectively.

And then, in 1996, the ICC committee of the LCSGJ started to work to establish a TNM classification of ICC. For the staging system, the patients with periductal infiltrating type and intraductal growth type were excluded because of the small number of patients. Thus this staging system for ICC was initially applied only to the mass-forming type tentatively. Several prognostic factors were investigated in 136 mass-forming type ICC samples by univariate and multivariate analyses.[18] Tumor size of 2 cm or less (hazard ratio [HR], 2.39; 95% confidence interval [CI], 18.06-0.32), lymph node metastasis (HR, 2.36; 95% CI, 4.33-1.28), number of nodules, solitary or multiple tumors (HR, 1.93; 95% CI, 3.18-1.17), serous membrane invasion (HR, 2.19; 95% CI, 3.60-1.33), portal vein invasion (HR, 1.68; 95% CI, 2.88-0.98), and hepatic vein invasion (HR, 1.18; 95% CI, 2.16-0.65) were significantly positive factors for predicting death. Based on these results, T factors were proposed as following: T1 is a tumor that is solitary, 2 cm or less in size, and without portal and hepatic vein and serous membrane invasion, T2 is a tumor with two of these three characteristics, T3 is a tumor with one of these three characteristics, and T4 is a tumor with none of these characteristics (Table 2).

There are three major routes of lymphatic spread in ICC: the hepatoduodenal route, the cardiac route, and the diaphragmatic route.[29] Lymph nodes were grouped

Table 2. TNM staging according to Liver Cancer Study Group of Japan (LCSGJ)

Stage	
T factor defined by 3 criteria	
Number of tumors: Solitary	
Size of tumor: 2 cm or less	
Negative invasion: Portal vein, hepatic vein, serous membrane	
T1	Fulfill all 3 criteria
T2	Fulfill 2 of 3 criteria
T3	Fulfill 1 of 3 criteria
T4	Fulfill none of 3 criteria
N0	No metastasis to lymph node
N1	Metastasis to any lymph node
M0	No distant metastasis
M1	Distant metastasis
Stage I	T1N0M0
Stage II	T2N0M0
Stage III	T3N0M0
Stage IVA	T4N0M0 / AnyTN1M0
Stage IVB	AnyTAnyNM1

Table 3. Japanese classification of lymph-nodes stations

Number	Site	Number	Site
1	Right cardial	12	Hepatoduodenal ligament
2	Left cardial	13	Retropancreatic
3	Lesser gastric curvature	14	Superior mesenteric artery
4	Greater curvature	15	Middle colic
5	Suprapyloric	16	Paraaortic
6	Infrapyloric	17	Superior pancreatic
7	Left gastric artery	18	Inferior pancreatic

according to the Classification of Primary Liver Cancer by the LCSGJ.[11] Lymph nodes are numbered as shown in Table 3.

In the 1st edition of LCSGJ,[10] the right and left lobes of the liver have different routes of lymphatic drainage according to the tumor location. Therefore the grouping of regional lymph nodes is distinguished by the tumor location (Fig. 2). LCSGJ

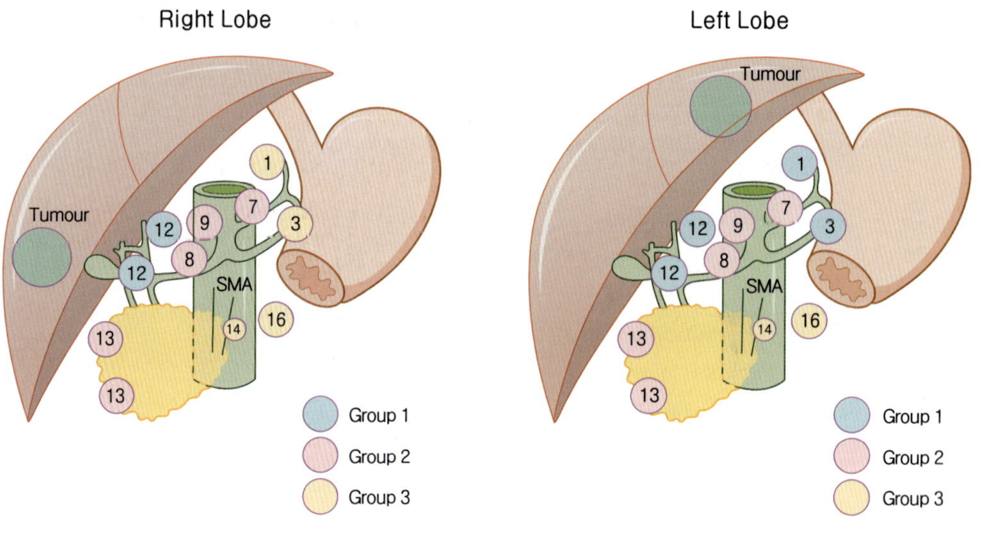

Fig. 2 The lymphatic drainage according to the tumor location.

defined regional lymph nodes in the 1st English edition[10] as following: for right lobe tumors, regional lymph nodes were defined as lymph nodes in the hepatoduodenal ligament, but for left lobe tumors, regional lymph nodes were defined as those in the right cardiac portion along the lesser curvature of the stomach and in the hepatoduodenal ligament.[10] Nozaki et al. reported that metastasis from left lobe tumors is often (50%) found in locations distant from the hepatoduodenal ligament without metastasis in the ligament.[27]

In the 2nd edition of the LCSGJ, the N category is no longer subdivided according to the tumor location.[11] This reflects clinical studies that did not show a significant difference of prognosis in patients with regional positive lymph nodes versus those with non-regional lymph nodes.[27,30] It has been suggested that lymph node metastasis is a strong prognostic factor for ICC.[20-22,24,25] As soon as lymph node metastases occur, positive lymph nodes are rarely limited to the regional lymph nodes.[31] It could not confirm the hypotheses that regional lymph nodes as defined by the UICC were the most frequent sites of metastases or that the prognosis of the patients with regional lymph node metastasis (N1) was better than that of patients with distant lymph node

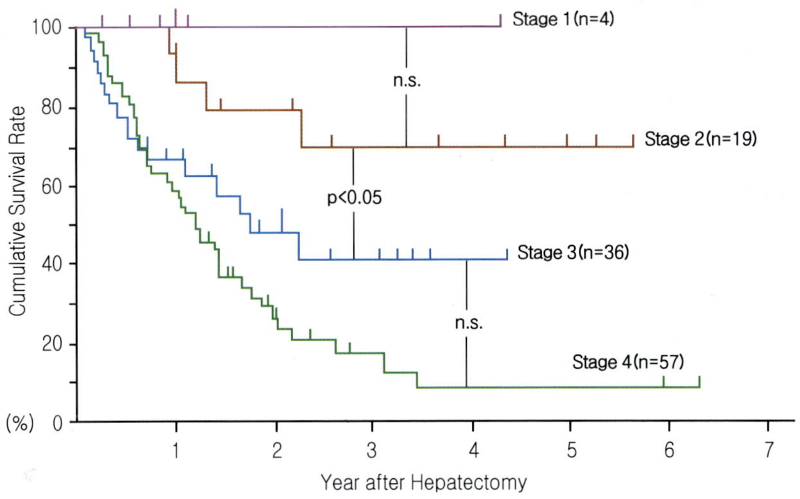

Fig. 3 Survival rate of ICC according to TNM classification of LCSGJ.[18]

metastasis (N2). However, the fact that any positive lymph node metastasis made the prognosis of the patient significantly worse than negative lymph node metastasis was confirmed.[18] These data were obtained from a nation-wide survey of 791 Japanese institutions. The results of 1,087 patients with ICC did not show significant differences in the 3-year survival of N1, N2, and N3 patients: 29%, 22%, and 12% respectively.[32] Without providing a proposal for further lymph-node grouping, the 2nd edition of the LCSGJ classification[11] subdivides the N category only according to lymph-node metastasis. The N category is therefore divided in two categories: N0 and N1 (Table 2). The M category is subdivided into the presence of distant metastasis to other organs or non-regional lymph nodes: M0 (without distant metastasis) and M1 (with distant metastasis).[11] The stage grouping is shown in Table 2.

The survival rates of ICC patients who underwent curative resection showed that the differences in survival rates between any two neighboring stages are not always significant[18] (Fig. 3). This is because the number of the subjects still was not enough to obtain a statistically significant difference even though it was a multi-institutional study. However, separation of the survival curves was found to be appropriate.

2. Extrahepatic Cholangiocarcinoma

1) Hilar cholangiocarcinoma

Extrahepatic cholangiocarcinomas are characterized by short or median survival times in the range of months. Cholangiocarcinoma arising from the bifurcation of the main intrahepatic ducts, or hilum, was described by Klatskin in 1965.[33] Perihilar tumors have been referred as Klatskin tumors from that time. Tumors arising from this site are 40 to 60% of all cholangiocarcinomas and have a worse prognosis than distal lesions or those arising from intrahepatic bile ducts.[34] Curative resection of the tumor offers the only chance for cure and long term survival to a patient.[35-37] The 5-year survival rates for patients with resection range from approximately 20 to 40%, and are significantly greater in patients who underwent a R0 resection.[38] Curative resection for hilar cholangiocarcinoma potentially requires a major hepatectomy with negative resection margins in almost every patient. Therefore, the evolution of staging systems for hilar cholangiocarcinoma has developed towards a system that measures resectability.

Several staging systems for hilar cholangiocarcinoma have been proposed. The Bismuth-Corlette classification system,[39] specific for Klatskin tumors, has been used widely. The AJCC TNM[9] and Japanese Society of Biliary Surgery (JSBS) classifications[40] for extrahepatic cholangiocarcinomas are also used for categorizing hilar cholangiocarcinomas. Bismuth-Corlette classification, AJCC TNM and JSBS classification have some limitation for predicting both survival and resectability. The Memorial Sloan-Kettering Cancer Center (MSKCC) group proposed the clinical T staging system for hilar cholangiocarcinoma that stratifies patients preoperatively into subgroups based on potential for resection. It is based on biliary ductal involvement, vascular involvement, and hepatic lobar atrophy.

(1) AJCC TNM classification[9]

The AJCC TNM system 6th edition was published in 2002 (Table 4). Both the UICC and the AJCC adopted the same TNM classification and staging systems. The new classification focuses on vascular invasion requiring vascular resection and reconstruction, as well as lymph node metastasis.

Invasion of the subepithelial fibromuscular connective tissue is classified as the T1 in the 6th edition. The T2 is defined as invasion beyond the wall of the bile duct. Actually, T1 and T2 categories are the same in 5th and 6th edition. The T3 group of the 5th edition is divided into two categories by the 6th edition (Table 5). The T3 tumor in the 6th edition invades liver, gallbladder, pancreas, and/or unilateral tributaries of the portal vein or hepatic artery. And the T4 tumor in 6th edition invades the main portal vein or its tributaries bilaterally, common hepatic artery, or adjacent structures such as the colon, stomach, duodenum, and abdominal wall.

Table 4. AJCC TNM staging system for extrahepatic cholangiocarcinoma (6th edition)

TNM	
Tx	Primary tumor cannot be assessed
T0	No evidence of primary tumor
Tis	Carcinoma in situ
T1	Tumor confined to the bile duct Histologically
T2	Tumor invades beyond the wall of the bile duct
T3	Tumor invades the liver, gallbladder, pancreas, and/or ipsilateral branches of the portal vein (right or left) or hepatic artery (right or left)
T4	Tumor invades any of the following: main portal vein or its branches bilaterally, common hepatic artery, or other adjacent structures, such as the colon, stomach, duodenum, or abdominal wall.
Nx	Regional lymph nodes cannot be assessed
N0	No metastasis to lymph node
N1	Regional lymph node metastasis
Mx	Distant metastasis cannot be assessed
M0	No distant metastasis
M1	Distant metastasis
Stage 0	Tis N0 M0
Stage IA	T1 N0 M0
Stage IB	T2 N0 M0
Stage IIA	T3 N0 M0
Stage IIB	T1-3 N1 M0
Stage III	T4 Any N M0
Stage IV	AnyT AnyN M1

Table 5. Comparison of the AJCC/UICC staging system between 5th and 6th editions

5th edition			6th edition	
		T category		
Tis	Carcinoma in situ	→	Tis	Carcinoma in situ
T1	Ductal wall		T1	Ductal wall
T2	Perifibromuscularconnective tissue	→	T2	Beyond ductal wall
T3	Adjacent structures	→	T3	Liver, GB, pancreas or unilateral vessels
		↘	T4	Other adjacent organs, or main or bilateral vessels
		N category		
N0	No regional LN metastasis	→	N0	No regional LN node metastasis
N1	Hepatoduodenal ligament LN	→	N1	Regional LN metastasis
N2	Other regional LN	↗		
		Staging system		
Stage	TNM	→	Stage	TNM
0	TisN0M0	→	0	TisN0M0
I	T1N0M0	→	IA	T1N0M0
II	T2N0M0		IB	T2N0M0
III	T1N1,2M0	↗	IIA	T3N0M0
	T2N1,2M0	↘ ↗	IIB	T1,2,3N1M0
IVA	T3AnyNM0	→	III	T4AnyNM0
IVB	AnyTAnyNM1	→	IV	AnyTAnyNM1

There is a potential for ambiguity in distinguishing T1 and T2 extrahepatic cholangiocarcinomas. Determining the border of the bile duct can be difficult to discern in some cases, even histologically.[42,43] However the outer border of the bile duct is defined by the outer smooth muscle layer. It is known that the distribution of the smooth muscle fibers varies along the extrahepatic bile duct. A continuous muscle layer may be seen in the distal extrahepatic bile duct, but only an interrupted or scattered muscle layer is present in the middle extrahepatic bile duct, and scanty muscle fibers are seen in the proximal extrahepatic bile duct.[42] The characteristics of bile duct and frequent desmoplastic stromal reaction accompanying extrahepatic cholangiocarcinoma may lead to confusion in the distinction between the T1 and T2 stages.

An analysis of 222 extrahepatic bile duct carcinomas by Hong et al.[44] demonstrated no differences in survival rates between patients with T2 tumors (stage IB) and patients with T3 tumors (stage IIA). This result can be explained by the different anatomic structures in the different regions of the extrahepatic bile duct. A middle common bile duct cancer with extended pericholedochal soft tissue can be staged as T2, while a tumor of the same depth of invasion may be staged as T3 in the distal bile duct because of minimal invasion of the pancreas.

The N factor was categorized into N0 (no lymph node metastasis) or N1 (regional lymph node metastasis). The regional lymph nodes include the hilar, celiac, periduodenal, peripancreatic, and superior mesenteric lymph nodes. The hilar nodes are the lymph nodes along the common bile duct, hepatic artery, portal vein, and cystic duct. The N1 (cystic duct, pericholedochal and/or hilar lymph nodes, e.g. those in the hepatoduodenal ligament) and N2 (peripancreatic, head only, periduodenal, periportal, celiac, superior mesenteric, and/or posterior pancreaticoduodenal lymph nodes) categories were distinguished by the location of invaded nodes in the 5th edition,[8] while in the 6th edition,[9] they were consolidated as the N1 group (regional lymph node metastasis). Optimal histologic examination of a regional lymphadenectomy specimen should include analysis of a minimum of three lymph nodes.[9] Nishio et al compared 166 patients with perihilar cholangiocarcinoma undergoing R0 resection according to the TNM classifications between 5th and 6th editions.[45] Although in the 5th edition, survival for pN0 patients was better than that of pN2 or pM1 patients, pN1 patients survived longer than pM1 patients with similar survival rates for pN1 and pN2 patients, and the differentiation between N1 and N2 did not affect the prediction of prognosis (Fig. 5a). In the 6th edition, the survival for pN0 patients was significantly better than that for newly defined pN1 and pM1 patients but the patients with pN1 in 6th edition (especially involved into the paraaortic lymph node) tended to survive longer than pM1 patients($p = 0.063$) (Fig 5b)).

Therefore the revision of new TNM classification for perihilar cholangiocarcinoma was proposed (Table 6).

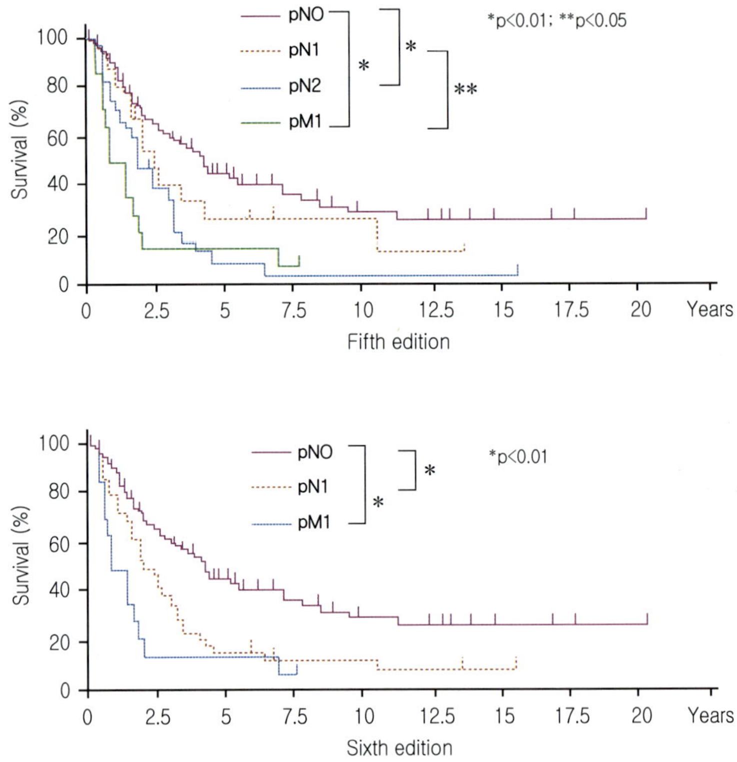

Fig. 5 Survival curvesw of 66 patients with perihilar cholangiocarcinoma, shown according to pN category based on AJCC system 5th ed (above(a)) & 6th ed. (below(b))

The M factor was categorized into M0 (no distant metastasis) and M1 (distant metastasis). Distant metastases usually occur late in the course of the disease, and are most often found in the liver, lungs, and peritoneum.

In the staging groupings, a single TNM classification must apply to both clinical and pathologic staging. With advances in imaging technology, integrated radiologic and pathologic staging of patients can be satisfactorily achieved. Clinical evaluation usually depends on the results of ultrasonography, CT, and/or MRCP (Magnetic Resonance Cholangiopancreatography) and PET (positron emission tomography). Clinical staging may also be based on findings from surgical exploration when the main tumor mass is not resected.[9]

Stage IA lesions are limited to the biliary mucosa or muscle wall, while stage IB

Table 6. The revising new TNM classification for perihilar cholangiocarcinoma by Nagoya Group

Stage		TNM
0	0	TisN0M0
I	IA	T1N0M0
	IB	T2N0M0
	IC	T3N0M0
II	IIA	T1-3N1M0
	IIB	T4N0M0
III	IIIA	T4N1M0
	IIIB	AnyTN2M0
IV		AnyTAnyNM1

T: category is the same as in the AJCC TNM classification (6th edition)
No: lymph node metastasis, N1: regional lymph node metastasis,
N2: more widespread lymph node metastasis
M0: No distant metastasis apart from lymph node metastasis,
M1: distant extradonal metastasis

tumors extend beyond the bile duct wall. Stage IIA lesions are metastatic to liver, gall bladder, pancreas, unilateral branches of the portal vein or hepatic artery, while stage IIB tumors involve regional lymph nodes. Stage III lesions are extensively invasive to the main portal vein or its branches, common hepatic artery, or adjacent organs, while stage IV tumors involve distant metastases. Nishio et al. reported that the 6th edition gave excessive value to cancer invasion of the portal bifurcation at the expense of regional lymph node metastasis. In that report, stage III tumors are composed of T4N0M0 and T4N1M0. Thus Nishio et al. proposed that cancer invasion to the portal bifurcation and regional lymph node metastasis should be weighted equally in the further revision of staging system.[45] As many as 50% of patients are stage III upon presentation, and 10~20% have stage IV disease.[46] Therefore the AJCC systems had the fewest early-stage patients with gross disease evident at the conclusion of surgery.[47]

The presence of residual tumors is also described although it is not a part of TNM staging. R0 describes a microscopically margin-negative resection, which means no gross or microscopic residual tumor existing in the tumor bed. R1 indicates removal of all macroscopic disease but with microscopic margins that are positive for tumor.

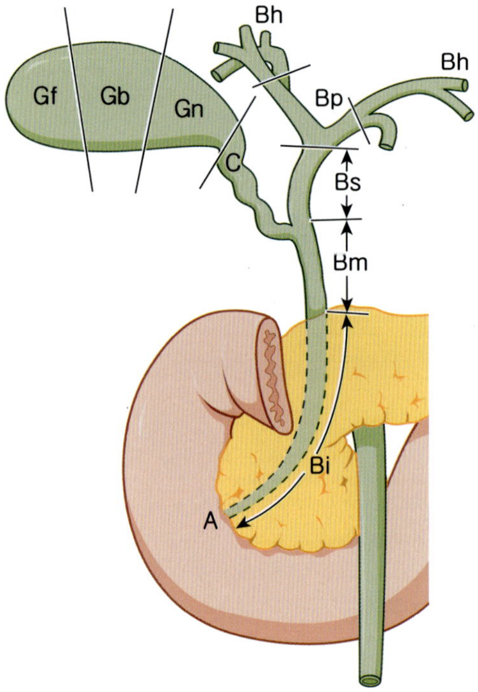

Fig. 6 Anatomical nomenclature of the biliary tract (Japanese Society of Biliary Surgery. Classification of biliary tract carcinoma.

Bh ; Intrahepatic bile ducts, Bp ; Portal (Hilar) bile duct, Bs ; Superior bile duct, Bm ; Middle bile duct, Bi ; Inferior bile duct, Gf ; Fundus of the gallbladder, Gb ; Body of the gallbladder, Gn ; Neck of the gallbladder, C ; Cystic duct

R2 indicates gross residual disease. R0 resection has been known to be a significant prognostic factor for survival in individuals with hilar cholangiocarcinoma.[41,48-50]

To assess the ability to predict survival according to 6th edition, Nishio et al. in Nagoya's group investigated 166 patients with perihilar cholangiocarcinoma undergoing R0 resection.[45] Survival rate was similar to patients with stages IA, IB, and IIA. Survival was significantly better in patients with stages IA and IB tumors than in those with stages IIB, III, and IV, and stage IIA patients survived longer than stage III or IV patients. Survival was longer for stage IIB patients than for stage IV patients. Hidalgo et al. reported on the survival outcomes of 44 hilar cholangiocarcinoma patients who underwent resections.[49] The 5-year survival rates of these individuals with stage IB, IIA, or IIB were 53%, 53%, and 34%, respectively. For those with stage III or IV tumors, the survival times at 1 and 3 years were 42% and 0%, and 25%

Table 7. JSBS (Japanese Society of Biliary Surgery) Classification of extrahepatic cholangiocarcinoma

The T category (primary tumor invasion)

T_1	S_0	$Hinf_0$	$Panc_0$	PV_0	A_0
T_2	S_1	$Hinf_1$	$Panc_1$	PV_0	A_0
T_3	S_2	$Hinf_1$	$Panc_1$	PV_0	A_0
T_4	Any	$Hinf_{2,3}$	$Panc_{2,3}$	$PV_{1,2,3}$	$A_{1,2,3}$
pT_1	m, fm	$pHinf_0$	$Panc_0$	pPV_0/PV_0	pA_0/A_0
pT_2	ss	$pHinf_{1a}$	$Panc_{1a}$	pPV_0/PV_0	pA_0/A_0
pT_3	se	$pHinf_{1b}$	$Panc_{1b}$	pPV_0/PV_0	pA_0/A_0
pT_4	Any	$pHinf_{2,3}$	$Panc_{2,3}$	$pPV_{1,2,3}/PV_{1,2,3}$	$pA_{1,2,3}/A_{1,2,3}$

m; mucosa, fm; fibromuscular layer, ss; subserosal se; serosal exposure and/or pancreas invasion

Serosa

S_0	No invasion of the serosa
S_1	Doubtful invasion of the serosa and/or serosal surface
S_2	Definite invasion of the serosa
S_3	Invasion of other organs or structures: the stomach, abdominal wall, colon, and inferior vena cava

Liver	$Hinf_0$: No direct invasion of the liver $Hinf_1$: Doubtful direct invasion of the liver $Hinf_2$: Definite direct invasion of portal bile ducts $Hinf_3$: Definite direct invasion beyond portal bile ducts
Gallbladder	$Ginf_0$: No direct invasion of the gallbladder $Ginf_1$: Doubtful direct invasion of the gallbladder $Ginf_2$: Definite invasion limited to the area of the cystic duct $Ginf_3$: Definite invasion of the gallbladder
Pancreas	$Panc_0$: No invasion of the pancreas $Panc_1$: Doubtful invasion of the pancreas $Panc_2$: Definite invasion of the bile duct around the pancreas $Panc_3$: Severe invasion of the pancreas
Duodenum	DU_0: No invasion of the duodenum DU_1: Doubtful invasion of the duodenum DU_2: Invasion of the duodenum around the bile duct DU_3: Definite invasion of the duodenum
Portal veins	PV_0: No invasion of portal veins PV_1: Doubtful invasion of portal veins PV_2: Definite invasion of portal veins PV_3: Severe invasion of portal veins (narrowing or obstruction)
Hepatic arteries	A_0: No invasion of hepatic arteries A_1: Doubtful invasion of hepatic arteries A_2: Definite invasion of hepatic arteries A_3: Severe invasion of hepatic arteries (narrowing or obstruction)

N category of JSBS Classification of extrahepatic cholangiocarcinoma

	Bp, Bs	Bm	Bi
N_1	12h, 12a1a2, 12p1p2, 12b1b2, 12	12b1b2, 12	12b2, 13a
N_2	8ap, 13	8ap, 12h, 12a1a2, 12p1p2, 13	8ap, 12a1a2, 12p1p2, 12b1, 12c, 14ab
N_3	1-7, 9-11, 13b, 14abcd, 15, 16a1a2, 16b1b2, 17ab, 18	1-7, 9-11, 13b,14abcd, 15, 16a1a2, 16b1b2, 17ab, 18	1-7, 9-11, 12h, 15, 16a1a2, 16b1b2, 17ab, 18

N_0	No evidence of lymph node metastasis
N_1	Metastasis to group 1 lymph nodes, but no metastasis to group 2 and 3 lymph nodes
N_2	Metastasis to group 2 lymph nodes ,but no metastasis to group 3 lymph nodes
N_3	Metastasis to group 3 lymph nodes

M category of JSBS Classification of extrahepatic cholangiocarcinoma	
Liver metastasis	H_0: No evidence of liver metastasis H_1: Metastasis limited to one lobe H_1(r): Metastasis limited to the right lobe H_1(l): Metastasis limited to the left lobe H_2: A few metastases to both lobes H_3: Numerous metastases to both lobes
Peritoneal metastasis	P_0: No evidence of peritoneal metastasis P_1: Metastasis to the peritoneum adjacent to extrahepatic bile ducts P_2: A few metastases to the distant peritoneum P_3: Numerous metastases to the distant peritoneum
distant metastasis	M(-): No evidence of distant metastasis other than peritoneal and/or liver metastases M(+): Distant metastases other than peritoneal and/or liver metastases

JSBS stage grouping

Surgical stage

	H_o, P_o, M(-)				$H_{1,2,3}$, $P_{1,2,3}$, M(+)
	N_o	N_1	N_2	N_3	
T_1	I	II		IVa	
T_2	II	III			IVb
T_3			IVa		
T_4	IVa				

Final stage

	H_0, P_0, M(-)				$H_{1,2,3}$, $P_{1,2,3}$, M(+)
	pN_0	pN_1	pN_2	pN_3	
PT_1	I	II		IVa	
PT_2	II	III			IVb
PT_3			IVa		
PT_4	IVa				

Curability (surgical or final)

HM; Proximal hepatic transection line

DM; Distal bile duct transection line

EM; Dissected periductal soft tissue

- DM_0, HM_0, EM_0: resection margin more than 5 mm
- DM_1, HM_1, EM_1: resection margin less than 5 mm
- DM_2, HM_2, EM_2: resection margin involved by tumor

	H	P	ND	DM	HM	EM	M
Cur A	H_0	P_0	N<D	DM_0	HM_0	EM_0	M(-)
Cur B	Not satisfying the criteria for Cur A and C						
Cur C	$H_{1,2,3}$	$P_{1,2,3}$	N>D	DM_2	HM_2	EM_2	M(+)

and 0%, respectively (p=0.07). The differences were more noticeable when disease stages I-II were compared with disease stages III-IV, with a median survival of 36.1 month and, 9 months, respectively (p=0.013).

(2) JSBS classification

In 2003, "The General Rules for Surgical and Pathological Studies on Cancer of the Biliary Tract of the Japanese Society of Biliary Surgery" (JSBS, 5th edition) was published (Table 7) to clarify the classification according to anatomical location of the extrahepatic bile duct[40]. The operative findings, operative results, and methods used to describe histopathological results were described and the concepts for the early bile duct were defined[40] but has not been broadly accepted until now[51]. The operative findings are subdivided and recorded as following: (1) tumor location, (2) tumor size and number, (3) gross type, (4) T category,

(5) lymph nodes, (6) liver metastasis, (7) peritoneal metastasis, (8) distant metastasis, (9) stones, (10) stage grouping, (11) operative procedures, (12) lymph node dissection, (13) invasion of surgical margin, and (14) resectability. Histopathologi-cal results are recorded as follows: (1) tumor location, (2) invasion of the tumor, (3) pT category, (4) lymph node metastasis, and (5) invasion of surgical margin.

The anatomical locations of the extrahepatic bile ducts are classified as shown in Fig. 6. The hilar bile duct (Bp) can be defined as following: The right side is limited to the junction of the anterior and posterior intrahepatic bile ducts. The left side is limited to the junction of the lateral and internal intrahepatic bile ducts. The lower side extends down to the upper margin of common hepatic duct (Bs).

The T category of extrahepatic bile duct carcinoma was subclassified according to the invasions of (1) serosa, (2) liver, (3) gallbladder, (4) pancreas, (5) duodenum, (6) portal veins, and (7) hepatic arteries. Of the seven factors, the invasion of the gallbladder and the duodenum does not influence the determin-

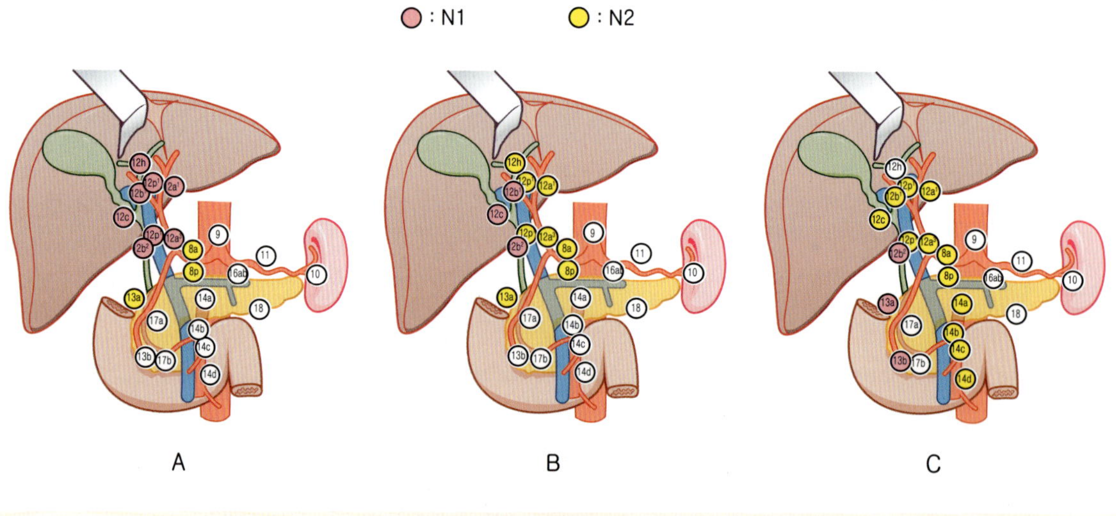

Fig. 7 Lymphatic drainage according to tumor location (JSBS)
A: Bp, Bs tumor (perihilar cholangiocarcinoma), B: Bm tumor (middle bile duct cancer), C: Bi tumor (distal bile duct cancer)

ation of T category or stage; however, they are associated with resectability and the extent of surgical procedures.

The regional lymph node groups of extrahepatic cholangiocarcinoma are subclassified by the location of the tumor (Fig. 7 and Table 7). The N1 stage has metastases to only group 1 lymph nodes without metastasis to group 2 and 3 lymph nodes. The N2 stage has metastases to group 2 lymph nodes without metastasis to group 3 lymph nodes. The N3 stage has metastases to group 3 lymph nodes. The M category is subclassified as liver metastasis, peritoneal metastasis, and distant metastasis. The stage grouping is concluded by surgical stage (sStage) according to operative findings and final stage (fStage) according to histopathological examination.

Sano et al. reported that among 126 hilar cholangiocarcinoma patients, 69 of them (54.8%) had stage III or IV disease according to JSBS classification. The 1-, 3-, 5-, and 10- year overall survival rates of these 126 patients were 82.4%, 43.9%, 35.2%, and 22.2%, respectively.[52]

(3) Bismuth-Corlette classification

The Bismuth-Corlette classification provides an anatomical extension of the tumor (Fig. 8).[39] Type I tumors are defined as a lesion confined below the confluence of the right and left hepatic ducts. Type II tumors extend to the confluence of the right and left hepatic ducts. Type IIIa tumors extend to the second confluence of the right hepatic duct, and type IIIb tumors extend to the second confluence of the left hepatic duct. Type IV tumors extend to the second confluences on both the right and left hepatic ducts.

Ikeyama et al. from the Nagoya group reported that 351 patients with hilar cholangiocarcinoma underwent resection-17 (4.8%) bile duct resections and 334 (95.2%) hepatectomies with or without portal vein resection and/or pancreatoduodenectomy.[53] According to the Bismuth classification criteria, tumors were distributed among types I, II, III, and IV with 24 (6.8%), 30 (8.5%), 148 (42.2%), and 149 (42.5%) patients in each group, respectively. Most of the hilar cholangiocarcinomas belonged to type III or IV.[48,53,54] The Bismuth-Corlette classification did not predict survival or prognosis.[48,54] This classification has been

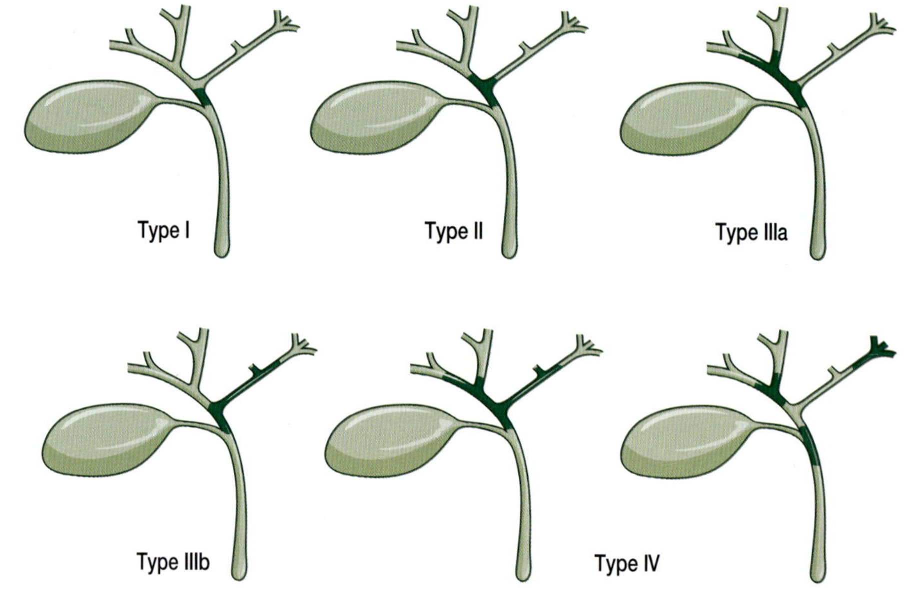

Fig. 8 Bismuth-Corlette classification of hilar cholangiocarcinoma.

a classical classification system for hilar cholangiocarcinoma, and is useful tool for determining resection or palliative treatment and the type of surgery; however, surgical candidates cannot be determined solely by this classification.[55] Therefore it is not adequate to determine resectability or predict the prognosis for the different subgroups.

(4) MSKCC Clinical T Stage Criteria

Currently, preoperative evaluation and determination of resectability is an important issue for hilar cholangiocarcinomas because patients with hilar cholangiocarcinomas commonly possess advanced disease that is not amenable to surgical treatments.[35,56] The modified Bismuth-Corlette classification stratifies patients based only on the extent of biliary involvement by the tumor, while the AJCC staging system is based largely on pathological criteria and has little applicability for preoperative staging to determine resectability. In 1998, Burke et al. in the MSKCC proposed the clinical T stage for hilar cholangiocarcinoma dividing the patients into four groups.[57] In 2001, Jarnagin et al. in the MSKCC group modified the clinical T staging system using data from preoperative imaging studies based on biliary ductal involvement, vascular involvement, and hepatic

Table 8. Memorial Sloan-Kettering T stage for hilar cholangiocarcinoma

Clinical Stage	Criteria
T1	Tumor involving biliary confluence±unilateral extension to 2° biliary radicles
T2	Tumor involving biliary confluence±unilateral extension to 2° biliary radicles and ipsilateral portal vein involvement±ipsilateral hepatic lobar atrophy
T3	Tumor involving biliary confluence+bilateral extension to 2° biliary radicles; or unilateral extension to 2° biliary radicles with contralateral portal vein involvement; or unilateral extension to 2° biliary radicles with contralateral hepatic lobar atrophy; or main or bilateral portal vein involvement

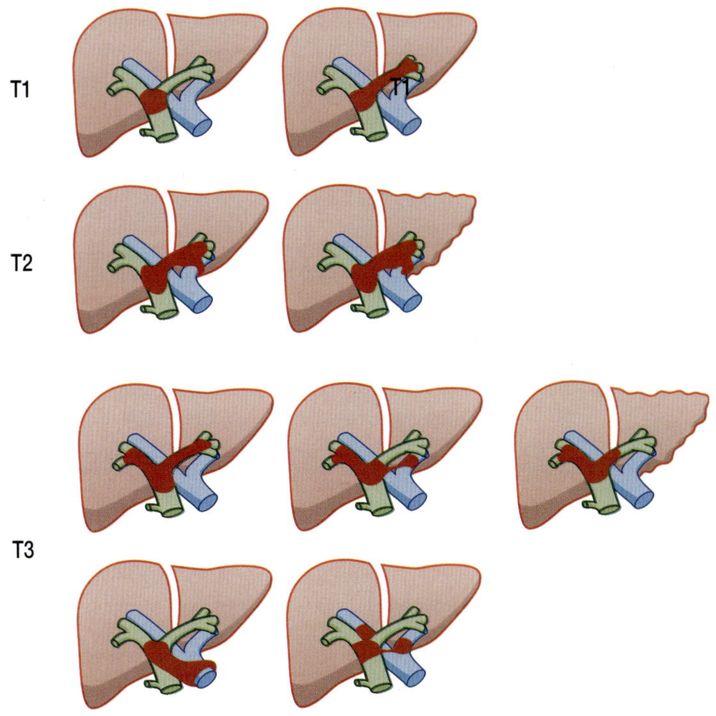

Fig. 9 Clinical T stage of the MSKCC criteria for resectability of hilar cholangiocarcinoma.

lobar atrophy irrespective of N and M factor.[41] The staging systems are shown in Table 8 and Fig. 9. Individuals with T3 tumors corresponding to the Bismuth-Corlette type 4, bilateral, or main portal vein invasion, or Bismuth-Corlette type 3 tumors with contralateral portal vein invasion or hepatic atrophy are considered poor candidates for surgery. However, some Bismuth type 4 tumors with favorable anatomy or short segmental invasion of the main portal vein may not be

Table 9. Resectability and incidence of negative margins stratified by MSKCC T staging system

T stage	No.	Explored with curative intent	Resected	(-) Margins	Hepatic resection	Portal vein resection	Metastatic disease	Median survival (mo)
1	87	73 (84%)	51 (59%)	38	33	2	18 (21%)	20
2	95	79 (83%)	29 (31%)	24	29	7	40 (43%)	13
3	37	8 (22%)	0	0	0	0	15 (41%)	8
Total	219	160 (71%)	80 (37%)	62	62	9	73 (33%)	16

* 6 patients had incomplete data and could not be accurately staged. The percentage indicates the proportion of patients within each stage grouping or of the total number of patients. Metastatic disease refers to metastases to N2 level lymph nodes or to distant sites. Median survival was calculated for all patients, including those who died perioperatively.

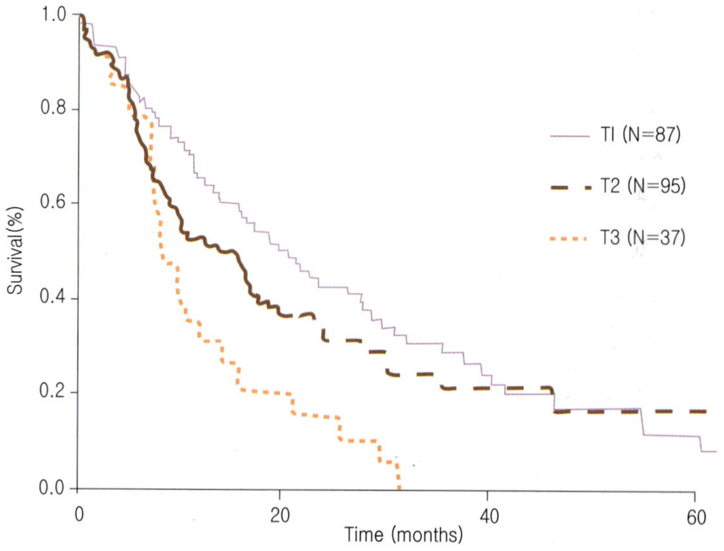

Fig. 10 Survival of all patients stratified by T stage.
Solid line indicates T1 tumors (n=87; median survival 20months). Dashed line indicates T2 tumors (n=95; median survival 13 months). Dotted line indicates T3 tumors (n=37; median survival 8months) p<0.0092 by Cox regression.

an absolute contraindication to attempt curative resection.[58-60]

The clinical T staging system accounts for local tumor extent and correlates closely with both resectability and survival rates. In an analysis of 225 patients with hilar cholangiocarcinoma, resectability was nearly 60% in T1 tumors and 31% in T2 tumors, but 0% in T3 tumors (Table 9). Survival also decreased with increasing clinical T stage (Fig. 10).[41] On the other hand, there was no correlation with survival and stage based on the AJCC classification. In addition, the likelihood of distant metastatic disease increased with more locally advanced lesions at higher clinical T stage.[41] Therefore, in hilar cholangiocarcinomas, the MSKCC clinical T stage is useful for assessing resectability and predicting prognosis. It has been reported, however, that the MSKCC staging system overestimates the potential for complete resection.[47] Additionally, Zervos et al. reported that none of the three staging systems (AJCC, Bismuth-Corlette, and MSKCC clinical T stage) does what that are purported to do as far as predicting survival.[47]

2) Distal common bile duct cancer

Twenty to 30% of all cholangiocarcinomas originate in the lower bile duct, and adenocarcinoma of the distal bile duct represents approximately 5 to 10% of all periampullary tumors.[61-63] Although there may be some overlap, tumors of the lower bile duct are classified according to their anatomical location. Mid-bile duct tumors arise below the confluence in the common bile duct between the upper border of the duodenum and the cystic duct; distal bile duct tumors are those that arise anywhere from the duodenum to the ampulla of Vater.[61] True mid-bile duct tumors are distinctly uncommon. It may be difficult preoperatively to distinguish distal bile duct cancer from ductal adenocarcinoma of the pancreatic head. In reality, it is unnecessary to pursue diagnostic studies to distinguish between these lesions because the operation is the same. Complete resection, generally requiring a pancreaticoduodenectomy, is the only effective therapy for cancers of the lower bile duct.[64-68] 5-year survival rates of 35 to 50% have been reported following surgical resection.[64-66,68]

Distal common bile duct cancers are staged according to the AJCC system for tumors of the extrahepatic bile ducts (Table 4). However this system is of limited clinical use, because it does not consider all of the factors that define resectability, especially the vascular involvement (portal vein, superior mesenteric artery/vein, and common hepatic artery). Involvement of major vascular elements would appear to occur less often with cholangiocarcinoma than with pancreatic adenocarcinoma.[69] Distal bile duct cancers are more often amenable to resection, have less microscopic disease at the resection margin, and less frequent spread of the tumor to adjacent lymph nodes than pancreatic adenocarcinomas.[61-63]

According to the AJCC T category, a tumor invading the pancreas is classified as a T3 tumor, while a tumor invading the duodenum is a T4 tumor. Ebata et al. analyzed 95 patients with distal bile duct cancers who underwent pancreatoduodenectomy. Those with T1 tumors (n=9) had very favorable prognoses with a 5-yr survival rate of 89%, and those with pT2 (n=24) tumors had the second most favorable prognoses with a 5-yr survival rate of 73%. In contrast, the survival rates of patients with pT3 (n=32) and pT4 (n=30) tumors were poor and almost similar, with 5-year survival rates of 31% and 29%, respectively, suggesting that distal bile duct cancer, irrespective of the middle or distal tumor, extends progressively to the pancreas, followed by the duodenum or the portal vein. Although duodenal invasion usually occurs after pancreatic invasion in distal bile duct cancer, the most significant prognostic factor is pancreatic invasion, not duodenal invasion. The pancreas is a key organ and a major determinant of T classification in distal bile duct cancer. Ebata et al. proposed a new T classification for distal bile duct cancer:[70] T1-T3 exactly correspond to the T classifications of the AJCC and T4 (other organ invasion including the hepatic artery invasion), a tumor with hepatic artery invasion, is a local factor leading to irresectability. They proposed that the AJCC T classification is not satisfactory for distal bile duct cancer and should be revised. Furthermore, they suggested that perihilar cholangiocarcinoma and distal bile duct cancer may need to be staged differently.[70]

In addition to curative resection, lymph node status appears to be a critical determinant of outcome.[64-68] The 5-year survival rate of the lymph node negative and lymph node positive groups have been reported to be 58 to 73%, and 17 to 31%, respectively.[64-66,68] In some reports, patients with up to two positive lymph nodes had a more favorable prognosis than other patients, although positive lymph node metastasis was present.[64,65]

In 43 patients with distal cholangiocarcinoma who underwent surgical resection, stage I patients (n=14, 5-year survival rate 77%) demonstrated a more favorable survival than stage II and III patients (n=27, 5-year survival rate 27%) (p=0.002).[58]

The JSBS classification is also used for staging of distal bile duct cancer, which is the same as previously stated (Table 7, Fig. 7).

Conclusion

Cholangiocarcinomas show different biological behavior according to the anatomical location of the tumors. The staging systems have been directed towards determining resectability and prognosis. However, an appropriate staging system for cholangiocarcinomas is still controversial. Although the biologic behaviors of ICC & HCC are quite different, the staging system of ICC proposed by AJCC was mainly developed from the stage of HCC, The staging system proposed by LCSGJ is specific for ICC. However, this classification refers only to the mass-forming type of cholangiocarcinoma. Therefore the staging system must be supplemented to allow staging of periductal infiltrative and intraductal growth types.

The staging systems for extrahepatic cholangiocarcinoma proposed by AJCC, JSBS, and MSKCC all consider the tumor location, and vascular and hepatic invasion to provide information on tumor resectability and to reflect prognosis. However, the superiority of these staging systems will need to be evaluated by future comparative studies.

Reference

1. http://www.cancer.gov/cancertopics/factsheet/Detection/staging.
2. Sano T, Shimada K, Sakamoto Y, et al. Prognosis of perihilar cholangiocarcinoma: hilar bile duct cancer versus intrahepatic cholangiocarcinoma involving the hepatic hilus. Ann Surg Oncol 2008;15:590-599

3. Vauthey J, Pawlik T, Abdalla E, et al. Is extended hepatectomy for hepatobiliary malignancy justified? Ann Surg 2004;239:722-730.
4. Killeen R, Harte S, Maguire D, Malone D. Achievable outcomes in the management of proximal cholangiocarcinoma: an update prepared using "evidence-based practice" techniques. Abd Imaging 2008;33:54-57.
5. Ristagno N, Knuth A, Pestalozzi B. Is an aggressive surgical approach worthwhile in biliary cancer? Int Semin Surg Oncol. 2007;4:26-35.
6. Sobin L, Wittekind C. TNM classification of malignant tumours 5th ed. New York: Wiley-Liss, 1997.
7. Sobin L, Wittekind C. TNM classification of malignant tumours. 6th ed. New York: Wiley-Liss, 2002.
8. Fleming I, Cooper J, Hensen D. AJCC cancer staging manual. 5th ed. Philadelphia: Lippincott-Raven, 1997.
9. Greene F, Page D, Fleming I. AJCC cancer staging manual. 6th ed. New York: Springer-Verlag, 2002.
10. Liver Cancer Study Group of Japan. The General rules for the clinical and pathological study of primary liver cancer. 1st ed. Tokyo: Kanehara, 1997.
11. Liver Cancer Study Group of Japan. The general rules for clinical and pathological study of primary liver cancer. 2nd English ed. Tokyo: Kanehara, 2003.
12. Japan LCSGo. Classification of primary liver cancer. 1st ed. Tokyo: Kanehara, 1997.
13. Harrison L, Fong Y, Klimstra D, et al. Surgical treatment of 32 patients with peripheral intrahepatic cholangiocarcinoma. Br J Surg 1998;85:1068-1070.
14. Shaib Y, El-Serag H. The epidemiology of cholangiocarcinoma. Semin Liver Dis 2004; 24:115-126.
15. Berthiaume E, Wands J. The molecular pathogenesis of cholangiocarcinoma. Semin Liver Dis 2004;24:127-138.
16. Broomé U, Olsson R, Lööf L, et al. Natural history and prognostic factors in 305 Swedish patients with primary sclerosing cholangitis. Gut 1996; 38:610-615.
17. Pitt H, Dooley W, Yeo C, Cameron J. Malignancies of the biliary tree. Curr Probl Surg 1995; 32:1-9.
18. Yamasaki S. Intrahepatic cholangiocarcinoma: macroscopic type and stage classification. J Hepatobiliary Pancreat Surg 2003;10:288-291.
19. Weber S, Jarnagin W, Klimstra D, et al. Intrahepatic cholangiocarcinoma: resectability, recurrence pattern, and outcomes. J Am Coll Surg 2001;193:384-391.
20. Hanazaki K, Kajikawa S, Shimozawa N, et al. Prognostic factors of intrahepatic cholangiocarcinoma after hepatic resection: Univariate and multivariate analysis. Hepato-Gastroenterology 2002;49:311-316.

21. Uenishi T, Yamazaki O, Yamamoto T, et al. Serosal invasion in TNM staging of mass-forming intrahepatic cholangiocarcinoma. J Hepatobiliary Pancreat Surg 2005;12:479-483.
22. Nakagohri T, Asano T, Kinoshita H, et al. Aggressive surgical resection for hilar-invasive and peripheral intrahepatic cholangiocarcinoma. World J Surg 2003;27:289-293.
23. Tajima Y, Kuroki T, Fukuda K, et al. An intraductal papillary component is associated with prolonged survival after hepatic resection for intrahepatic cholangiocarcinoma. Br J Surg 2004;91:99-104.
24. Shimada K, Sano T, Sakamoto Y, et al. Clinical impact of the surgical margin status in hepatectomy for solitary mass-forming type intrahepatic cholangiocarcinoma without lymph node metastases. J Surg Oncol 2007;96:160-165.
25. Nakagawa T, Kamiyama T, Kurauchi N, et al. Number of lymph node metastases is a significant prognostic factor in intrahepatic cholangiocarcinoma. World J Surg 2005;29:728-733.
26. Ohtsuka M, Ito H, Kimura F, et al. Results of surgical treatment for intrahepatic cholangiocarcinoma and clinicopathological factors influencing survival. Br J Surg 2002;89:1525-1531.
27. Nozaki Y, Yamamoto M, Ikai I, et al. Reconsideration of the lymph node metastasis pattern (N factor) from intrahepatic cholangiocarcinoma using the International Union Against Cancer TNM staging system for primary liver carcinoma. Cancer 1998;83:1923-1929.
28. Song G, Lee S, Lee Y, et al. Analysis of survival and factors affecting the survival after surgical resection of peripheral cholangiocarcinoma: 318 cases in single institute. Korean J Hepatol 2007;13:208-221.
29. Tsuji T, Hiraoka T, Kanemitsu K, et al. Lymphatic spreading pattern of intrahepatic cholangiocarcinoma. Surgery 2001;129:401-407.
30. Yamamoto M, Takasaki K, Yoshikawa T. Lymph node metastasis in intrahepatic cholangiocarcinoma. Jpn J Clin Oncol 1999;29:147-150.
31. Shimada M, Yamashita Y, Aishima S, et al. Value of lymph node dissection during resection of intrahepatic cholangiocarcinoma. Br J Surg 2001;88:1463-1466.
32. Ikai I, Itai Y, Okita K, et al. Report of the 15th follow-up survey of primary liver cancer. Hepatol Res 2004;28:21-29.
33. Klatskin G. Adenocarcinoma of the hepatic duct at its bifurcation within the porta hepatic. An unusual tumor with distinctive clinical and pathological features. Am J Med 1965;38:241-256.
34. Nakeeb A, Pitt H, Sohn T, et al. Cholangiocarcinoma. A spectrum of intrahepatic, perihilar, and distal tumors. Ann Surg Oncol 1996;224:463-475.
35. Pichlmayr R, Lamesch P, Weimann A, et al. Surgical treatment of cholangiocellular carcinoma. World J Surg 1995;19:83-88.

36. Kawasaki S, Imamura H, Kobayashi A, et al. Results of surgical resection for patients with hilar bile duct cancer: application of extended hepatectomy after biliary drainage and hemihepatic portal vein embolization. Ann Surg 2003;238:84-92.

37. Baer H, Stain S, Dennison A, et al. Improvements in survival by aggressive resections of hilar cholangiocarcinoma. Ann Surg 1993;217:20-27.

38. Jarnagin W, Shoup M. Surgical management of cholangiocarcinoma. Semin Liver Dis 2004;24:189-199.

39. Bismuth H, Corlette M. Intrahepatic cholangioenteric anastomosis in carcinoma of the hilus of the liver. Surg Gynecol Obstet 1975;140:170-178.

40. Japanese Society of Biliary Surgery. The general rules for surgical and pathological studies on cancer of the biliary tract. 2nd ed. Tokyo: Kanehara, 2004.

41. Jarnagin W, Fong Y, DeMatteo R, et al. Staging, resectability, and outcome in 225 patients with hilar cholangiocarcinoma. Ann Surg 2001;234:507-519.

42. Hong S, Kang G, Lee H, Ro J. Smooth muscle distribution in the extrahepatic bile duct: histologic and immunohistochemical studies of 122 cases. Am J Surg Pathol 2000;24:660-667.

43. Hong S, Presley A, Stelow E, et al. Reconsideration of the histologic definitions used in the pathologic staging of extrahepatic bile duct carcinoma. Am J surg pathol 2006;30:744-749.

44. Hong S, Kim M, Pi D, et al. Analysis of extrahepatic bile duct carcinomas according to the New American Joint Committee on Cancer staging system focused on tumor classification problems in 222 patients. Cancer 2005;104:802-810.

45. Nishio H, Nagino M, Oda K, et al. TNM classification for perihilar cholangiocarcinoma: comparison between 5th and 6th editions of the AJCC/UICC staging system. Langenbecks Arch Surg 2005;390:319-327.

46. Khan S, Davidson B, Goldin R, et al. Guidelines for the diagnosis and treatment of cholangiocarcinoma: Consensus document. Gut 2002;51 (suppl VI): vi1-vi9.

47. Zervos E, Osborne D, Goldin S, et al. Stage does not predict survival after resection of hilar cholangiocarcinomas promoting an aggressive operative approach. Am J Surg 2005; 190:810-815.

48. Otani K, Chijiiwa K, Kai M, et al. Outcome of surgical treatment of hilar cholangiocarcinoma. J Gastrointest Surg 2008;12:1033-1040.

49. Hidalgo E, Asthana S, Nishio H, et al. Surgery for hilar cholangiocarcinoma: The Leeds experience. Eur J Surg oncol 2008;34:787-794.

50. Nishio H, Nagino M, Nimura Y. Surgical management of hilar cholangiocarcinoma: the Nagoya experience. HPB 2005;7:259-262.

51. Cha J, Kim M, Lee S, et al. Clinicopathological review of 61 patients with early bile duct cancer. Clin Oncol 2006;18:669-677.

52. Sano T, Shimada K, Sakamoto Y, et al. Changing trends in surgical outcomes after major hepatobiliary resection for hilar cholangiocarcinoma: a single-center experience over 25 years. J Hepatobiliary Pancreat Surg 2007;14:455-462.

53. Ikeyama T, Nagino M, Oda K, et al. Surgical approach to Bismuth type I and II hilar cholangiocarcinomas. Ann Surg 2007;246:1052-1057.

54. Konstadoulakis M, Roayaie S, Gomatos I, et al. Aggressive surgical resection for hilar cholangiocarcinoma: is it justified? Audit of a single center's experience. Am J Surg 2008; 196:160-169.

55. Bold RJ, Goodnight JE Jr. Hilar cholangiocarcinoma: surgical and endoscopic approaches. Surg Clin North Am 2004;84:525-542.

56. Pitt H, Nakeeb A, Abrams R, et al. Perihilar cholangiocarcinoma. Postoperative radiotherapy does not improve survival. Ann Surg 1995;221:788-797.

57. Burke E, Jarnagin W, Hochwald S, et al. Hilar cholangiocarcinoma:patterns of spread, the importance of hepatic resection for curative operation, and a presurgical clinical staging system. Ann Surg 1998;228:385-394.

58. Lee H, Kim S, Lee J, et al. Preoperative assessment of resectability of hepatic hilar cholangiocarcinoma: combined CT and cholangiography with revised criteria. Radiology 2006;239:113-121.

59. Muñoz L, Roayaie S, Maman D, et al. Hilar cholangiocarcinoma involving the portal vein bifurcation: long-term results after resection. J Hepatobiliary Pancreat Surg 2002;9:237-241.

60. Neuhaus P, Jonas S, Bechstein W, et al. Extended resections for hilar cholangiocarcinoma. Ann Surg 1999;230:808-818.

61. Tompkins R, Thomas D, Wile A, Longmire W. Prognostic factors in bile duct carcinoma. Analysis of 96 cases. Ann Surg 1981;194:447-457.

62. Fong Y, Blumgart L, Lin E, et al. Outcome of treatment for distal bile duct cancer. Br J Surg 1996;83:1712-1715.

63. Yeo C, Cameron J, Sohn T, et al. Six hundred fifty consecutive pancreatii-coduodenectomies in the 1990s: pathology, complications, and outcomes. Ann Surg 1997; 226:248-257.

64. Yoshida T, Matsumoto T, Sasaki A, et al. Prognostic factors after pancreatoduodenectomy with extended lymphadenectomy for distal bile duct cancer. Arch Surg 2002;137:69-73.

65. Murakami Y, Uemura K, Hayashidani Y, et al. Pancreatoduodenectomy for distal cholangiocarcinoma: prognostic impact of lymph node metastasis. World J Surg 2007;31: 337-342.

66. Kayahara M, Nagakawa T, Ohta T, et al. Role of nodal involvement and the periductal soft-tissue margin in middle and distal bile duct cancer. Ann Surg 1999;229:76-83.

67. Bortolasi L, Burgart L, Tsiotos G, et al. Adenocarcinoma of the distal bile duct. Dig Surg 2000;17:36-41.

68. Murakami Y, Uemura K, Hayashidani Y, et al. Prognostic significance of lymph node metastasis and surgical margin status for distal cholangiocarcinoma. J Surg Oncol 2007;95: 207-212.

69. Jarnagin W. Cholangiocarcinoma of the extrahepatic bile ducts. Semin Surg Oncol 2000; 19:156-176.

70. Ebata T, Nagino M, Nishio H, et al. Pancreatic and duodenal invasion in distal bile duct cancer: paradox in the tumor classification of the American Joint Committee on Cancer. World J Surg 2007;31:2008-2015.

VIII • Diagnosis

VIII · I
Clinical and Laboratory Assessment

1. Clinical Features

1) Symptoms

Cholangiocarcinoma is a rare neoplasm, which accounts for approximately 3% of gastrointestinal cancers worldwide.[1] Cholangiocarcinomas usually become symptomatic when the tumor obstructs the biliary drainage system, causing painless jaundice. Rarely, an asymptomatic cholangiocarcinoma is found during the evaluation of abnormal liver tests. The pain is generally described as a constant dull ache in the right upper quadrant but cholangitis is an unusual presentation. Fever, night sweats and weight loss may occur in addition to right upper quadrant abdominal pain.[2,3] The presentation of cholangiocarcinoma depends on the anatomical location of the cancer. Intrahepatic cholangiocarcinoma typically presents as a mass lesion detected by abdominal imaging or with nonspecific symptoms; obstructive symptoms are rare. In contrast, hilar or extrahepatic lesions will often present with jaundice, acholic stool, pruritus, weight loss and abdominal pain.[2-4]

2) Signs

Physical signs include jaundice, hepatomegaly, or a right upper quadrant mass. A palpable gallbladder, caused by obstruction distal to the take off of the cystic duct

(Courvoisier's sign), occurs rarely.[2-5] The diagnosis of perihilar or extrahepatic cholangiocarcinoma can be established by cholangiography.[5]

2. Laboratory Assessment

Abnormal laboratory-test results in biliary tract cancer can be divided into those due to interference with normal physiologic processes, resulting from inhibition of normal bile flow or tumor invasion, and those due to the secretion of abnormal products.[6]

1) Liver function test

The limitations of conventional laboratory test such as the liver function test are well recognized. Elevated conjugated bilirubin would mean extrahepatic cholestasis. Alkaline phosphatase and gamma-glutamyl transpeptidase usually rises in conjunction with bilirubin. Aminotransferases may be normal or minimally elevated, but high elevations typically do not occur until the tumor is advanced and progressive liver damage has occurred.[2]

2) Serum tumor markers

Serologic testing is supportive and in most instances done prior to or concurrent with imaging studies, though not necessary for the diagnosis of cholangiocarcinoma. CA 19-9, CEA, and CA 125 are the most studied tumor associated markers with cholangiocarcinomas. Of all three, CA 19-9 has the most utility.[7] CEA and CA 125 are non-specific as they are elevated in patients with cholangiocarcinoma and other gut-derived malignancies, and they have a low sensitivity as well.[8] The caveat to the interpretation of an elevated CA 19-9 is the coexistence of bacterial cholangitis, which may not always be overt. Hepatolithiasis also commonly leads to increased levels of CA 19-9, and also CEA and CA 125. Therefore, cholangiocarcinoma should not be diagnosed on the basis of these tests alone except in patients with known risk factors or virtually diagnostic imaging studies.

3) Screening with tumor markers

In an unrelated at-risk population, a study from Thailand demonstrated the utility of testing serum interleukin-6 levels in conjunction with CA 19-9 in patients with chronic biliary parasitosis. A CA 19-9 value >100 U/ml combined with an IL-6 value >50 pg/ml had a sensitivity of 80% and accuracy of 76%.[9]

The patients with PSC are at a higher risk for cholangiocarcinoma and the diagnosis of malignancy is clinically challenging. The presentation and cholangiographic findings in biliary tract strictures in PSC are similar to those of cholangiocarcinoma.[5] However, screening biliary instrumentation in stable, asymptomatic PSC patients is not recommended due to the concurrent risk of pancreatitis (>7% in patients with PSC), however, when clinically indicated advanced testing should be utilized to diagnose early cancers in PSC patients.[10,11] Asymptomatic high risk patients may be surveyed non-invasively, such as with a serum CA 19-9 value and MRCP annually to achieve early cancer detection, although there are no outcome studies or cost-effectiveness information to advocate this approach. In patients with PSC a value of CA 19-9 >100 U/ml has a sensitivity of 89% and specificity of 86%, and in patients without PSC the sensitivity is 53%, for the diagnosis of cholangiocarcinoma.[10,12] Increasing the cut off to >129 U/ml in patients PSC provided a sensitivity of 78.6%, and improved the specificity to 98.5%, and a positive predictive value of 56.6%.[11] In patients with advanced disease, the level may be strikingly elevated, though not universally.

4) Novel serum tumor markers

Proteomic profiling using surface-enhanced laser desorption/ionization time-of-flight mass spectrometry has been used to identify proteomic profiles with a high sensitivity and specificity for cholangiocarcinoma.[13] The specific proteins are unknown, but this approach holds promise for identifying new serum biomarkers of cholangiocarcinoma. The human mucin 5, subtypesA and C (MUC5AC) have been evaluated as a biomarker. The use of a sandwich enzyme-linked immunosorbent assay for MUC5AC showed 71% sensitivity and 90% specificity with an area under the curve of a receiver operating characteristic curve of 0.8141, which is comparable to other biomarkers. This simple test may be useful for some but not all cholangiocarcinomas, but warrants further evaluation.[14] Other less well studied biomarkers that have been recently described include real-time-PCR for hTERT mRNA in serum and the use of C-reactive protein for the diagnosis of hilar lesions.[15,16]

Reference

1. Vauthey JN, Blumgart LH. Recent advances in the management of cholangiocarcinomas. Semin Liver Dis 1994;14:109-114.
2. Nagorney DM, Donohue JH, Farnell MB, Schleck CD, Ilstrup DM. Outcomes after curative resections of cholangiocarcinoma. Arch Surg 1993;128:871-879.
3. Nakeeb A, Pitt HA, Sohn TA, Coleman J, Abrams RA, Piantadosi S, Hruban RH, Lillemoe KD, Yeo CJ, Cameron JL. Cholangiocarcinoma. A spectrum of intrahepatic, perihilar, and distal tumors. Ann Surg 1996;224:463-475.
4. Woo SM, Ryu JK, Lee SH, Yoo JW, Park JK, Kim YT, Jang JY, Kim SW, Kang GH, Yoon YB. Recurrence and prognostic factors of ampullary carcinoma after radical resection: comparison with distal extrahepatic cholangiocarcinoma. Ann Surg Oncol 2007;14:3195-201.
5. Patel T, Singh P. Cholangiocarcinoma: emerging approaches to a challenging cancer. Curr Opin Gastroenterol 2007;23:317-323.
6. de Groen PC, Gores GJ, LaRusso NF, Gunderson LL, Nagorney DM. Biliary tract cancers. N Engl J Med 1999;341:1368-1378.
7. Malhi H, Gores GJ. Cholangiocarcinoma: modern advances in understanding a deadly old disease. J Hepatol 2006;45:856-867.
8. Chen CY, Shiesh SC, Tsao HC, Lin XZ. The assessment of biliary CA 125, CA 19-9 and CEA in diagnosing cholangiocarcinoma—the influence of sampling time and hepatolithiasis. Hepatogastroenterology 2002;49:616-620.
9. Tangkijvanich P, Thong-ngam D, Theamboonlers A, Hanvivatvong O, Kullavanijaya P, Poovorawan Y. Diagnostic role of serum interleukin 6 and CA 19-9 in patients with cholangiocarcinoma. Hepatogastroenterology 2004;51:15-19.
10. Nichols JC, Gores GJ, LaRusso NF, Wiesner RH, Nagorney DM, Ritts RE, Jr. Diagnostic role of serum CA 19-9 for cholangiocarcinoma in patients with primary sclerosing cholangitis. Mayo Clin Proc 1993;68:874-879.
11. Levy C, Lymp J, Angulo P, Gores GJ, Larusso N, Lindor KD. The value of serum CA 19-9 in predicting cholangiocarcinomas in patients with primary sclerosing cholangitis. Dig Dis Sci 2005;50:1734-1740.

12. Lim JH, Park CK. Pathology of cholangiocarcinoma. Abdom Imaging 2004;29:540-547.

13. Chalasani N, Baluyut A, Ismail A, Zaman A, Sood G, Ghalib R, McCashland TM, Reddy KR, Zervos X, Anbari MA, Hoen H. Cholangiocarcinoma in patients with primary sclerosing cholangitis: a multicenter case-control study. Hepatology 2000;31:7-11.

14. Bamrungphon W, Prempracha N, Bunchu N, Rangdaeng S, Sandhu T, Srisukho S, Boonla C, Wongkham S. A new mucin antibody/enzyme-linked lectin-sandwich assay of serum MUC5AC mucin for the diagnosis of cholangiocarcinoma. Cancer Lett 2007;247:301-308.

15. Leelawat K, Leelawat S, Ratanachu-Ek T, Trubwongchareon S, Wannaprasert J, Tripongkaruna S, Chantawibul S, Tepaksorn P. Circulating hTERT mRNA as a tumor marker in cholangiocarcinoma patients. World J Gastroenterol 2006;12:4195-4198.

16. Gerhardt T, Milz S, Schepke M, Feldmann G, Wolff M, Sauerbruch T, Dumoulin FL. C-reactive protein is a prognostic indicator in patients with perihilar cholangiocarcinoma. World J Gastroenterol 2006;12:5495-5500.

VIII·II

Radiologic Imaging (US, CT, MR)

Ultrasound sonography (US) is being commonly used as the first diagnostic modality for evaluation of jaundice or intrahepatic mass. US can accurate differentiate obstructive or nonobstructive jaundice and can predict the level of obstruction. US has high accessibility and does not have radiation exposure problem. But detection and characterization of tumor may be limited on US, especially in infiltrative hilar cholangiocarcinoma or small intrahepatic tumor, due to poor tissue contrast, overlying structures, and obesity and operator dependency. Use of high-resolution equipment may increase sensitivity and specificity of US up to 86~96%.[1-3] Recently introduced contrast enhanced US and intraductal US have a potential to improve diagnostic information.[4-6] Computed tomography (CT) can be performed in suspected patients for evaluation and determination of accurate tumor extension. Location and extent of tumor, adjacent organ or vessel invasion, and metastasis can be evaluated accurately by CT.[7-9] Multidetector-row CT (MDCT) provides faster scanning allowing less motion and respiratory artifacts, as well as thinner scanning allowing the acquisition of isotropic images which can provide various imaging reformation such as multiplanar reformation (MRP), curved reformation, and 3-D volume rendering.[8,10-12] MR and MRCP are useful imaging modality for cholangiocarcinoma. MR has an excellent soft tissue contrast which allows accurate prediction of tumor extent and vessel invasion by evaluating preservation or obliteration of fat plane between tumor and vessel. MRCP can evaluate entire biliary tree non-invasively including distal bile duct to the tumor and also useful in predicting tumor extent.[13-15] Cholangiocarcinomas can be classified into intrahepatic, hilar and distal according to their locations and into mass-forming, periductal-infiltrating and intraductal according to their morphology.

1. Intrahepatic Cholangiocarcinoma

1) Mass-forming intrahepatic cholangiocarcinoma (MFICA)

MFICA is characterized by a homogenous mass with an irregular margin and is frequently associated with peripheral bile duct dilatation. On US, MFICA usually shows a homogenous hyperechoic mass.[16] On contrast enhanced US (CEUS), about 70% of MFICA reveals hypervascular mass compared with the adjacent liver in the arterial phase. On delayed phase, most of MFICA shows hypoechoic mass compared with the surrounding liver.[4] This enhancement pattern is different from findings seen on contrast enhanced dynamic CT scan. This difference of enhancement pattern is due to the different distribution of the sonographic and CT contrast agents. The US contrast agent is intravascular and it does not flow outside the vessel, whereas the CT contrast agent can flow into the interstitium until it reaches the equilibrium state.[4,17] On precontrast CT, MFICA shows homogenous low attenuating mass with irregular but well defined margins. On dynamic contrast enhanced CT, it appears irregular peripheral rim enhancement in the arterial phase and gradual centripetal fill-in in the

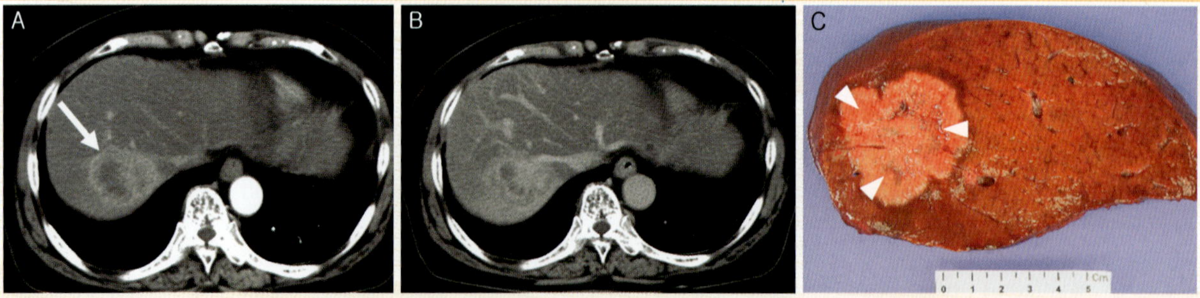

Fig. 1 67 year-old female with mass-forming cholangiocarcinoma.

A: An axial arterial phase CT scan shows low attenuating mass with peripheral rim enhancement (arrow) B: On delayed phase, the periphery of tumor which shows arterial enhancement reveals washout of contrast media. The central portion of the tumor shows no enhancement which may consist of coagulative necrosis. C: Photograph of gross specimen reveals multilobulated mass with central necrosis (arrow head).

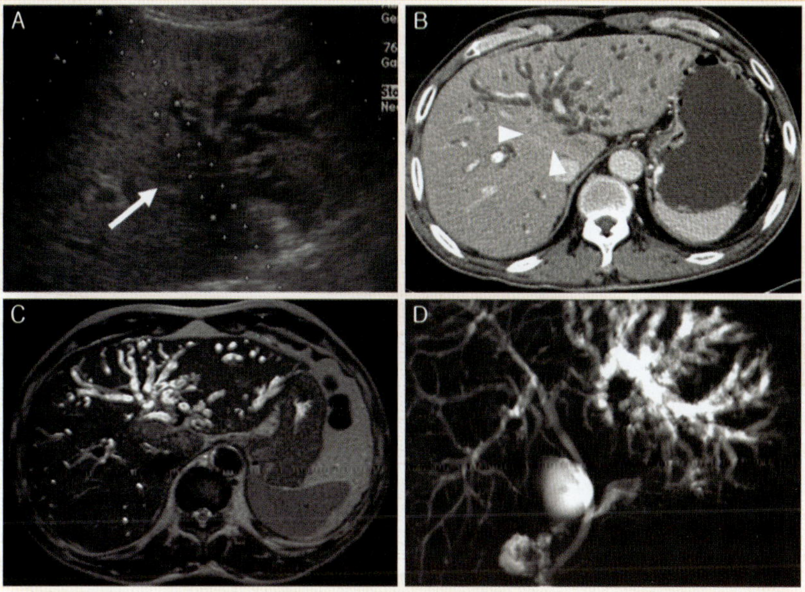

Fig. 2 64 year-old male with cholangiocarcinoma.

A: US shows hypoechoic mass (arrow) with peripheral bile duct dilatation. B: Contrast enhanced portal venous phase CT scan shows lobulated mass (arrow heads) with peripheral duct dilatation. C: On T2-weighted image and D: MRCP, diffuse peripheral bile duct dilatation is seen in the entire liver, which is suggestive finding of *clonorchiasis sinensis* sequelae.

delayed phase (Fig. 1).[16,18] Retraction of the liver capsule and presence of satellite nodules adjacent to the tumor are frequently seen.[19,20] Intratumoral calcification also can be seen, especially in tumors with high mucin content.[16] Some imaging findings may be seen associated with a specific etiology of cholangiocarcinoma. Intrahepatic peripheral ductal dilatation in the remote liver can be seen in patients with underlying clonorchiasis (Fig. 2).[21] About 10% of intrahepatic stone disease is complicated by cholangiocarcinoma and 70% of cholangiocarcinoma presents with intrahepatic stone. In case of patients with underlying liver cirrhosis, MFICA especially less than 3 cm in diameter, the enhancement pattern on dynamic CT scan can be similar to hepatocellularcarcinoma which shows arterial enhancement and delayed washout.[22] In that case, HCC should be considered as a differential diagnosis. The MR imaging findings of MFICA are similar to those on CT scan.[23-25] MFICA appears hypointense on T1-weighted image, and hyperintense on T2-weighted image. Central hypointensity can be seen on T2-weighted image. This area may consist of fibrosis or coagulative necrosis which may show prolonged contrast pooling on delayed

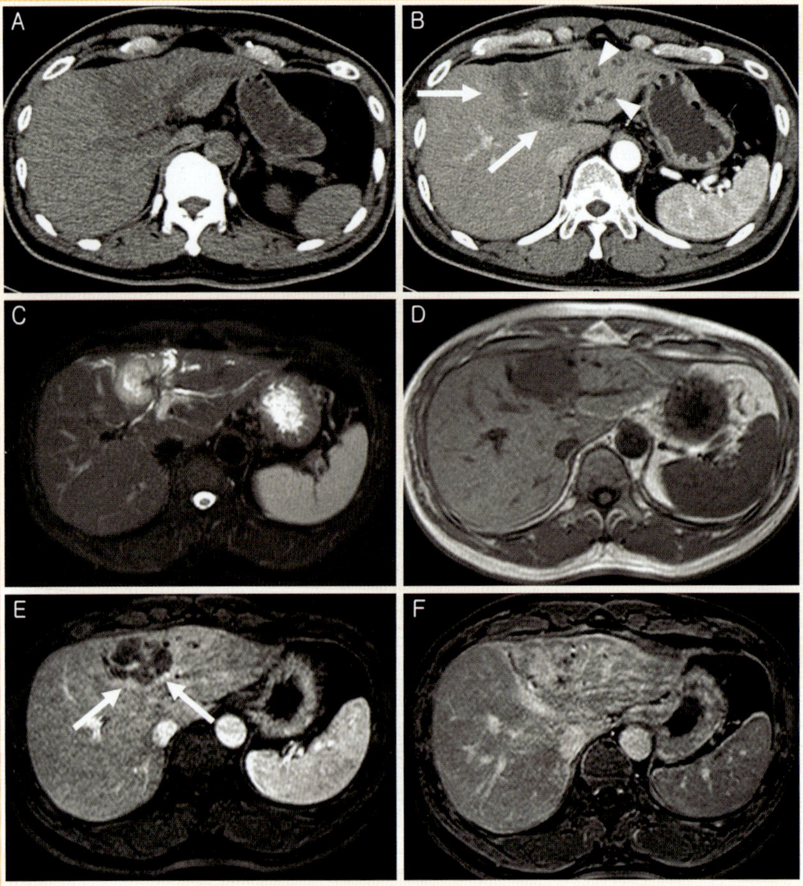

Fig. 3 52 year-old male with mass forming cholangiocarcinoma.

A: On precontrast CT scan, low attenuting mass is seen in the left lobe of the liver. B: Contrast enhanced arterial phase CT scan reveals low attenuating mass with peripheral rim like enhancement (arrow) and peripheral bile duct dilatation (arrow head). The mass shows high signal intensity C: on T2-weighted image and low signal intensity D: on T1-weighted image. E: Contrast enhanced arterial phase T1-weighted image shows peripheral rim enhancement (arrow). F: On contrast enhanced delay phase T1-weighted image, the central portion of the tumor shows delayed enhancement.

phase.[23,24] On gadolinium enhanced T1-weighted MR images, tumor shows peripheral enhancement with progressive central fill-in similarly in contrast enhanced CT.[18,23] The peripheral area that has early enhancing and is rapidly washout consists of actively growing tumor cells (Fig. 3).[26] Differential diagnoses of MFICA include sclerosing hepatocellular carcinoma (HCC), hepatic metastasis, organizing abscess and hepatic tuberculosis. Sclerosing HCC and combined hepatocellular carcinoma-cholangiocarcinoma appear nearly identical to cholangiocarcinoma.[27-29] An abscess and hepatic tuberculosis may mimic mass forming cholangiocarcinoma, but can be distinguished from cholangiocarcinoma by peripheral multilayered wall and central cystic change. Hepatic metastasis sometimes mimics mass forming cholangiocarcinoma and hard to differentiate both in imaging study and even in biopsy because both tumor are pathologically adenocarcinoma. In that case, search for primary tumor can be helpful for differential diagnosis.

2) Periductal infiltrating cholangiocarcinoma

Periductal infiltrative type is rare in intrahepatic cholangiocarcinoma. This type of tumor appears diffuse periductal thickening and increased enhancement with dilated or irregularly narrowed duct on CT and MR.[30,31] Within the liver, the periductal infiltrating tumor combined with mass-forming is more common than a purely periductal growing type (Fig. 4). The differential diagnosis includes a periportal lymphangitic metastasis from the extrahepatic tumors and peribiliary cysts.[32] These may be distinguished from periductal infiltrating cholangiocarcinoma by the absence of ductal dilatation.

3) Intraductal papillary cholangiocarcinoma

Intraductal cholangiocarcinoma can be classified into macroscopic papillary lesions and microscopic papillary tumor without gross papillary structure. The former shows grossly papillary tumor or polypoid lesions within the intrahepatic bile duct and

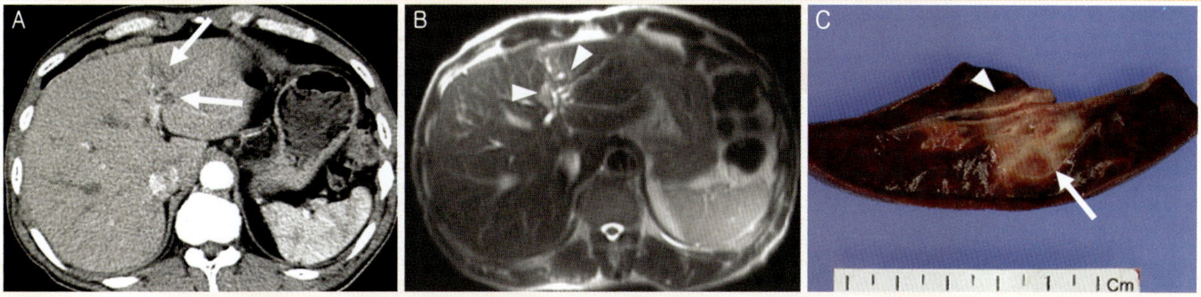

Fig. 4 67 year-old male with periductal infiltrating and mass-forming cholangiocarcinoma.

A: On arterial phase CT scan, periductal low attenuating lesion (arrow) with mild peripheral bile duct dilatation is seen. B: T2-weighted MR image reveals diffuse periductal thickening (arrow head). C: Photograph of gross specimen shows periductal infiltrating (arrow head) and mass-forming tumor (arrow).

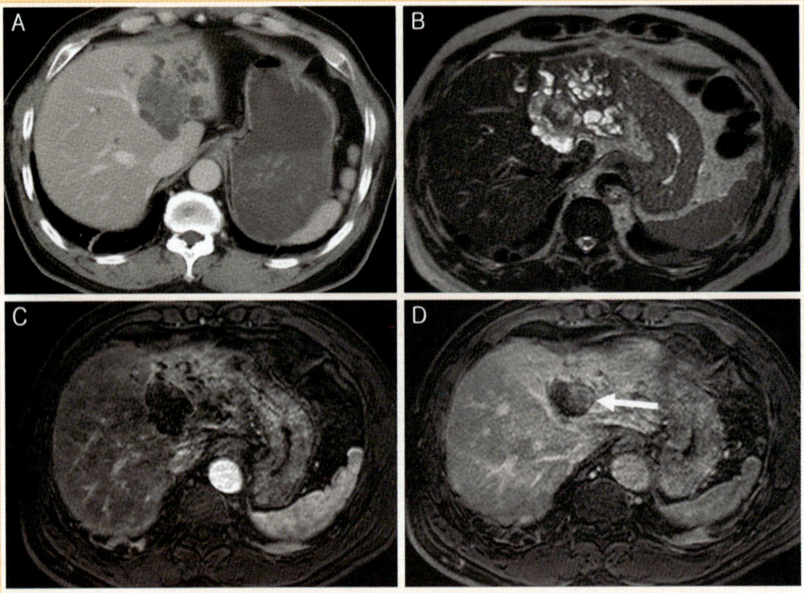

Fig. 5 62 year-old male with intraductal cholangiocarcinoma.

A: On contrast enhanced CT scan and B: T2-weighted MR image, polypoid mass is seen within the bile duct. Peripheral intrahepatic duct dilatation is also noted. On contrast enhanced C: arterial phase and D: portal venous phase T1-weighted MR image, polypoid mass shows delayed enhancement (arrow).

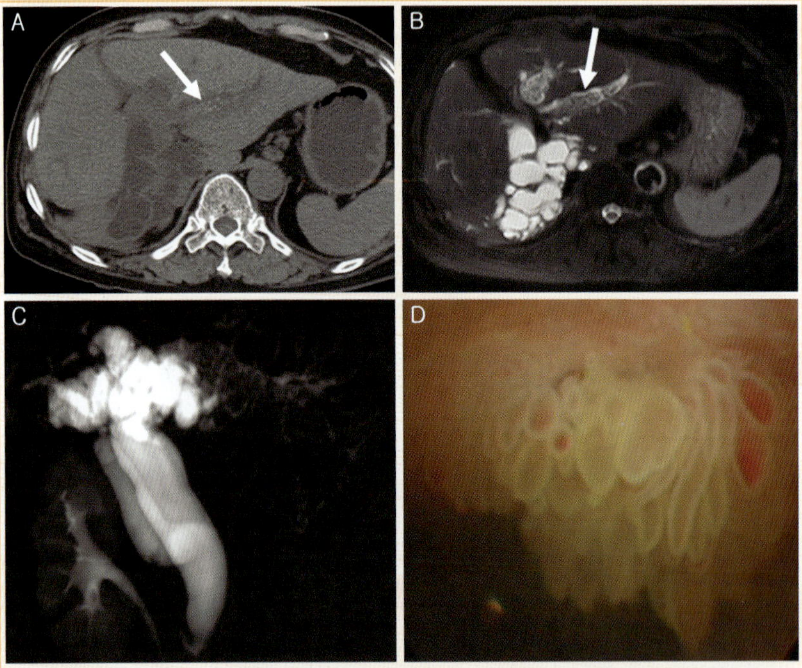

Fig. 6 67 year-old female with intraductal biliary neoplasm.

A: On precontrast CT scan and B: T2-weighted image, right posterior segmental duct shows marked dilatation. Intrahepatic stone is seen in the left intrahepatic duct (arrow). C: MRCP shows marked dilatation of intrahepatic and extrahepatic bile duct. D: Choledocoscopy shows polypoid lesion within the duct .

currently thought to be the counter part of the intraductal papillary mucinous neoplasm of the pancreas. The latter appears flat or micropapillary growth associated with a biliary intraepithelial neoplasia (BilIN), which is thought to be a precursor of cholangiocarcinoma in a multistep carcinogenesis and a counterpart of pancreatic intraepithelial neoplasia (PanIN).[33-36] Macroscopic papillary tumors reveal multiple superficial spreading papillary or plaque-like masses with ductal dilatation on imaging studies. On US, an intraductal mass shows echogenic lesion. Because this lesion usually confined to the wall, bile duct wall reveals intact. On CT, an intraductal mass shows hypo- or iso-attenuating lesion within the dilated bile duct, compared to adjacent liver parenchyma. After contrast enhancement, the tumor shows enhancement (Fig. 5). When the tumor is small and isoattenuating to the liver, a tumor may not be seen.[37-39] Some intraductal papillary tumors produce mucin.[40] Imaging study reveals severe dilatation of bile duct (Fig. 6). Bile duct dilatation may be seen in both proximal and distal to the tumor because it secretes mucin. It is hard to detect mucin itself, because mucin shows echo-free on US and isoattenuation to the liver on precontrast CT.[38] In case of BilIN, only diffuse ductectasia or focal stricture may be seen without grossly demonstrable intraductal polypoid lesion. In that case, differential diagnosis includes benign structure with or without ductal dilatation due to intrahepatic stone or longstanding clonorchiasis.

2. Extrahepatic Cholangiocarcinoma

1) Hilar cholangiocarcinoma

Hilar cholangiocarcinomas or Klatskin tumors refer to tumors arising from the confluence of the right and left ducts within the porta hepatis.[41] Periductal infiltrating type is the most common hilar cholangiocarcinoma. Peirductal infiltrating cholangiocarcinoma is characterized by growth along the dilated or narrowed bile duct without a definite mass formation and presents as an elongated, spiculated or branch-like abnormality. Hilar cholangiocarcinoma usually shows isoechoic or hypoechoic to the adjacent liver parenchyma.[3,42] Intrahepatic bile duct dilatation and nonunion of the right and left hepatic duct is the most common US findings in Klatskin tumors. In case of papillary or nodular type cholangiocarcinoma, intraluminal or nodular lesion can be seen within the bile duct.[1,2,42] Contrast enhanced US improves the detection and determination of the extent of the tumor.[5] On CT scan, infiltrating hilar cholangiocarcinoma shows focal thickening of ductal wall with obliterating the lumen.[19] For evaluation of operability or determination of surgical plan, longitudinal tumor spread as well as lateral tumor extension is important. Previous reports showed that detection rate was only 40-69% and the accuracy of resectability evaluation was only 54% on conventional CT scan.[7,43,44] In the era of multidetector CT (MDCT), the accuracy of tumor involvement evaluation increased 84~100%.[7,45] In the evaluation of resectability, both horizontal involvement of tumor that includes adjacent vessel and organ invasion and vertical tumor extent is important. Vascular occlusion, ipsilateral hepatic atrophy, stenosis or contour deformity, or tumor contact where more than 50% of the perimeter of the vessel suggest vascular invasion by the tumor (Fig. 7).[45,46] Accuracy of portal vein invasion and hepatic artery invasion are reported 85.5% and 92.7%, respectively. Accuracy of vertical tumor extension is reported 84~100%.[7,45] The overall accuracy of resectability reached 74.5~91.7%.[9,45] The CT criteria for identification of metastatic lymph node are as follows: larger than 10 mm in short-axis diameter, presence of central necrosis, and hyperattenuating compared with liver parenchyma in the portal phase.[45,46] But, lymph node evaluation is still limited and the overall accuracy of lymph node metastasis evaluation has been reported 73%.[7,47] Recently, three-dimensional image,

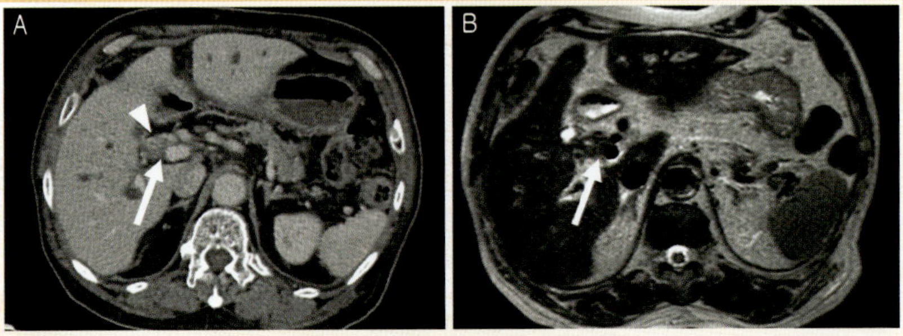

Fig. 7 82 year-old male with hilar cholangiocarcinoma.

A: On contrast enhanced CT scan and B: T2-weighted MR image, focal thickening of hilar bile duct is seen (arrow head). The tumor abuts the main portal vein with loss of fat plane (arrow), suggesting portal vein invasion.

multiplanar reformatted image, curved reformatted image and CT cholangiography are introduced and these methods could be helpful for diagnosis and planning of operation.[8,11,48,49] On MR, tumor appears hypointense to the liver on T1-weighted image and moderate hyperintense on T2-weighted image. On contrast enhanced MR, most tumors are hypovascular compared with adjacent liver and show a heterogeneous enhancement on delayed phase.[23,50] On MR cholangiopancreatography (MRCP), tumor reveals irregular thickening of the bile duct wall with symmetrical upstream bile duct dilatation.[23] The accuracy of vertical tumor spread is 81.5~90.7%. T2-weighted MR image is especially useful to determine the preserved fat plane between the tumor and vascular structure, which may be difficult to identify on contrast enhanced dynamic image.[46] Accuracy of hepatic artery and portal vein invasion was 82.7~90.1% and 95.1~97.5%, respectively. These results were comparable with accuracy of MDCT. Accuracy of prediction of lymph node metastasis is still not sufficient and has been reported about 74%.[23,51] MRCP has also benefit for evaluation of biliary anatomy. For surgical planning, variations of the bile duct anatomy are important. Common anatomical variation includes insertion of the right posterior or posterior duct to the left hepatic duct and trifurcation of the right anterior, posterior and left hepatic ducts. In cases of favorable anatomy such as the right anterior duct and right posterior duct drains separately into the common bile duct(trifurcation) or the right posterior duct drains to the left bile duct, Bismuth-Corlette type IV tumor can still be operable (Fig. 8).[46]

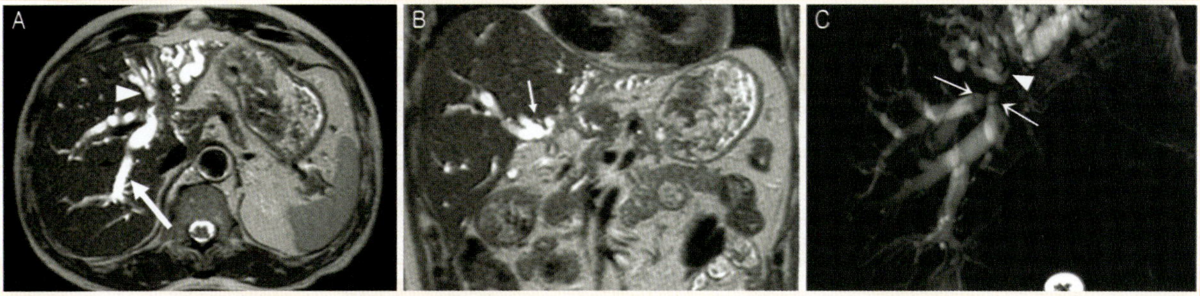

Fig. 8 67 year-old male with hilar cholangiocarcinoma.

A: On axial T2-weighted image, right posterior duct (arrow) drains to the left bile duct (arrow head). Tumor invades the confluence of right posterior duct and left intrahepatic bile duct. B: On T2-weighted coronal image, right anterior duct (small arrow) drains directly into the common bile duct. C: MRCP shows separation of right posterior duct (arrow), right anterior duct (small arrow) and left bile duct (arrow head), suggesting Bismuth Corlette type V tumor. But this patient underwent left lobectomy including segment 4 and caudate lobe because of the bile duct variation.

2) Distal CBD cancer

Periductal infiltrating type is the most common type of distal CBD cancer. US reveals dilatation of the CBD and/or pancreatic duct. Primary tumor itself is usually not seen in the transabdominal US. Endoscopic US or intraductal US can help to detect the tumor and to define the invasion and extent of tumor.[52-54] On CT or MR image, the dilated CBD shows abrupt luminal narrowing with ductal wall thickening.[19,55] The involved segment reveals delayed enhancement on contrast enhanced CT or MR images (Fig. 9).[55-57] On MRCP, tumor reveals abrupt bile duct narrowing with irregular margins in the distal narrowed segment. MRI with MRCP can add more diagnostic accuracy due to the high sensitivity of MRCP.[58] Sometimes differential diagnosis of benign and malignant CBD stricture is difficult. Malignant stricture shows longer involved segment, a wall thicker than 1.5 mm, and strong enhancement on the arterial or portal venous phase on CT or MR. Among these imaging findings, enhancement during portal venous phase is the most important characteristics of malignant stricture.[56]

Conclusion

Recent development of cross sectional imaging has markedly improved the diagnostic accuracy of the evaluation of cholangiocarcinoma. Sonography is accurate to identify biliary and also can be useful to determine the level of obstruction. However, longitudinal extension of tumor can be better evaluated by using MRCP, which can be used with routine MR examinations for better evaluation of extraductal structures as well as vascular abnormality combined with contrast enhanced dynamic MR imaging. MDCT has become popular and useful to evaluate biliary and vascular anatomy for the assessment of tumor extent and determination of resectability of a tumor by utilizing its excellent spatial and temporal resolution providing various postprocessing techniques that improves the visualization and assessment of the cholangiocarcinomas.

Reference

1. Bloom CM, Langer B, Wilson SR. Role of US in the detection, characterization, and staging of cholangiocarcinoma. Radiographics 1999;19:1199-218.
2. Robledo R, Muro A, Prieto ML. Extrahepatic bile duct carcinoma: US characteristics and accuracy in demonstration of tumors. Radiology 1996;198:869-873.
3. Looser C, Stain SC, Baer HU, Triller J, Blumgart LH. Staging of hilar cholangiocarcinoma by ultrasound and duplex sonography: a comparison with angiography and operative findings. Br J Radiol 1992;65:871-877.
4. D'Onofrio M, Vecchiato F, Cantisani V, Barbi E, Passamonti M, Ricci P, Malago R, Faccioli N, Zamboni G, Pozzi Mucelli R. Intrahepatic peripheral cholangiocarcinoma (IPCC): comparison between perfusion ultrasound and CT imaging. Radiol Med (Torino) 2008;113: 76-86.
5. Khalili K, Metser U, Wilson SR. Hilar biliary obstruction: preliminary results with Levovist-enhanced sonography. AJR Am J Roentgenol 2003;180:687-693.
6. Kawashima H, Hirooka Y, Itoh A, Hara K, Kanamori A, Uchida H, Goto J, Nonogaki K, Matsumoto Y, Ohmiya N, Niwa Y, Goto H. Progress of endoscopic ultrasonography and intraductal ultrasonography in the diagnosis of malignant biliary diseases. J Hepatobiliary Pancreat Surg 2006;13:69-74.
7. Unno M, Okumoto T, Katayose Y, Rikiyama T, Sato A, Motoi F, Oikawa M, Egawa S, Ishibashi T. Preoperative assessment of hilar cholangiocarcinoma by multidetector row computed tomography. J Hepatobiliary Pancreat Surg 2007;14:434-440.
8. Choi JY, Lee JM, Lee JY, Kim SH, Lee MW, Han JK, Choi BI. Assessment of hilar and extrahepatic bile duct cancer using multidetector CT: value of adding multiplanar reformations to standard axial images. Eur Radiol 2007;17:3130-3138.
9. Chen HW, Pan AZ, Zhen ZJ, Su SY, Wang JH, Yu SC, Lau WY. Preoperative evaluation of resectability of Klatskin tumor with 16-MDCT angiography and cholangiography. AJR Am J Roentgenol 2006;186:1580-1586.
10. Cody DD. AAPM/RSNA physics tutorial for residents: topics in CT. Image processing in CT. Radiographics 2002;22:1255-1268.
11. Endo I, Shimada H, Sugita M, Fujii Y, Morioka D, Takeda K, Sugae S, Tanaka K, Togo S, Bourquain H, Peitgen HO. Role of three-dimensional imaging in operative planning for hilar cholangiocarcinoma. Surgery 2007;142:666-675.
12. Choi JY, Kim MJ. Hilar Cholangiocarcinoma: Current Role of Preoperative Imaging Using State-of-the-art US, MDCT, MR, and Direct Cholangiography. AJR Am J Roentgenol; In press.
13. Kim JY, Lee JM, Han JK, Kim SH, Lee JY, Choi JY, Kim SJ, Kim HJ, Kim KH, Choi BI. Contrast-enhanced MRI combined with MR cholangiopancreatography for the evaluation of patients with biliary strictures: differentiation of malignant from benign bile duct strictures. J Magn Reson Imaging 2007;26:304-312.

14. Masselli G, Manfredi R, Vecchioli A, Gualdi G. MR imaging and MR cholangiopancreatography in the preoperative evaluation of hilar cholangiocarcinoma: correlation with surgical and pathologic findings. Eur Radiol 2008.

15. Masselli G, Gualdi G. Hilar cholangiocarcinoma: MRI/MRCP in staging and treatment planning. Abdom Imaging 2008;33:444-451.

16. Ros PR, Buck JL, Goodman ZD, Ros AM, Olmsted WW. Intrahepatic cholangiocarcinoma: radiologic-pathologic correlation. Radiology 1988;167:689-693.

17. Burns PN, Wilson SR. Focal liver masses: enhancement patterns on contrast-enhanced imagesconcordance of US scans with CT scans and MR images. Radiology 2007;242:162-174.

18. Zhang Y, Uchida M, Abe T, Nishimura H, Hayabuchi N, Nakashima Y. Intrahepatic peripheral cholangiocarcinoma: comparison of dynamic CT and dynamic MRI. J Comput Assist Tomogr 1999;23:670-677.

19. Han JK, Choi BI, Kim AY, An SK, Lee JW, Kim TK, Kim SW. Cholangiocarcinoma: pictorial essay of CT and cholangiographic findings. Radiographics 2002;22:173-187.

20. Kim TK, Choi BI, Han JK, Jang HJ, Cho SG, Han MC. Peripheral cholangiocarcinoma of the liver: two-phase spiral CT findings. Radiology 1997;204:539-543.

21. Choi BI, Park JH, Kim YI, Yu ES, Kim SH, Kim WH, Kim CY, Han MC. Peripheral cholangiocarcinoma and clonorchiasis: CT findings. Radiology 1988;169:149-153.

22. Kim SJ, Lee JM, Han JK, Kim KH, Lee JY, Choi BI. Peripheral mass-forming cholangiocarcinoma in cirrhotic liver. AJR Am J Roentgenol 2007;189:1428-1434.

23. Manfredi R, Barbaro B, Masselli G, Vecchioli A, Marano P. Magnetic resonance imaging of cholangiocarcinoma. Semin Liver Dis 2004;24:155-164.

24. Maetani Y, Itoh K, Watanabe C, Shibata T, Ametani F, Yamabe H, Konishi J. MR Imaging of Intrahepatic Cholangiocarcinoma with Pathologic Correlation. Am J Roentgenol 2001;176:1499-1507.

25. Vilgrain V, Van Beers BE, Flejou JF, Belghiti J, Delos M, Gautier AL, Zins M, Denys A, Menu Y. Intrahepatic cholangiocarcinoma: MRI and pathologic correlation in 14 patients. J Comput Assist Tomogr 1997;21:59-65.

26. Valls C, Guma A, Puig I, Sanchez A, Andia E, Serrano T, Figueras J. Intrahepatic peripheral cholangiocarcinoma: CT evaluation. Abdom Imaging 2000;25:490-496.

27. Zuo HQ, Yan LN, Zeng Y, Yang JY, Luo HZ, Liu JW, Zhou LX. Clinicopathological characteristics of 15 patients with combined hepatocellular carcinoma and cholangiocarcinoma. Hepatobiliary Pancreat Dis Int 2007;6:161-165.

28. Nishie A, Yoshimitsu K, Asayama Y, Irie H, Aibe H, Tajima T, Shinozaki K, Nakayama T, Kakihara D, Shimada M, Aishima S, Yoshida K, Honda H. Detection of combined hepatocellular and cholangiocarcinomas on enhanced CT: comparison with histologic findings. AJR Am J Roentgenol 2005;184:1157-1162.

29. Lee WJ, Lim HK, Jang KM, Kim SH, Lee SJ, Lim JH, Choo IW. Radiologic spectrum of cholangiocarcinoma: emphasis on unusual manifestations and differential diagnoses.

Radiographics 2001;21:S97-S116.

30. Lim JH, Park CK. Pathology of cholangiocarcinoma. Abdom Imaging 2004;29:540-547.

31. Han JK, Lee JM. Intrahepatic intraductal cholangiocarcinoma. Abdom Imaging 2004;29:558-564.

32. Tada H, Morimoto M, Shima T, Hirana H, Nakagawa Y, Shimamoto K, Nagano N. Progressive jaundice due to lymphangiosis carcinomatosa of the liver: CT appearance. J Comput Assist Tomogr 1996;20:650-652.

33. Zen Y, Adsay NV, Bardadin K, Colombari R, Ferrell L, Haga H, Hong SM, Hytiroglou P, Kloppel G, Lauwers GY, van Leeuwen DJ, Notohara K, Oshima K, Quaglia A, Sasaki M, Sessa F, Suriawinata A, Tsui W, Atomi Y, Nakanuma Y. Biliary intraepithelial neoplasia: an international interobserver agreement study and proposal for diagnostic criteria. Mod Pathol 2007;20:701-709.

34. Zen Y, Aishima S, Ajioka Y, Haratake J, Kage M, Kondo F, Nimura Y, Sakamoto M, Sasaki M, Shimamatsu K, Wakasa K, Park YN, Chen MF, Atomi Y, Nakanuma Y. Proposal of histological criteria for intraepithelial atypical/proliferative biliary epithelial lesions of the bile duct in hepatolithiasis with respect to cholangiocarcinoma: preliminary report based on interobserver agreement. Pathol Int 2005;55:180-188.

35. Zen Y, Fujii T, Itatsu K, Nakamura K, Minato H, Kasashima S, Kurumaya H, Katayanagi K, Kawashima A, Masuda S, Niwa H, Mitsui T, Asada Y, Miura S, Ohta T, Nakanuma Y. Biliary papillary tumors share pathological features with intraductal papillary mucinous neoplasm of the pancreas. Hepatology 2006;44:1333-1343.

36. Kloppel G, Kosmahl M. Is the intraductal papillary mucinous neoplasia of the biliary tract a counterpart of pancreatic papillary mucinous neoplasm? J Hepatol 2006;44:249-250.

37. Lim JH. Cholangiocarcinoma: morphologic classification according to growth pattern and imaging findings. AJR Am J Roentgenol 2003;181:819-827.

38. Lim JH, Yi CA, Lim HK, Lee WJ, Lee SJ, Kim SH. Radiological spectrum of intraductal papillary tumors of the bile ducts. Korean J Radiol 2002;3:57-63.

39. Lee JW, Han JK, Kim TK, Kim YH, Choi BI, Han MC, Suh KS, Kim SW. CT features of intraductal intrahepatic cholangiocarcinoma. AJR Am J Roentgenol 2000;175:721-725.

40. Kim HJ, Kim MH, Lee SK, Yoo KS, Park ET, Lim BC, Park HJ, Myung SJ, Seo DW, Min YI. Mucin-hypersecreting bile duct tumor characterized by a striking homology with an intraductal papillary mucinous tumor (IPMT) of the pancreas. Endoscopy 2000;32:389-393.

41. Klatskin G. Adenocarcinoma of the Hepatic Duct at Its Bifurcation within the Porta Hepatis. An Unusual Tumor with Distinctive Clinical and Pathological Features. Am J Med 1965;38:241-256.

42. Hann LE, Greatrex KV, Bach AM, Fong Y, Blumgart LH. Cholangiocarcinoma at the hepatic hilus: sonographic findings. AJR Am J Roentgenol 1997;168:985-989.

43. Choi BI, Lee JH, Han MC, Kim SH, Yi JG, Kim CW. Hilar cholangiocarcinoma: comparative study with sonography and CT. Radiology 1989;172:689-692.

44. Nesbit GM, Johnson CD, James EM, MacCarty RL, Nagorney DM, Bender CE. Cholangiocarcinoma: diagnosis and evaluation of resectability by CT and sonography as procedures complementary to cholangiography. AJR Am J Roentgenol 1988;151:933-938.

45. Lee HY, Kim SH, Lee JM, Kim SW, Jang JY, Han JK, Choi BI. Preoperative assessment of resectability of hepatic hilar cholangiocarcinoma: combined CT and cholangiography with revised criteria. Radiology 2006;239:113-121.

46. Chung YE, Kim MJ, Park YN, Lee YH, Choi JY. Staging of extrahepatic cholangiocarcinoma. Eur Radiol 2008;18:2182-2195.

47. Roche CJ, Hughes ML, Garvey CJ, Campbell F, White DA, Jones L, Neoptolemos JP. CT and pathologic assessment of prospective nodal staging in patients with ductal adenocarcinoma of the head of the pancreas. AJR Am J Roentgenol 2003;180:475-480.

48. Kim HJ, Kim AY, Hong SS, Kim MH, Byun JH, Won HJ, Shin YM, Kim PN, Ha HK, Lee MG. Biliary ductal evaluation of hilar cholangiocarcinoma: three-dimensional direct multidetector row CT cholangiographic findings versus surgical and pathologic results—feasibility study. Radiology 2006;238:300-308.

49. Nino-Murcia M, Jeffrey RB, Jr., Beaulieu CF, Li KC, Rubin GD. Multidetector CT of the pancreas and bile duct system: value of curved planar reformations. AJR Am J Roentgenol 2001;176:689-693.

50. Soyer P, Bluemke DA, Reichle R, Calhoun PS, Bliss DF, Scherrer A, Fishman EK. Imaging of intrahepatic cholangiocarcinoma: 2. Hilar cholangiocarcinoma. AJR Am J Roentgenol 1995;165:1433-1436.

51. Park HS, Lee JM, Choi JY, Lee MW, Kim HJ, Han JK, Choi BI. Preoperative evaluation of bile duct cancer: MRI combined with MR cholangiopancreatography versus MDCT with direct cholangiography. AJR Am J Roentgenol 2008;190:396-405.

52. Mittelstaedt CA. Ultrasound of the bile ducts. Semin Roentgenol 1997;32:161-171.

53. Oikarinen H. Diagnostic imaging of carcinomas of the gallbladder and the bile ducts. Acta Radiol 2006;47:345-358.

54. Palazzo L. Staging of ampullary carcinoma by endoscopic ultrasonography. Endoscopy 1998;30 Suppl 1:A128-131.

55. Kim JH, Kim MJ, Chung JJ, Lee WJ, Yoo HS, Lee JT. Differential diagnosis of periampullary carcinomas at MR imaging. Radiographics 2002;22:1335-1352.

56. Choi SH, Han JK, Lee JM, Lee KH, Kim SH, Lee JY, Choi BI. Differentiating malignant from benign common bile duct stricture with multiphasic helical CT. Radiology 2005;236:178-183.

57. Guarise A, Venturini S, Faccioli N, Pinali L, Morana G. Role of magnetic resonance in characterising extrahepatic cholangiocarcinomas. Radiol Med (Torino) 2006;111:526-538.

58. Andersson M, Kostic S, Johansson M, Lundell L, Asztely M, Hellstrom M. MRI combined with MR cholangiopancreatography versus helical CT in the evaluation of patients with suspected periampullary tumors: a prospective comparative study. Acta Radiol 2005;46:16-27.

VIII · III
Endoscopic Assessment

1. Endoscopic Retrograde Cholangiography (ERC)

Introduction

Cholangiocarcinoma is an adenocarcinoma that originates primarily from epithelial cells of the bile duct and is the second most common cause of liver cancer, after hepatocellularcarcinoma. Cholangiocarcinomas are traditionally classified into intrahepatic and extrahepatic cholangiocarcinomas. Intrahepatic cholangiocarcinomas are often observed as a parenchymal mass, and most show a progressed state. Extrahepatic cholangiocarcinomas commonly appear as obstructions of the left and right bile ducts, the common hepatic duct, and the common bile duct. There are many similarities between the two conditions, but they also show differences in epidemiology and clinical patterns; furthermore, the mechanisms are believed to be different.[1]

Cholangiocarcinoma is a rare tumor, but its incidence has been increasing over the last 30 years.[2] In Korea, the occurrence and death rate of cholangiocarcinoma in the 2000s showed an increasing trend, and registered numbers of cholangiocarcinoma in 2007 were 13321 (8225 males and 5066 females).[3] The death rate due to intrahepatic cholangiocarcinoma has been increasing worldwide. The 5 year survival rate has continued to be very low and has not changed much over the last 20 years, despite earlier diagnosis, improvements in surgical techniques, and new treatment modalities, including bile duct stenting and photodynamic therapy.[4]

Endoscopic retrograde cholangiography (ERC) enables accurate diagnoses of bile duct disease by providing endoscopic information regarding the major papilla and radiological information regarding the bile duct, gall bladder, and pancreatic tract. However, noninvasive diagnostic methods such as contrast-enhanced CT, MRCP, and endoscopic ultrasound (EUS) have recently begun to replace ERC in the diagnosis and staging of cholangiocarcinomas. ERC is still applied when additional information is required regarding the state of the bile duct in a patient diagnosed with cholangiocarcinoma through abdominal ultrasound and radiological studies such as CT. ERC is especially useful when cholangiocarcinoma is suspected in a patient having sclerosing cholangitis and is an informative test in determining the extent of the cancer.[5] ERC also has the advantage of allowing diagnosis and treatment of biliary drainage to be carried out at the same time in patients with obstructive jaundice.

There are almost no absolute contraindications for ERC in cholangiocarcinoma, and diagnosis and therapies are possible. It is now widely used for acute cholangitis, which has been considered a contraindication in the past, and even for cholangiocarcinomas with biliary pancreatitis. Relative contraindications include uncorrectable coagulopathy, patient refusal, and severe acute pancreatitis.

The technique of ERC is difficult and complex. It should be performed by an endoscopist with experience in both diagnostic and therapeutic endoscopy to avoid unnecessary risk. Good results can be obtained with the cooperation of well-trained gastrointestinal endoscopy nurses or associates and radiologists.

1) Classification of cholangiocarcinoma by ERC

According to Seifert et al.[6] extrahepatic cholangiocarcinomas are classified by cholangiography into three forms: obstructive-type, stricture-type, and bulging-type cholangiocarcinomas.

The obstructive-type cholangiocarcinoma (Fig. 1) is known as the most common form, but until recently, this form was as rare as 10% of cases. A biliary catheter,

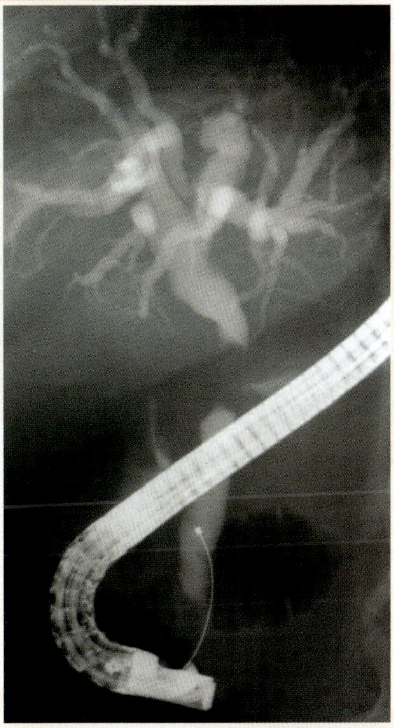

Fig. 1 Obstructive-type Cholangiocarcinoma
ERC shows abrupt filling defect at the mid-portion of CBD.

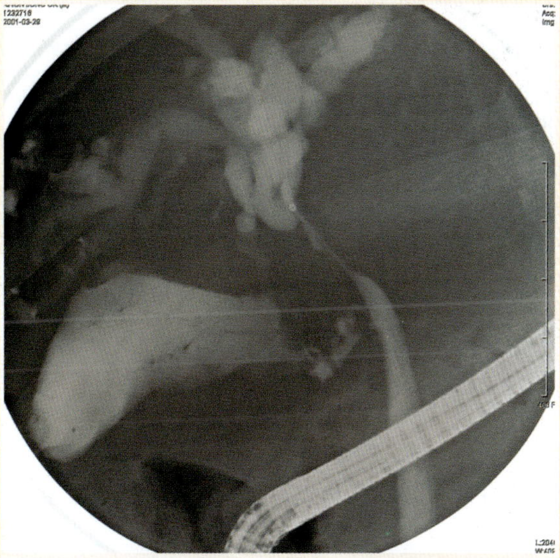

Fig. 2 Obstructive-type Cholangiocarcinoma
ERC shows irregular filling defect at the proximal portion of CBD.

which can be U-shaped, V-shaped, or inverted, should be inserted deeply to check for obstruction. Obstruction of the proximal bile duct may be contrasted using a balloon catheter and may be observed with percutaneous transhepatic cholangiography. It is necessary to distinguish between obstructive-type cholangiocarcinoma and bile duct stones or benign strictures. The obstructive cholangiocarcinoma can appear as a nodal type to the naked eye. The infiltrates are relatively short-range but form a mass that blocks the bile duct. Jaundice typically appears at an early stage and is readily diagnosed. Surgery is usually possible, and the prognosis is relatively good.

The stricture-type cholangiocarcinoma (Fig. 2) may appear similar to the infiltration type by observation of the bile duct with the naked eye. The stricture can be short or long. In the case of a hilum, the stricture length may be short; the cholangiocarcinoma can spread in a circle, with a lumen showing dilatation of the proximal part and an irregular stricture. Alternatively, a stricture can be long, tortuous, and irregular, with a "rat tail" shape. The stricture-type cholangiocarcinoma is characterized by tumor infiltration and growth in the submucosal layer along the bile duct wall surface, rather than in the luminal cavity, and tends to be diagnosed only after many tumors have developed; thus, the prognosis is typically not good. When stricture-type extrahepatic cholangiocarcinoma is suspected, the differential diagnosis should include strictures due to benign diseases (Fig. 3) of various causes, because benign strictures can often close the bile duct lumen, showing signs of local stricture and increased thickness of the bile duct wall similar to that seen in malignant strictures. Careful diagnosis is necessary to reduce unnecessary surgery; 8~13% of cases that were diagnosed as malignant strictures by ultrasound, CT, or cholangiography before surgery were actually found to be strictures due to fibrosis. Characteristics that suggest malignant (Fig. 4) rather than benign strictures in cholangiography include rapidly, irregularly, or asymmetrically narrowed bile ducts

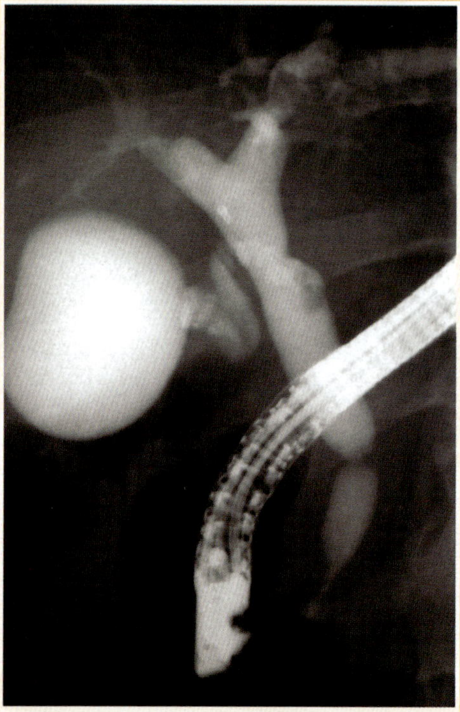

Fig. 3 Benign stricture of bile duct

ERC shows localized ring-like filling defect at the mid-portion of CBD.

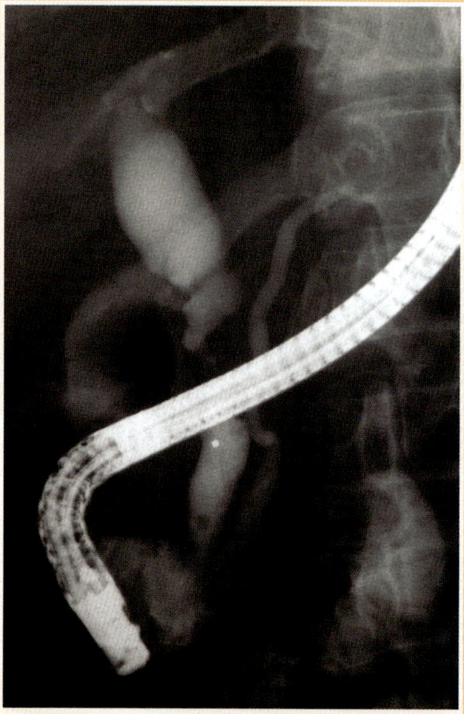

Fig. 4 Malignant stricture of bile duct

ERC shows irregular, asymmetrical filling defect.

accompanying double duct signs. According to Park et al., the length of the stricture can be helpful in discerning whether it is malignant: malignant strictures were significantly longer (average, 30.0±8.5 mm) than benign strictures (14.9±5.5 mm).[7] An infiltrating cholangiocarcinoma can also look like a stricture; it may spread under the epithelial layer of the bile duct and induce severe fibrosis and desmoplastic reactions without forming a mass, showing a long stricture. A recent report concluded that MRCP is similar to ERC in differentiating between malignant and benign strictures, but that ERC affords higher resolution, making it more helpful in determining the malignancy of stricture lesions.[8]

The bulging-type cholangiocarcinoma (Fig. 5) appears grossly as a papillary type and accounts for 30% of all extrahepatic cholangiocarcinomas. It appears as a filling defect on cholangiography; the margin is ambiguous and is typically observed fixed to the bile duct. Bulging-type characteristics include tumor progression up and down, following the surface level of the bile duct wall. There are many cases in which the longitudinal infiltration range of the tumor is much larger than the depth of tumor infiltration, and there are many cases in which the accurate determination of mass is difficult, even with high-resolution cholangiography. Thus, when considering curative surgery, preoperative cholangiography should be performed. Cholangiography typically shows this tumor as a long shape, attached slightly to the bile duct, and tending to be brittle.

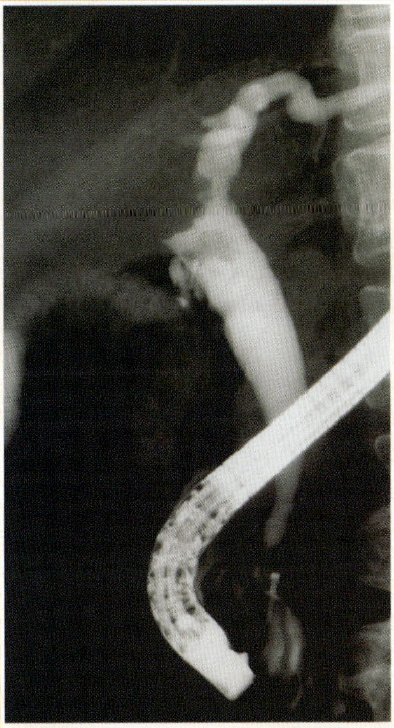

Fig. 5 Bulging-type Cholangiocarcinoma

ERC shows nodular filling defect at the bifurcation of bile duct.

Extrahepatic cholangiocarcinomas are also classified into three types, depending on their location in the bile duct: hilar, mid, and peripheral. Hilar cholangiocarcinomas account for about 60% of all extrahepatic cholangiocarcinomas and can be typed according to the Bismuth-Corlette classification. Type I shows no obstruction at the merger of the left and right bile ducts; type II has closure limited to the merger site and no infiltration of the second bifurcation, and type III has an obstruction at the merger site and a shape at the second bifurcation, with greater invasion of the left or right bile duct bifurcation (right invasion, type IIIa; left invasion, type IIIb). In type IV, both sides are invaded, to the second bifurcation or beyond. MRCP (Fig. 6) is preferred for examining hilar cholangiocarcinomas, because the spread of the lesion outside the bile duct (e.g., vascular invasion), lymph node enlargement, and a missing bile duct with no connection to the main bile duct can be evaluated. Nevertheless, ERC is sometimes essential for assessing the definite range of tumor invasion.

Furthermore, ERC is helpful in the diagnosis of hilar and intrahepatic cholangiocarcinomas. In such tumors, the proximal bile duct does not appear clearly by cholangioscopy owing to the stricture. Although the proximal portion of stricture could be contrasted by using excessive contrast agent, this is not advisable; the contrast medium will not readily wash out after the examination, and thus the risk of cholangitis and sepsis is increased. If it is necessary to inject a large amount of contrast medium into the proximal portion of the obstruction, an appropriate drainage technique should be considered.

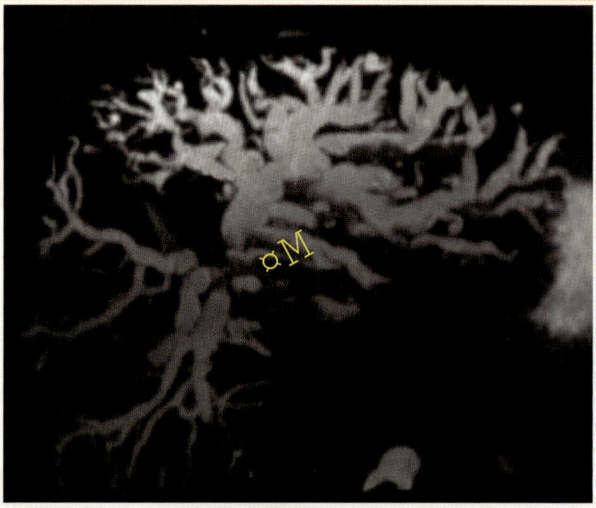

Fig. 6 MRCP shows significant dilatation of left IHD and cut-off signal at the bifurcation area of IHD(Arrow)
IIIb type of Bismuth-Corlette classification.

2) Role of ERC in cholangiocarcinoma

ERC has been used for more than 30 years in the diagnosis and treatment of bilopancreatic disease; however, because of complications, the safer and non-invasive MRCP has recently been preferred. Nevertheless, ERC can provide diagnostic information and allow tissue collection. It can also be used to perform drainage and stent insertion in bile duct obstructions. Therefore, ERC remains an important technique in the diagnosis and treatment of cholangiocarcinoma.

3) Role of ERC in the diagnosis of cholangiocarcinoma

ERC is a powerful method for diagnosing cholangiocarcinoma, but it is an invasive examination and is therefore associated with some risk. However, it is possible to systematically diagnose cholangiocarcinoma by brush cytology of the bile duct and forceps biopsy.

(1) Brush cytology and forceps biopsy

Cytology can be performed by scraping the surface of the cholangiocarcinoma with an endoscopic brush to obtain cancer cells (Fig. 7). Foutch et al. reviewed the literature regarding this examination and reported that the overall sensitivity of brush cytology was 59%, with greater sensitivity in cholangiocarcinomas than in pancreatic head cancer.[9] However, extrahepatic cholangiocarcinomas have severe desmoplasia and fibrosis, which decrease the positive predictive value of histological examination. In one study, only about one-third of patients showed positive results on brush cytology, although when accompanied by forceps biopsy, the positive predictive value was increased to 40-70% (Fig. 8).[10] Jailwala et al. performed triple tissue collection from 133 patients by using brush cytology, fine needle aspiration, and forceps biopsy.[11] The overall sensitivity was 77%, and these authors recommended using two or more methods in diagnosing cholangiocarcinomas.

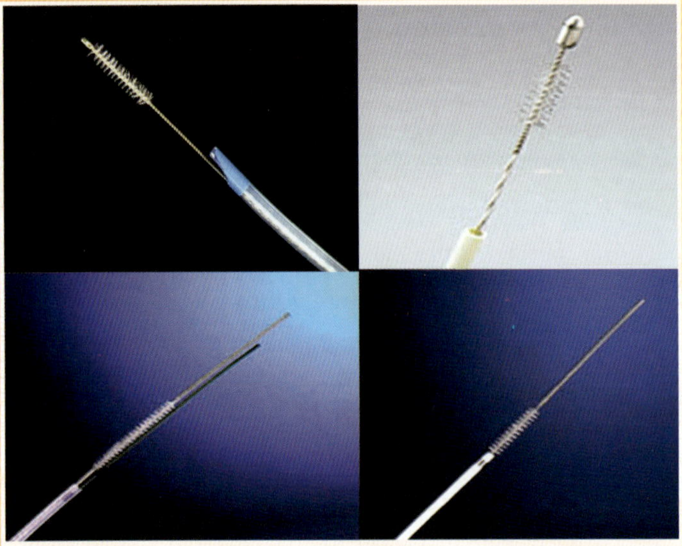
Fig. 7 Various types of brush cytology devices

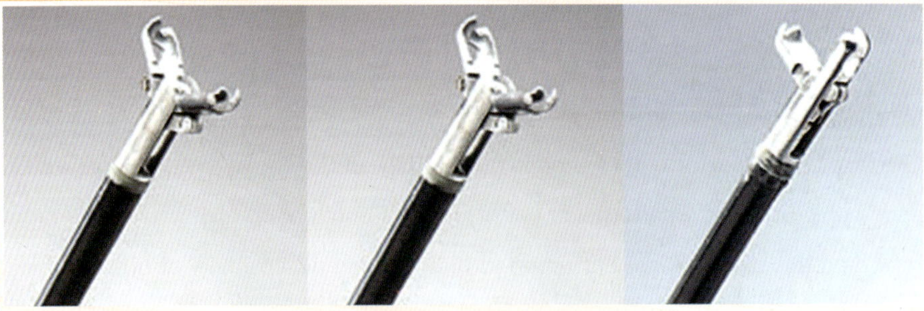
Fig. 8 Various types of forceps biopsy for obtaining tissues from bile duct

(2) FISH and DIA

As diagnostic techniques in cholangiocarcinomas, fluorescence in situ hybridization (FISH) and digitized image analysis (DIA) have recently been used in combination with specimens acquired through ERC. These tests evaluate aneuploidy and chromosomal abnormalities in cells and may be useful in the diagnosis of extrahepatic cholangiocarcinomas in the future.[12] According to one study, the sensitivity of FISH in diagnosing extrahepatic cholangiocarcinomas was 34%, and that of brush cytological examination was 15%. FISH examination has high sensitivity and specificity (91%), similar to brush cytology.[13] In a comparative study of DIA and brush cytological examination in cholangiocarcinoma patients, the sensitivity of DIA was 39.3%, and that of brush cytology was 17.9%; the specificity of DIA was 77.3%; and that of brush cytology was 97.7%.[14]

4) Role of ERC in the treatment of cholangiocarcinoma by bile duct stent insertion

The insertion of an endoscopic stent is a palliative treatment method for malignant bile duct obstructions; it improves clinical symptoms and quality of life in obstructive jaundice patients, but it does not extend the survival period.[4] Issues to evaluate when considering bile duct stent placement as a palliative treatment include the location and extent of the obstruction, contraction of the hepatic lobes, type of stent, number of stents, and life expectancy. It is also important to perform a tomographic analysis before ERC in order to increase the success rate of bile duct stent surgery, to avoid contracted hepatic lobes, and to prevent bile duct infection that can occur after surgery.[15] The type and number of stents in palliative treatment of cholangiocarcinoma depends on the individual case, but a single bile duct stent treatment is typically sufficient for hilar cholangiocarcinoma Bismuth type I. There is no consensus in Bismuth types 2, 3, and 4. A recent report regarding bile duct stent treatment in patients with Bismuth types 1, 2, and 3 found that a bile duct stent was sufficient to improve malignant bile duct closure symptoms and that the frequency of bile duct inflammation was low; however, the survival rate was not improved.[16]

Conclusion

MRCP has some advantages over ERC in diagnosing cholangiocarcinoma: it is permits the evaluation of the proximal and distal bile duct in a malignant stricture, and it facilitates defining the spread of extra-biliary lesions such as vascular infiltration and lymph node enlargement. MRCP can also be helpful in determining a treatment plan, and it avoids the complication of cholangitis due to inefficient removal of the contrast agent used in cholangiography.[17] In its opinion issued in 2002 on endoscopic retrograde cholangiography in diagnosis and treatment, the National Institutes of

Health recommended MRCP as the examination for evaluating cholangiocarcinoma .[5]

On the other hand, ERC affords better resolution than MRCP and can clearly determine the range of cholangiocarcinoma, which can be ambiguous on MRCP examination. Systematic diagnosis is also possible using ERC in patients with an ambiguous diagnosis of cholangiocarcinoma. In cholangiocarcinoma patients who are not good candidates for conventional surgery, ERC enables treatments, including the insertion of bile duct stents, that improve the symptoms and quality of life for the patient. Although ERC, the previous gold-standard diagnostic method for cholangiocarcinoma, is currently being replaced by MRCP, ERC will continue to have important and useful application in the diagnosis and treatment of cholangiocarcinomas.

2. Peroral Cholangioscopy

1) History

Great advances have been made in the diagnosis and treatment of biliopancreatic disease since the introduction of endoscopic retrograde cholangioscopy (ERC) and sphincterotomy in the early 1970s. However, distinguishing between a filling defect and a stricture using ERC alone can be difficult, and when the first attempts to observe the bile and pancreatic ducts directly were undertaken in the mid-1970s, they were constrained by technical difficulties.[18] Recent technological advances leading to the development of fine, flexible, durable endoscopes with a working channel have resolved these problems, and observing abnormalities, obtaining specimens, and performing interventions while observing the bile ducts directly can now be achieved. Consequently, peroral cholangioscopy has become an important endoscopic procedure with broader clinical indications.

2) Introduction of peroral cholangioscopy

Peroral cholangioscopy is performed using a "mother-baby" scope system. This involves a trained endoscopist inserting a fine cholangioscope through a therapeutic duodenoscope.[19] The standard baby cholangioscope has an outer diameter of 4.5 mm and requires a larger duodenoscope as the mother scope. Recently, fine cholangioscopes with outer diameters of 2.0 to 3.5 mm have been developed that can be inserted through a standard duodenoscope (Fig. 9). Consequently, they are easy to operate and are more cost-effective.

The newest peroral cholangioscope has a distal end that can be shifted in two directions and it can be used for biopsies, cytology, needle aspiration, and catheter insertion through a 1.2~1.7-mm working channel. Some cholangioscopes can be inserted into the far end of the bile duct and used to examine the second and third branches of the intrahepatic ducts.

The peroral cholangioscopic approach to the biliary tree is safer and faster than PTCS and requires no percutaneous drainage. However, use of this technique is more difficult for lesions above the hilum because of significant limitations in the retroflexion capability of the babyscope tip after insertion into the bile duct. Biopsy study can be ineffective due to the limited maneuverability of the long baby scope, and the durability of the babyscope is less satisfactory. The specimens are small if a 3-

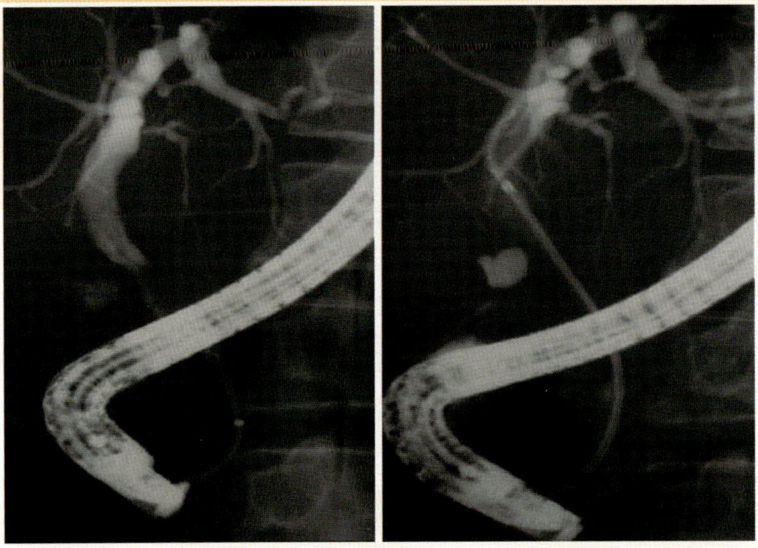

Fig. 9 'Mother-baby' scope system of peroral cholangioscopy

ERC shows fine cholagioscopy is inserted through therapeutic duodenoscope(left). Peroral cholangioscopic imaging of cholangiocarcinoma(Right).(Courtesy K.Yasuda, 2nd Red Cross Hospital, Kyoto, Japan)

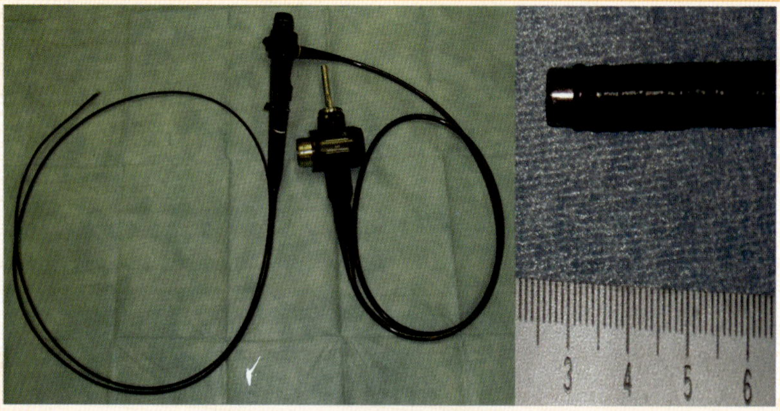

Fig. 10 Recent model of electronic babyscope(Olympus CHF-BP260)
(Courtesy K. Yasuda, 2nd Red Cross Hospital, Kyoto, Japan)

Fr biopsy forceps has to be used via the 1.2-mm working channel of microscopes with an outer diameter of 2.9 or 3.0mm (Fig. 10).[20]

3) Imaging of cholangiocarcinoma

Endoscopic retrograde cholangioscopy can clearly diagnose choledocholithiasis and bile leakage, but has difficulty in clearly distinguishing a biliary stricture from a filling defect. A filling defect appears in choledocholithiasis or with a polypoid tumor, while a stricture may appear when the biliary tract wall becomes thick or when the biliary tract is compressed by external disease.

Cholangiocarcinoma can lead to increased thickness of the bile duct wall, causing a stricture, and the abnormal mucosa can be observed directly using cholangioscopy. Conversely, when the bile duct is compressed by external disease, such as a metastatic lymph node, a stricture results, but the intraluminal mucosa of the bile duct appears normal. Moreover, the cancer cells of some cholangiocarcinomas can infiltrate along the submucosa so that the mucosa of the biliary tract may appear normal. Consequently, limits exist in diagnosing cholangiocarcinoma using cholangioscopy alone. Here, we review the literature, and present the cholangioscopic findings of malignant and benign strictures.

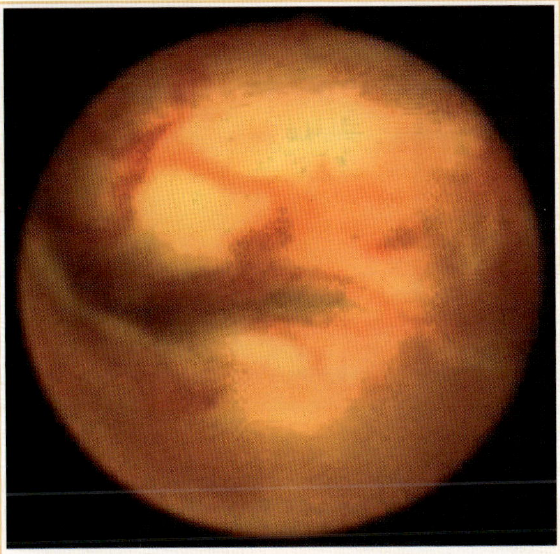

Fig. 11 Cholangioscopic imaging of malignant stricture
Cholangioscopy shows irregularly dilated, tortuous vessels and irregular surface of obstructing bile duct.

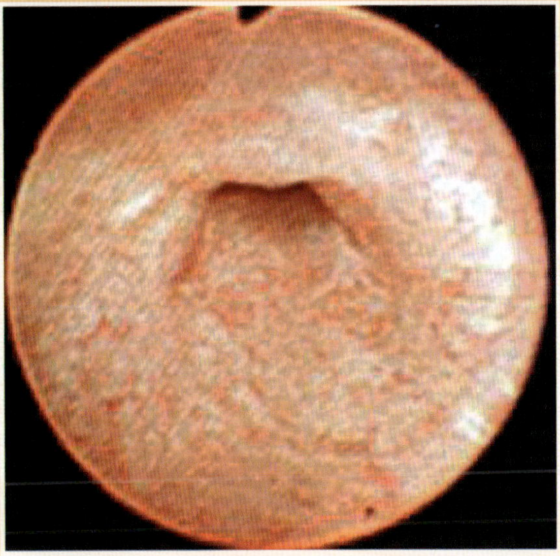

Fig. 12 Cholangioscopic imaging of benign stricture
Cholangioscopy shows smooth mucosal surface without neovascularization

At cholangioscopy, a malignant stricture contains irregularly dilated, tortuous tumor vessels (Fig. 11), oozes readily, and has an irregular surface.[21,22] In contrast, a benign stricture (Fig. 12) has a smooth surface mucosa without definite neovascularization, and lower homogenous papillogranular mucosa without a primary mass. Using peroral cholangioscopy, cholangiocarcinoma can be classified into nodular, papillary, and infiltrative types.

The nodular type consists of a nodular mass that compresses the intraluminal space of the biliary tract. A nodular mass bulging from one side of the biliary tract wall is characteristically found as a narrowed lumen skewed to one side. This can be observed more clearly with cholangiography than with cholangioscopy because cholangioscopy shows only the side of the mass that caused the obstruction, while cholangiography clearly shows both sides of the mass, as well as its shape. Marked neovascularization often occurs on the irregular mucosal surface of a nodular mass, and these abnormal vessels are called tumor vessels. The neovascularization facilitates the rapid growth of tumor cells. The vessels are usually irregular and observed as tortuous vessels on the surface of tumor, while the vascular structure of the normal

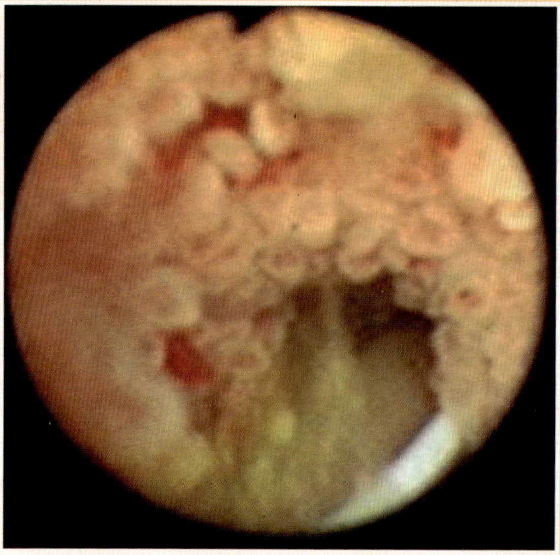

Fig. 13 Papillary type of cholangiocarcinoma.
Cholangioscopy shows irregular, serrated papillary mucosal surface.

biliary tract is not seen, and radial vessels cover or surround the bulging mass. In comparison to the infiltrative type, in most cases, the area of infiltration is limited.

The papillary type (Fig. 13) is observed as numerous papillary mucosal processes and appears as a superficial spreading lesion. These lesions are larger than the nodular type. On cholangiography, the papillary type has an irregular, serrated margin on the biliary tract wall. The growth of the mucosa may induce obstruction, cholestasis, and recurrent cholangitis. Cholangioscopy shows a papillary mass with a mixture of abscesses and sludge. Cleaning the site with a saline solution is necessary to improve the cholangioscopic view and to identify the papillary mass. The degree of papillary growth varies markedly, and definite papillary tumors are typically found in papillary adenocarcinoma, while small papillary processes can be seen in papillary adenoma. For papillary adenocarcinoma, cholangioscopy is required for two reasons. First, it is difficult to determine the extent of the tumor with cholangiography alone due to sludge and cholelithiasis found in the biliary tract in papillary adenocarcinoma. Second, fine protruding processes are not observed well with cholangioscopy. Therefore, when a fine protruding lesion is observed separate from the main lesion, it should be checked with cholangioscopy to determine whether many other lesions are present in the biliary tract. Finally, the pathological observations can be confirmed with a biopsy obtained using cholangioscopy.

In the infiltrative type, no obvious mass is observed, and the tumor appears as a stricture of the smoothly narrowing lumen. In this kind of adenocarcinoma, the cancer cells spread into the submucosa, and changes in the mucosal vessels are not obvious, while the neovascularization of the superficial layer is not as remarkable as in the nodular type. Nevertheless, the mucosa appears whiter, and minimal protrusion may be observed at the margin of the tumor vessels. The change in mucosa color is related to the spread of the cancer cells into the submucosa. This form of adenocarcinoma can infiltrate deep into the biliary tract and is difficult to differentiate from a benign stricture clinically, as a benign stricture also shows smooth narrowing and does not show tortuous neovascularization. For the differential diagnosis, the size of the stricture and changes in the surrounding biliary tract are important. When the expansion does not get progressively more severe, as in the diffuse type, but shows varying amounts of scarring, contracture, irregularity, and changes in lumen size, it suggests a benign stricture.

The differential diagnosis includes biliary papillomatosis, mucin-hypersecreting cholangiocarcinoma, biliary cystadenocarcinoma, and biliary papillomatosis, which is similar to papillary cholangiocarcinoma, except that multiple lesions occur on normal mucosa. A mucin-hypersecreting cholangiocarcinoma is similar to a papillary cholangiocarcinoma, except the biliary tract is dilated and filled with mucus.

4) Diagnostic accuracy in cholangiocarcinoma

In 1989, based on the observation of tumor neovascularization, a dense papillary pattern, and friable nodularity on cholangioscopy, the reported diagnostic accuracy for distinguishing benign and malignant strictures was 95%.[23] In a study of 97 patients examining whether oral cholangioscopy was effective in improving the low sensitivity of ERC and tissue sampling for diagnosing cholangiocarcinoma, ERC and tissue sampling had an accuracy of 78.0%, sensitivity of 57.9%, and specificity of 100%.[24] The addition of oral cholangioscopy, however, gave an accuracy of 93.4%, sensitivity of 100%, and specificity of 86.8%, leading to the conclusion that peroral cholangioscopy increased the diagnosis rate.[24] In that report, peroral cholangioscopy actually reduced the specificity because it indicated irregularly dilated, tortuous vessels, easy oozing, and an irregular surface in five patients, which led to a diagnosis of chronic pancreatitis in two patients and primary sclerosing cholangitis, autoimmune pancreatitis, and a peribiliary cyst in one patient each. Therefore, on peroral cholangioscopy, inflammatory benign biliary tract disease can give findings similar to cholangiocarcinoma during the active period.

5) Future prospects

The current problems with peroral cholangioscopy are the fragile scope, need for two different light sources, limited flexion of the tip, small instrument channel, and limited size of the biopsy specimens. As limitations exist regarding the maneuverability of the scope, performing a targeted biopsy using peroral cholangioscopy is often difficult. A future peroral cholangioscope with a large instrument channel related to suction apparatus and a built-in balloon to increase the image resolution will be helpful in diagnosing biliary tract disease, including cholangiocarcinoma.

Reference

1. Gores GJ. Cholangiocarcinoma: current concepts and insights. Hepatology 2003;37: 961-969.
2. Shaib Y, El-Serag HB. The epidemiology of cholangiocarcinoma. Semin Liver Dis 2004; 24:115-125.
3. 2008 Disease statistical data from NHIC, Health Insurance Research Institute. Korea.
4. Lazaridis KN, Gores GJ. Cholangiocarcinoma. Gastroenterology 2005;128:1655-1667.
5. NIH state-of-the-science statement on endoscopic retrograde cholangiopancreatography (ERCP) for diagnosis and therapy. NIH Consens State Sci Statements 2002;19:1-26.
6. Liguory C, Canard JM. Tumours of the biliary system. Clin Gastroenterol 1983;12:269-295.
7. Park MS, Kim TK, Kim KW, Park SW, Lee JK, Kim JS, Lee JH, et al. Differentiation of

extrahepatic bile duct cholangiocarcinoma from benign stricture: findings at MRCP versus ERCP. Radiology 2004;233:234-240.

8. Kim MJ, Mitchell DG, Ito K, Outwater EK. Biliary dilatation: differentiation of benign from malignant causes--value of adding conventional MR imaging to MR cholangiopancreatography. Radiology 2000;214:173-181.
9. Foutch, PG. Diagnosis of cancer by cytologic methods performed during ERCP. Gastrointest Endosc 1994; 40:249.
10. Khan SA, Davidson BR, Goldin R, Pereira SP, Rosenberg WM, Taylor-Robinson SD, Thillainayagam AV, et al. Guidelines for the diagnosis and treatment of cholangiocarcinoma: consensus document. Gut 2002;51 Suppl 6:VI 1-9.
11. Jailwala J, Fogel EL, Sherman S, Gottlieb K, Flueckiger J, Bucksot LG, Lehman GA. Triple-tissue sampling at ERCP in malignant biliary obstruction. Gastrointest Endosc 2000;51:383-390.
12. Gores GJ. Early detection and treatment of cholangiocarcinoma. Liver Transpl 2000;6: S30-34.
13. Kipp BR, Stadheim LM, Halling SA, Pochron NL, Harmsen S, Nagorney DM, Sebo TJ, et al. A comparison of routine cytology and fluorescence in situ hybridization for the detection of malignant bile duct strictures. Am J Gastroenterol 2004;99:1675-1681.
14. Baron TH, Harewood GC, Rumalla A, Pochron NL, Stadheim LM, Gores GJ, Therneau TM, et al. A prospective comparison of digital image analysis and routine cytology for the identification of malignancy in biliary tract strictures. Clin Gastroenterol Hepatol 2004; 2:214-219.
15. Levy MJ, Baron TH, Gostout CJ, Peterson BT, Farnell MB. Palliation of malignant extrahepatic biliary obstruction with plastic versus expandable metal stents: An evidence-based approach. Clin Gastroenterol Hepatol 2004;2:273-285.
16. De Palma GD, Galloro G, Siciliano S, Iovino P, Catanzano C. Unilateral versus bilateral endoscopic hepatic duct drainage in patients with malignant hilar biliary obstruction: results of a prospective, randomized, and controlled study. Gastrointest Endosc 2001; 53: 547-553.
17. Baillie J, Paulson EK, Vitellas KM. Biliary imaging: a review. Gastroenterology 2003; 124: 1686-1699.
18. Ponchon T, Valette PJ, Bory R, Bret PM, Bretagnolle M, Chavaillon A. Evaluation of a combined percutaneous-endoscopic procedure for the treatment of choledocholithiasis and benign papillary stenosis. Endoscopy 1987;19:164-166.
19. Pitt HA, Venbrux AC, Coleman J, Prescott CA, Johnson MS, Osterman FA, Jr., Cameron JL. Intrahepatic stones. The transhepatic team approach. Ann Surg 1994;219:527-535; discussion 535-527.
20. Shim CS, Neuhaus N, Tamada K. Direct Cholangioscopy. Endoscopy 2003;35:752-758

21. Seo DW, Lee SK, Yoo KS, Kang GH, Kim MH, Suh DJ, Min YI. Cholangioscopic findings in bile duct tumors. Gastrointest Endosc 2000;52:630-634.

22. Nimura Y. Staging of biliary carcinoma: cholangiography and cholangioscopy. Endoscopy 1993;25:76-80.

23. Nimura Y, Kamiya J, Hayakawa N, Shionoya S. Cholangioscopic differentiation of biliary strictures and polyps. Endoscopy 1989;21 Suppl 1:351-356.

24. Fukuda Y, Tsuyuguchi T, Sakai Y, Tsuchiya S, Saisyo H. Diagnostic utility of peroral cholangioscopy for various bile-duct lesions. Gastrointest Endosc 2005;62:374-382.

3. Percutaneous Transhepatic Cholangio-Scopy (PTCS)

A cholangioscope can be introduced into the biliary tree via several routes. The first approach is peroral insertion of cholangioscope via esophagus, the stomach, the duodenum and finally into the bile duct. The motherscope and babyscope are commonly used for this approach. The second approach is percutaneous transhepatic insertion of cholangioscope. The third approach is the use of the postoperative T-tube tract. The fourth approach is percutaneous transhepatic insertion of cholangioscope into the gallbladder directly. Other approaches such as intraoperative cholangioscopy or transpapillary cholecystoscopy are also tried.

1) Techniques of PTCS

Percutaneous transhepatic cholangioscopy is commonly used in Southeast Asian countries where intrahepatic stones are prevalent. This technique needs a newly made percutaneous transhepatic tract and the tract made for percutaneous transhepatic biliary drainage can be used for this purpose. In general, three steps are required for PTCS; percutaneous transhepatic biliary drainage, dilation of the tract, and cholangioscopic examination.

(1) Percutaneous transhepatic biliary drainage (PTBD) & tract dilation

The technique, PTBD has been usually used to relieve obstructive jaundice, drain infected bile, and to prevent or control cholangitis and sepsis. This technique can be an initial step for creating a percutaneous tract. PTBD can be performed under fluoroscopic or ultrasonographic guidance. For PTCS, the site of PTBD is very important. If the puncture site of PTBD to drain intrahepatic duct is inadequate, there can be an acute angulation during the course to the target lesion. Acute angulation is an important factor causing PTCS failure. Before selection of a PTBD site, cholangioscopist or interventional radiologist should be familiar with the anatomy of the biliary tree. The ideal PTBD site can be selected after meticulous review of several imaging studies such as ultrasonography, CT scan, endoscopic retrograde

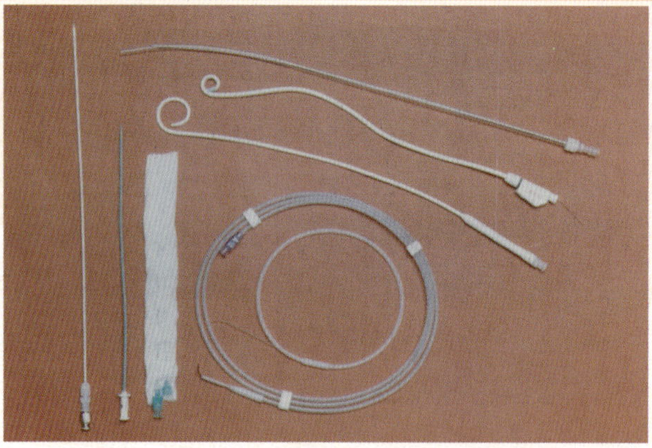

Fig. 1 PTBD kit. A set of intrument for PTBD includes Chiba needles for puncture, a guidewire, dilators and pigtail drainage cathters.

cholangiography or magnetic resonance cholangiography. A PTBD kit is composed of puncture needles, guides, a dilator and pigtail drainage tubes (Fig. 1). The usual diameter of initial PTBD tube is around 6~8 Fr. For initial puncture, peripheral duct selection is important because the insertion of PTBD tube into central duct carries significant risk of bleeding. Ultrasonography guided puncture or fluoroscopy guided puncture is commonly adopted method for initial peripheral duct selection. After selective puncture of a peripheral duct, a guidewire is inserted and a bougienage dilator is inserted over the guidewire. After dilation of the tract, a pigtail catheter can be introduced into the biliary tree. In cases with non-dilated intrahepatic duct, PTBD can be a risky procedure. To prevent several complications, the insertion of a endoscopic nasobiliary drainage tube and cholangiography using this tube are helpful for accurate targeting of intrahepatic duct.

For cholangioscopic examination of biliary tree, the diameter of percutaneous transhepatic tract should be larger than that of cholangioscope. The diameter of cholangioscope varies around 3.0~5.2 mm. Therefore the diameter of the percutaneous tract should be dilated at least up to 11~12 Fr when 11 Fr cholangioscope is considered to use. In the centers where 16 Fr cholangioscope is used, the tract should be dilated up to 16~18 Fr.

(2) Percutaneous transhepatic cholangioscopic examination

After full dilation of percutaneous transhepatic tract, seven to 10 days are usually required for the maturation of the sinus tract. Cholangioscopic examination can be performed after complete maturation of sufficiently dilated percutaneous transhepatic tract (Fig. 2). Premedication is required to relieve pain and anxiety. Meperidine is used for pain control and midazolam or diazepam can be used for

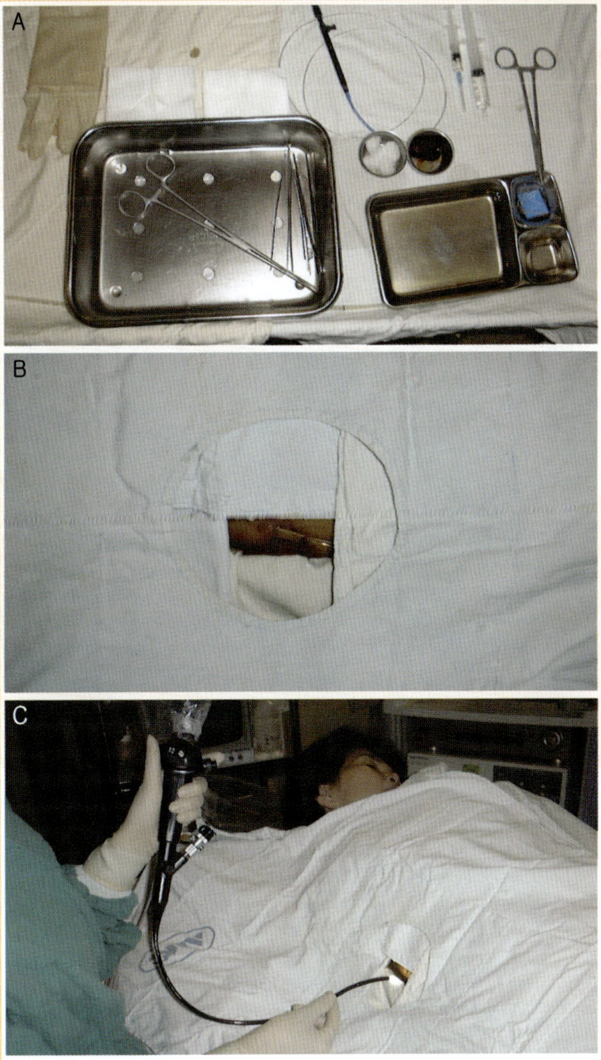

Fig. 2 Percutaneous transhepatic cholangioscopic examination.

A: Dressing set for PTCS. B: Draping was done before cholangioscopic examination. An 18 Fr PTCS catheter is visible and the tube is tied to skin to prevent migration. C: Checking of light source and saline irrigation before insertion of the cholangioscope into the body.

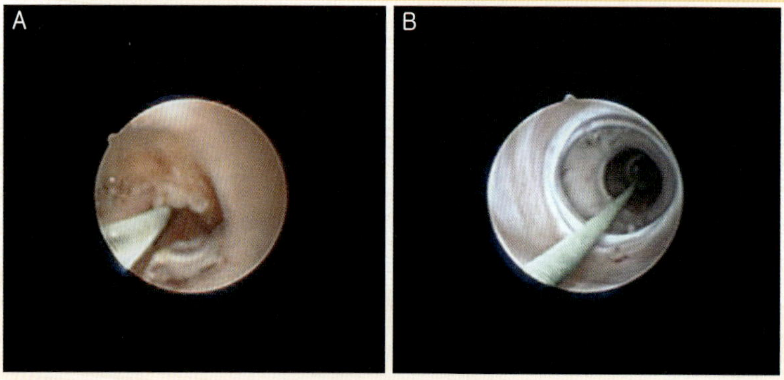

Fig. 3 A guidewire guidance into biliary tree.

At the first examination, the tract may not be maturated fully and there is a possibility of sinus tract collapse after removal of dilation tube. In order not to lose the tract, it is safe to insert a guidewire into the bile duct before removal of dilation tube. This guidewire helps to trace the collapsed tract.

anxiolysis and conscious sedation.The insertion of cholangioscope into fully dilated tract is not difficult. However, if the waiting period between the tract dilation and cholangioscopic examination is short, the insertion of cholangioscope can be difficult or sometimes traumatic. The tract may be collapsed after removal of dilation tube, especially at the first cholangioscopic examination. To guide smooth insertion of cholangioscope into the biliary tree, a guidewire which is inserted before removal of dilation tube can be used (Fig. 3). In the patient with severe jaundice, the maturation time should be long enough to obtain the complete epithelialization of the sinus tract. The free space between parietal peritoneum and liver capsule should be sealed off before cholangioscopic examination. In the patient with jaundice, the maturation time is rather slow and there is a risk of erroneous insertion of cholangioscope into peritoneal cavity through the afore mentioned free space. Bile leakage can occur through this space and bile peritonitis can develop as a possible complication.

When compared to other routes, percutaneous transhepatic cholangioscopy has several advantages. This approach enables us to evaluate both intrahepatic ducts and common bile duct and it is the shortest distance approach to the biliary tree (Fig. 4). The angulation maneuver of the tip of instrument and handling is easier than that of peroral cholangioscopy. The application of various techniques such as biopsy, suction

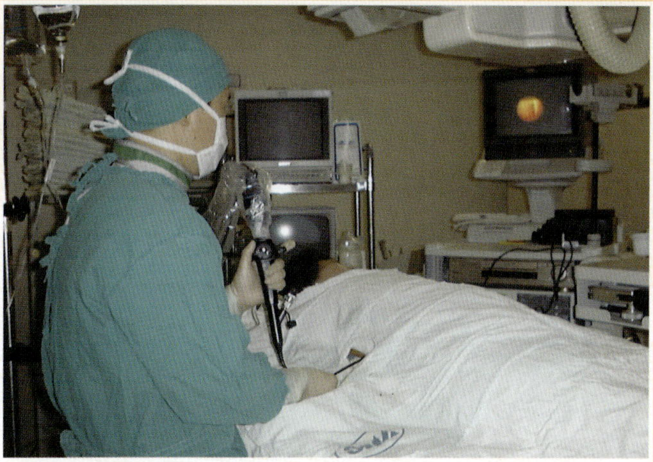

Fig. 4 Location of cholangioscopic video moniter and fluoroscopic moniter.

These two moniter should be located on the opposite side of the cholangioscopists and assistant so as to see the two monitor simultaneously without excessive head turning.

or dye spraying during cholangioscopic examination is not so difficult. Insertions of a balloon or a catheter under cholangioscopic guidance or application of biopsy forceps or electrohydraulic lithotripsy are much easier than peroral approach.

During cholangioscopic evaluation of biliary tree, irrigation is required to get the better view of the bile duct. In the biliary tree, pus, sludges or oozed blood can cause blurring of vision. Sometimes thick bile may prevent us from meticulous examination of the bile duct wall. To get a clear view of bile duct, continuous saline irrigation is recommended, and this is usually achieved by hanging a bottle of normal saline and letting the saline flow continuously into the instrumental channel of cholangioscope washing the bile duct.

2) Cholangioscopic findings of bile duct tumors

With the improvement of the skills of cholangioscopists, along with the development of newer instruments, more and more cholangioscopic examinations are performed to make the differentiation of benign and malignant lesions of the bile duct and for the evaluation of their extents.[1,2] There are several types of neoplasms within the bile duct. In this chapter, their typical cholangioscopic findings and characteristics according to their histology will be discussed.

(1) Bile duct adenoma

Benign bile duct tumors are quite rare. There are only several anecdotal reports in the literature.[3] Bile duct adenoma can be categorized into simple adenoma, tubular adenoma, or papillary adenoma, so called papilloma. Papillary adenoma or papilloma is more frequently observed than tubular adenoma. Papillary adenoma can be characterized by multiple papillary mucosal projections (Fig. 5). This lesion can occur with multiple mucosal projections at a single site or at multifocal sites. If it is noted at multifocal areas of the biliary tree, the diagnosis of biliary papillomatosis can be made. Papillary mucosal projections can be the cause of bile duct obstruction, bile stasis, and recurrent cholangitis. Upon cholangio-scopic examination, a lot of sludge material can be identified covering the papillary mass or between the papillary projections. Water irrigation is required to have a clear cholangio-scopic view to identify the papillary projections.

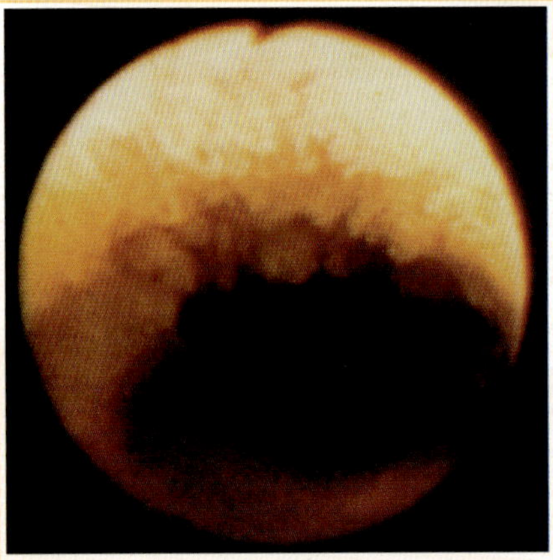

Fig. 5 Papillary adenoma.

A papillary adenoma or papilloma shows characteristic papillary mucosal projections upon cholangioscopic examination. These are superficial lesions and sometimes show multifocal lesions.

(2) Bile duct adenocarcinoma

Bile duct adenocarcinoma is the most common biliary malignancy. Based on cholangioscopic findings, bile duct adenocarcioma can be classified into three different types: nodular, papillary, and infiltrative.[4] Other types of bile duct adenocarcinoma, such as the nodular-infiltrative type or the papillo-infiltrative type, have also been described in the literature. However, these classifications can be confusing because the differential points are sometimes obscure and based on cholangiographic findings, not on cholangioscopic findings. Upon cholangioscopic examinations, the aforementioned three types show their unique appearances and can be easily differentiated.

a. Nodular type

In the nodular type, cholangioscopic examination reveals a nodular mass with luminal obstruction (Fig. 6). The nodular mass protrudes from one side of the bile duct wall; the luminal aperture is usually located eccentrically. The entire nodular mass can be identified more clearly by cholangiography than cholangioscopy. This is because the percutaneous cholangioscopic view shows only the upper side of the obstructing mass, while cholangio-graphy can

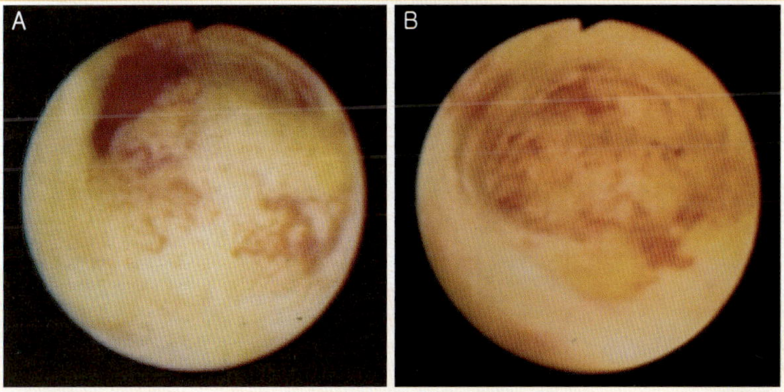

Fig. 6 Nodular tumor.
The typical cholangioscopic findings of nodular tumors are a nodular obstructing mass, surface neovascularization, eccentrically located luminal aperture.

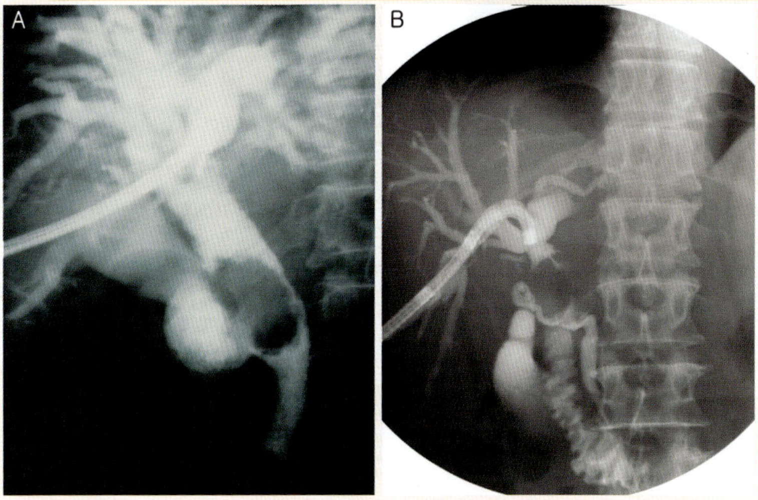

Fig. 7 Cholangiogram of nodular tumor.
A nodular tumor reveals a nodular filling defect upon cholangiography and the involved segment is usually short.

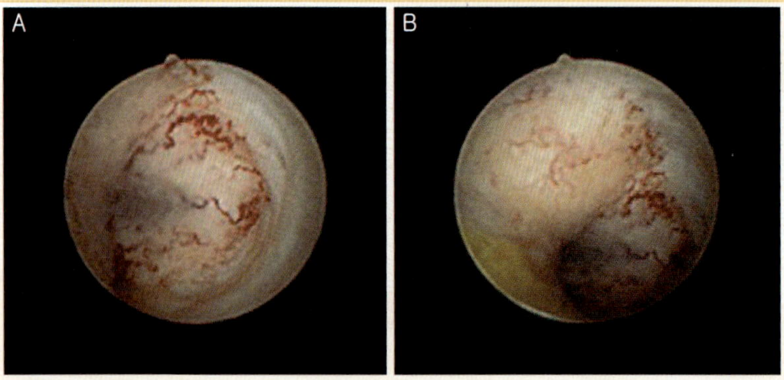

Fig. 8 Characteristic neovascularization on the surface of a nodular tumor.

A serpigenous tumor vessel is visible on the mucosal surface of a nodular tumor. The tumor cell shows rapid proliferation and neovascularization seems to be required to supply nutrients for rapidly growing tissue. These neovacularizations are characterized by irregular tortuosity.

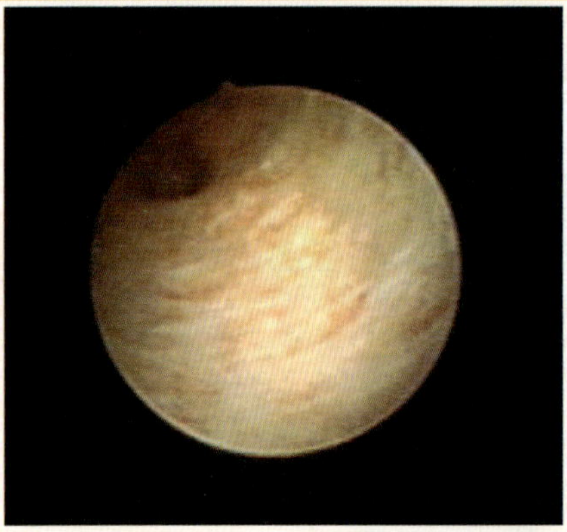

Fig. 9 Vasculature of the normal common bile duct.

Normal bile duct wall does not show prominent vasculature and the vascular network is faintly visible only when the cholangioscope is closely attached to the bile duct wall. The normal vasculature of a common bile duct shows sharp networking and a branching pattern. The course is rather straight, unlike a tumor vessel.

delineate the upper and lower side of the mass, which shows the nodular contour more clearly (Fig. 7).

A nodular tumor usually shows an irregular mucosal surface and marked neovascularization (Fig. 8). These abnormal vessels are called "tumor vessels". These neovascularizations seem to supply nutrients to the rapidly proliferating tumor cells. When compared to an infiltrative type tumor, the extent of a nodular tumor is usually limited to a short segment.

The characteristics of neovascularization are tortuous, irregular, serpiginous, and usually it does not show the networking pattern of the normal vasculature of a bile duct (Fig. 9). Instead, it shows a radially projecting pattern that surrounds or covers the elevated nodular tumor.

b. Papillary type

Papillary type bile duct cancer is characterized by multiple papillary mucosal projections (Fig. 10). This type of tumor shows a superficial spreading pattern, and the extent of the tumor is usually larger than that of a nodular tumor. Upon cholangiography, papillary type shows an irregular, serrated border of bile duct wall (Fig. 11). The papillary projections cause an obstruction to bile flow. And upon cholangioscopic examination, a large amount of sludge material, intermingled with pus, is frequently observed (Fig. 12). The height of the papillary projections can vary. A prominent papillary tumor is usually

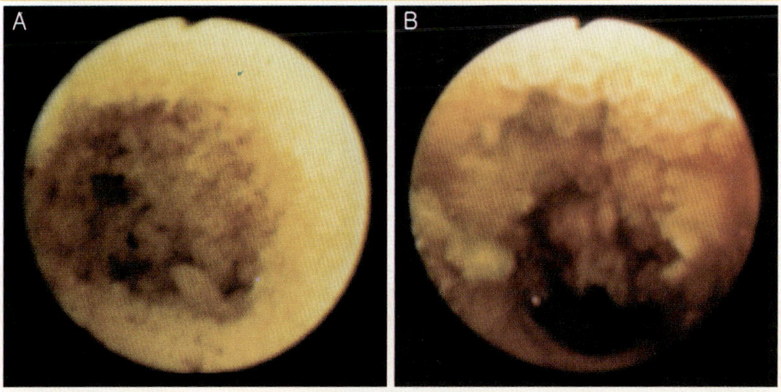

Fig. 10 Papillary adenocarcinoma.

A, B: The cholangioscopic characteristics of papillary adenocarcinoma are the numerous intraluminal papillary projections and the variable height of the papillary lesions.

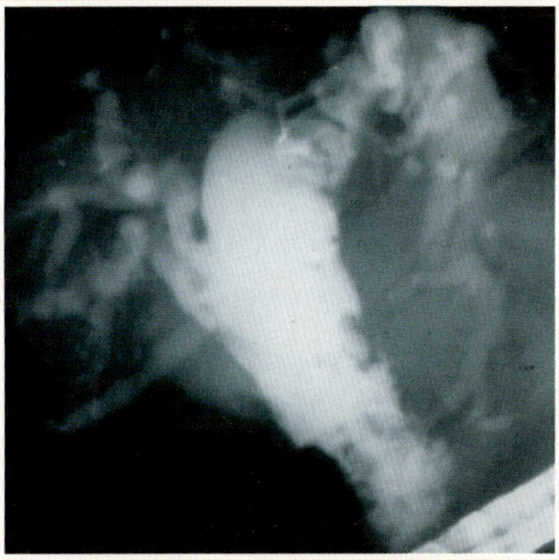

Fig. 11 Cholangiographic characteristics of papillary adenocarcinoma.

Upon cholangiography, papillary adenocarcinoma shows an irregular, serrated border of the bile duct wall or a ragged appearance. These changes seem to be caused by numerous papillary mucosal lesions and/or sludge material.sometimes show multifocal lesions.

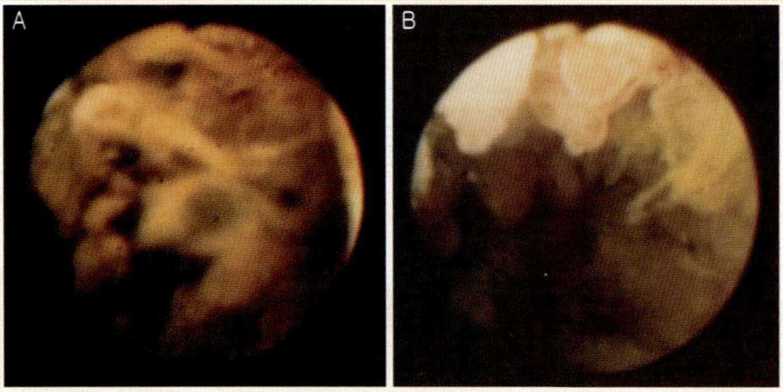

Fig. 12
A: Papillary adenocarcinoma covered with sludge materials and pus. Another case of papillary adenocarcinoma shows a large amount of sludge materials intermingled with pus. B: To get a clear view of mucosal changes, saline irrigations are frequently required. After saline irrigation, papillary tumors are visible on the upper part of the figure.

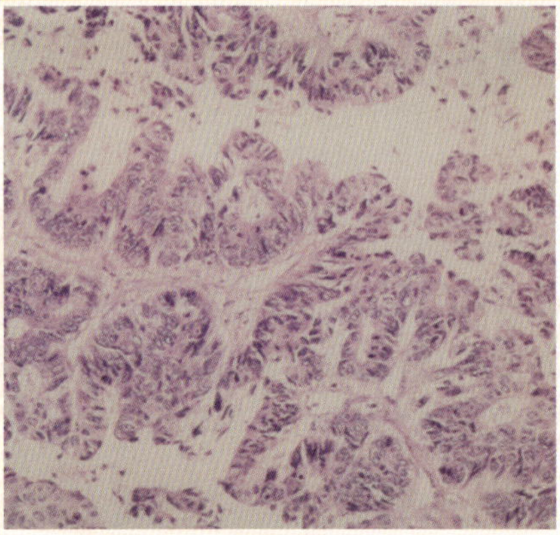

Fig. 13 Pathology of papillary adenocarcarcinoma.
A histologic examination of a papillary tumor shows multiple papillary mucosal changes, and cellular atypism, nuclear hyperchromatism, and stratification of the cell layer compartible with papillary adenocarcinoma.

identified in the region of a papillary adenocarcinoma (Fig. 13), while tiny villous projections are noted in the region of a papillary adenoma. For patients with papillary adenocarcinoma, a cholangioscopic examination is an indispensible procedure for several reasons. First, cholangiography alone is not usually sufficient to determine the extent of tumor. There can be a lot of sludge materials, pus or small stones in the biliary tree of patients with papillary tumors. These materials can erroneously appear on a cholangiogram as multiple filling defects. Second, the area of tiny villous projections are not clearly identifiable by cholangiography (Fig. 14, 15). As these tiny lesions can be noted unexpectedly at a site distant from the main lesion, cholangioscopic evaluation of the entire right and left biliary tree is required for the detection of multicentric occurrence.[5,6] Third, cholangioscopic biopsy can reveal the clear pathologic nature of the lesion (Fig. 16).

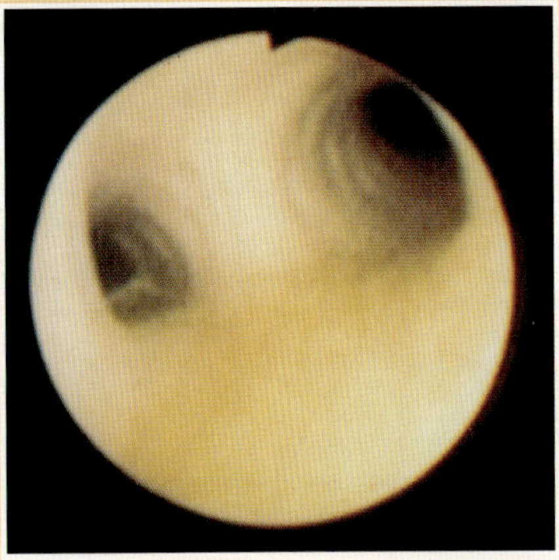

Fig. 14 Villous mucosal lesions.

A cholangioscopic examination of a papillary adenocarcinoma sometimes reveals minute villous mucosal changes. These villous changes usually correspond to adenoma instead of carcinoma.

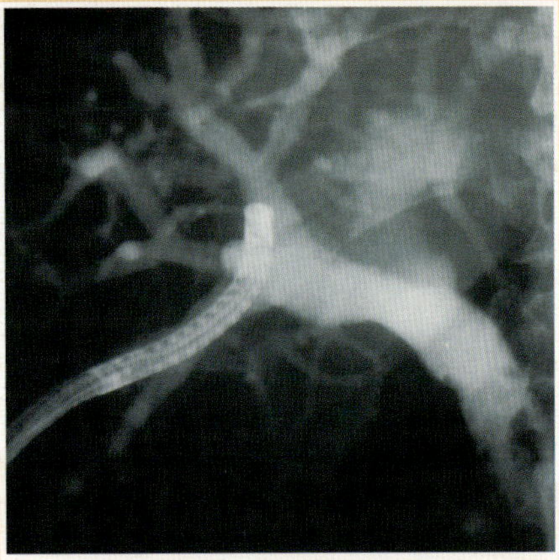

Fig. 15 A cholangiogram of the corresponding cholangioscopic area of villous mucosal changes.

The cholangioscopic examination in Fig. 13 clearly showed villous mucosal changes. However, these changes are hardly detectable with cholangiography.

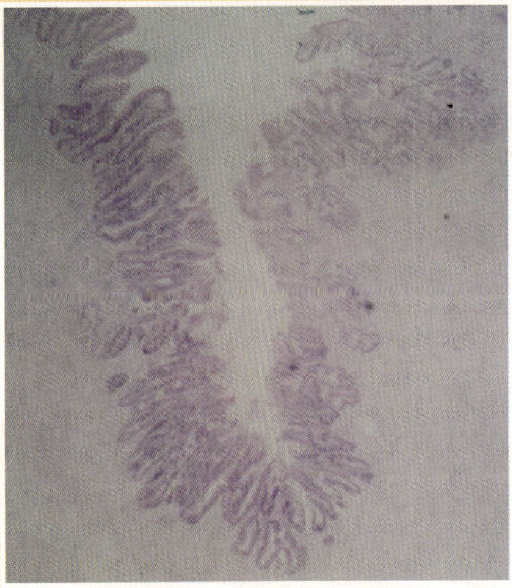

Fig. 16 Histological findings of villous projection.

C. Infiltrative type

In this type of tumor, the definite mucosal mass is not clearly visible and a smooth-tapered, luminal narrowing is present (Fig. 17). The mucosal change is not so prominent because this type of tumor shows intramural spreading pattern. The surface neovascularization is less conspicuous than a nodular tumor (Fig. 18), but whitish mucosal discoloration and subtle elevation is visible on the margin of the tumor vessel. The whitish mucosal discoloration seems to be associated with the intramural spreading of the tumor (Fig. 19, 20). This type of tumor usually involves a long segment of the bile duct (Fig. 21).

The problem of this type tumor is the difficulty of making a differential diagnosis from a benign stricture. A benign bile duct stricture also shows a

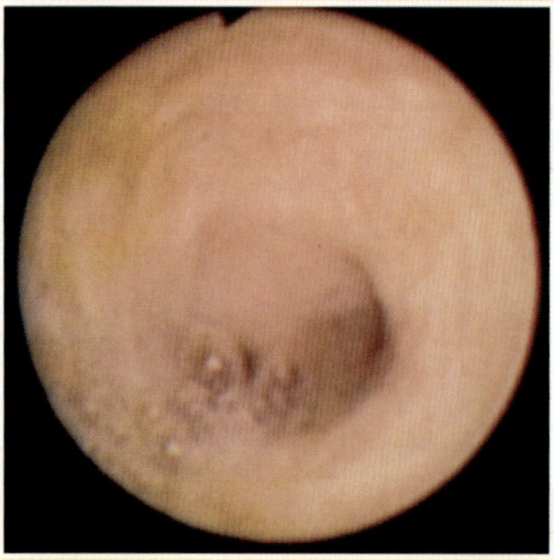

Fig. 17 Infiltrative type tumor.

This type of tumor shows a smooth tapered, luminal narrowing, and the surface mucosal change is not prominent.

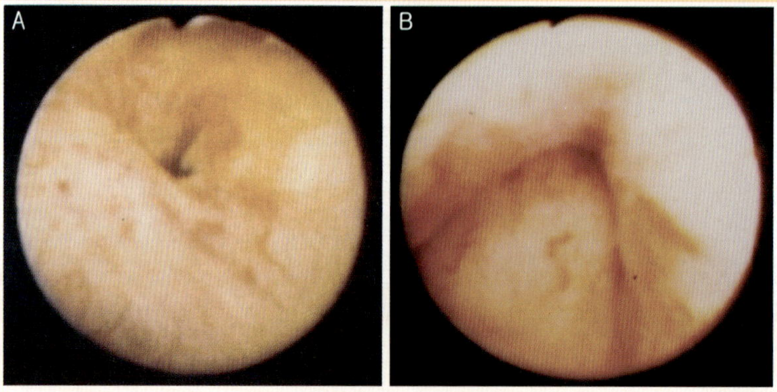

Fig. 18 Tumor vessel of infiltrative type tumor.

A, B: An infiltrative type tumor can reveal irregular surface neovascularizations. However, this change is not so prominent when compared to that of nodular tumors and is usually identifiable only in the close-up view.

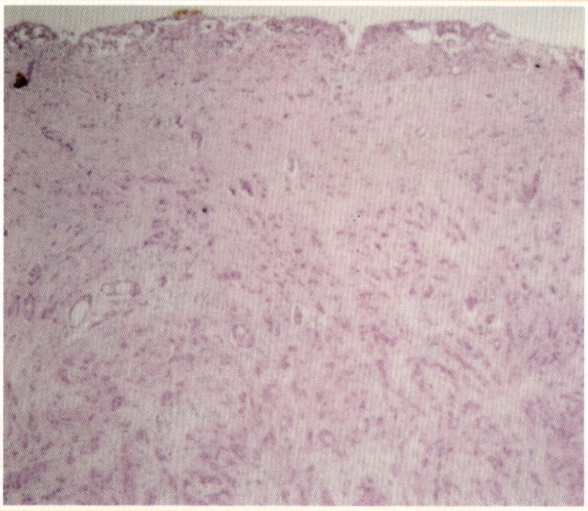

Fig. 19 Mucosal surface change in infiltrative type tumor.

The cancer cells are mainly located in the intramural submucosal layer. The surface epithelial layer is denuded and has mild dysplastic changes. Therefore, in this type of tumor, it is very difficult to get a sufficient amount of cancer cells by cholangioscopic biopsy.

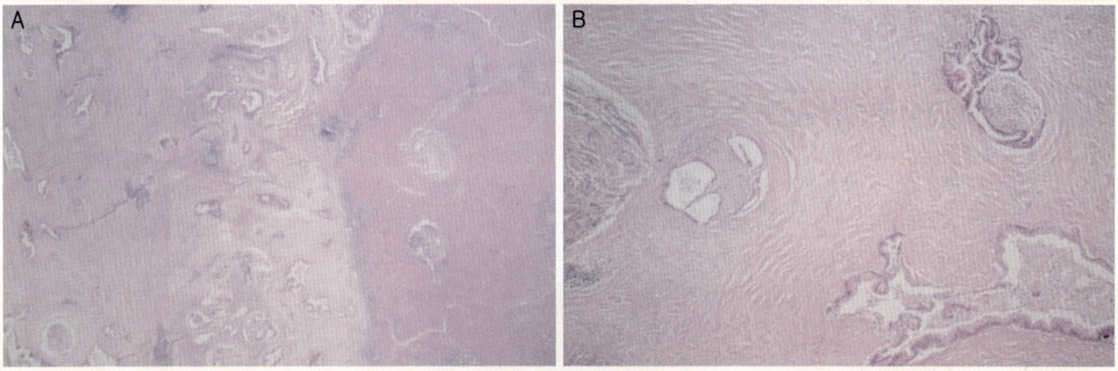

Fig. 20 Pathology of infiltrative type cancer.

A, B: Poorly differentiated adenocarcinoma cells are interspersed between fibrous tissue, and the cancer cells do not show clustering.

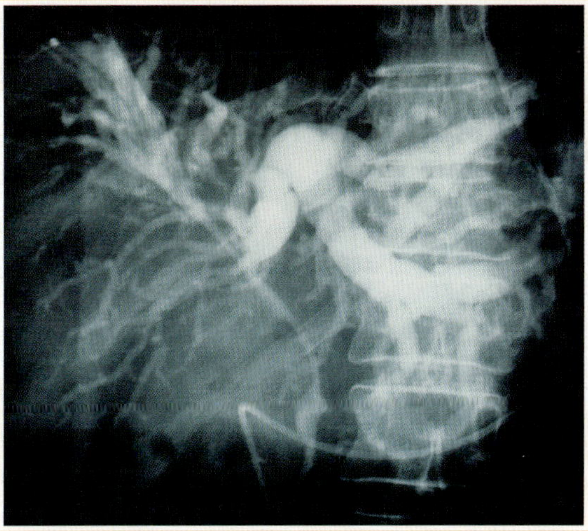

Fig. 21 Cholangiogram of infiltrative type tumor.

The characteristic cholangiographic findings of an infiltrative type tumor are a long segment luminal narrowing without irregularity of ductal margin.

smooth tapered narrowing, but surface neovascularization is usually not visible. For a differential diagnosis, not only the stricture segment, but also surrounding ductal changes are important. Scar contractures, angulations, or various shapes of luminal caliber changes, instead of diffuse proportional dilation or narrowing, favor a benign bile duct stricture.

(3) Biliary papillomatosis

Biliary papillomatosis is characterized by multicentric papillary tumors in the biliary tract.[7] A diagnosis of this entity can be made based on the following histological criteria: macroscopically, multifocal papillary growing tumors in the extrahepatic bile duct, with or without intrahepatic bile duct involvements (Fig. 22), and microscopically, branching papillary fronds, covered by columnar epithelium and supported by delicate fibrovascular stalks (Fig. 23). Biliary papillomatosis is a

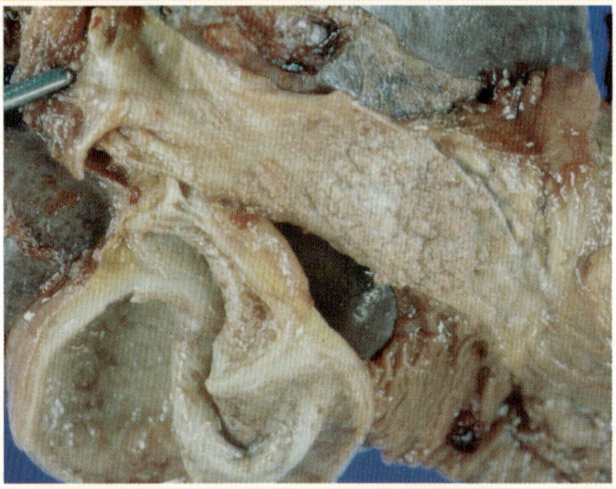

Fig. 22 Resected specimen of biliary papillomatosis.

A gross finding shows multiple, small, round or slightly ovoid-shaped tumors in the extrahepatic bile duct (small arrows), and small tiny lesions in the gallbladder (large arrows).

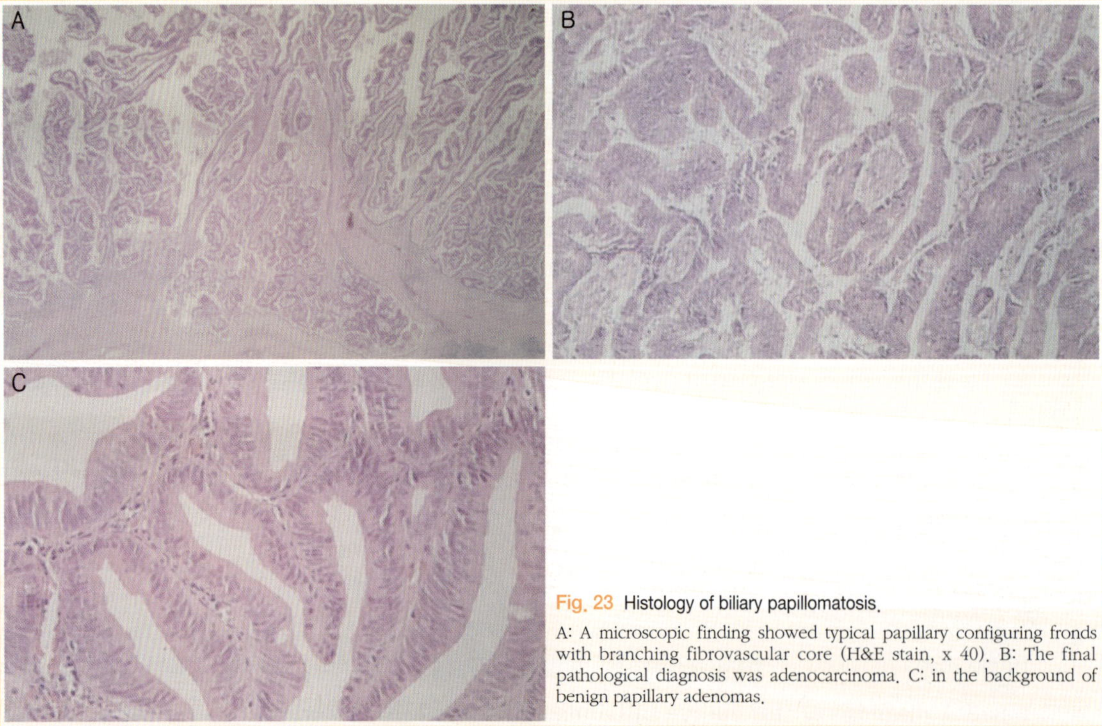

Fig. 23 Histology of biliary papillomatosis.

A: A microscopic finding showed typical papillary configuring fronds with branching fibrovascular core (H&E stain, x 40). B: The final pathological diagnosis was adenocarcinoma. C: in the background of benign papillary adenomas.

collection of benign papillary adenomas. However, these lesions can be transformed into papillary adenocarcinoma. Radiologic and cholangioscopic findings reflect these histological characteristics. Upon abdominal ultrasonography and computed axial tomography, dilatation of the extra- and/or intrahepatic bile duct are the most common findings (Fig. 24). Thickening of the bile duct wall can also be seen. Cholangiographic findings are multiple, round-to-ovoid filling defects in the dilated ducts, and ragged irregularity of the bile duct wall (Fig. 25). A cholangioscopic examination of biliary papillomatosis shows multiple or numerous papillary masses in the biliary tree (Fig. 26). The masses are soft and friable, and the surface color is

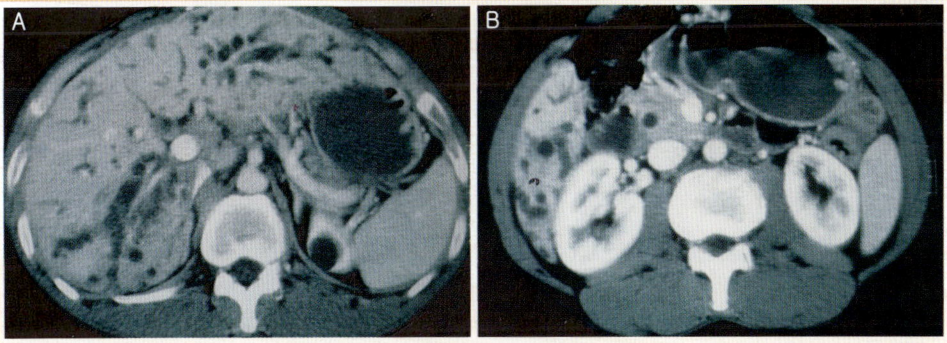

Fig. 24 CT finding of biliary papillomatosis.

This patient shows diffuse dilation of the intrahepatic duct (A) and the extrahepatic ducts (B). The extrahepatic bile duct wall is mildly thickened, but no definite mass obstructing the bile duct is visible.

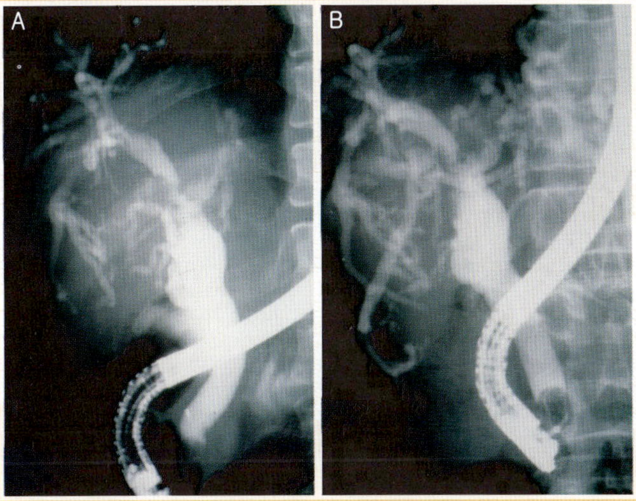

Fig. 25 Cholangiograms of biliary papillomatosis.

A: Endoscopic retrograde cholangiography shows multiple, small filling defects, and irregular luminal narrowing of the intrahepatic ducts. B: Balloon occlusion cholangiography shows serrated ductal wall in common hepatic duct and left intrahepatic duct (arrows) and these wall irregularities seems to be highly characteristic of papillary tumors.

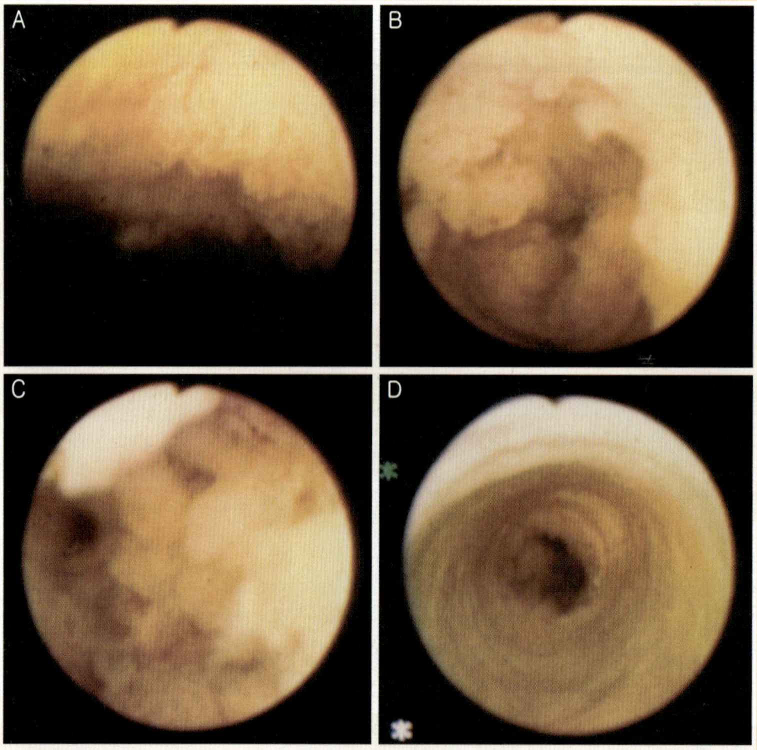

Fig. 26 Cholangioscopic findings of biliary papillomatosis.

A: A cholangioscopic examination of a common bile duct shows small papillary projections. These lesions were papillary adenoma. B: A distal common bile duct also shows relatively small sized papillary lesions. These lesions were also proved to be papillary adenoma upon cholangioscopic biopsy. C: A cholangioscopic examination of a left intrahepatic duct revealed numerous irregularly protruded papillary masses and the lumen were nearly obliterated. The papillary tumors were highly friable and easily detached from the bile duct wall. These papillary lesions were papillary adenocarcinoma. D: A mid-portion of the common bile duct. This area showed a normal smooth surface and papillary lesions were not visible.

usually bright yellow or pinkish. Since papillary lesions are multifocal in biliary papillomatosis, the normal intervening mucosa can be seen between lesions. Histologically, this normal looking area shows mild inflammatory changes. In the patient with biliary papillomatosis, the main papillary masses are usually located in the extrahepatic bile duct. However, the cholangioscopist should be careful about intrahepatic small or minute papillary lesions which are remote from the main extrahepatic tumors. A careful cholangioscopic examination is indispensable for the determination of the exact extent of the tumor and the type of surgery.[8]

(4) Mucin hypersecreting bile duct cancer

Mucin hypersecreting bile duct cancer is a rarely encountered entity and is similar to intraductal papillary mucinous neoplasm (IPMN) of the pancreas.[9,10] The fundamental similarity is a mucin over-producing property. This overproduced mucin is relatively viscous, and causes ductal obstruction and upstream duct dilatation (Fig. 27). Mucin hypersecreting bile duct cancer shows diffuse bile duct dilatation and mucinous ductal ectasia, similar to pancreatic duct ectasia in the patient with an IPMN (Fig. 28). Another similarity is the pathologic findings. Mucin hypersecreting bile duct cancer shows villous or papillary mucosal projections on histologic examination, as IPMN of the pancreas shows papillary or villous mucosal tumors. Mucin hypersecreting cancer causes frequent attacks of obstructive cholangitis by

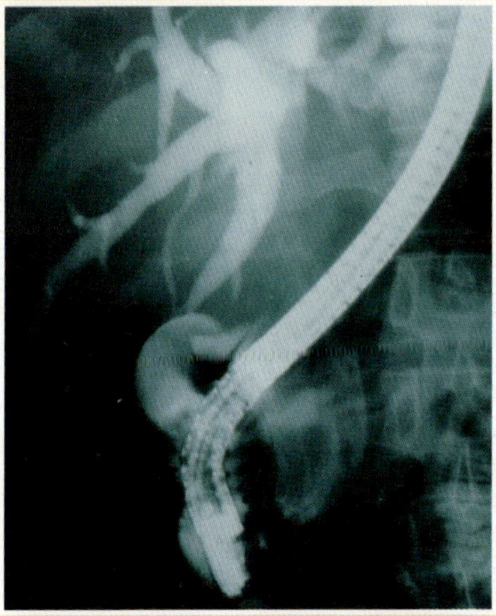

Fig. 27 A cholangiogram of mucin hypersecreting tumor.

An endoscopic retrograde cholangiography of mucin hypersecreting bile duct cancer shows diffuse biliary tree dilation and amorphous filling defect in the biliary tree. These ductectatic changes can be noted in the pancreatic duct of a patient with an intraductal papillary mucinous tumor. Downstream ductectasia is usually caused by mucin plugging. Amorphous filling defects are also caused by intraductal mucin.

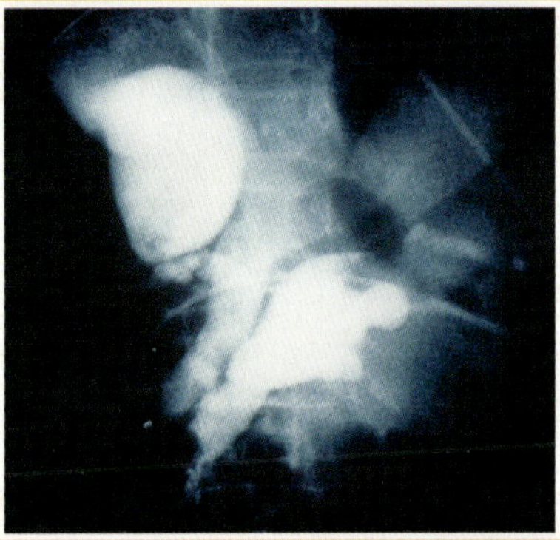

Fig. 28 A pancreatogram in a patient with intraductal papillary mucinous tumor.

The pancreatogram reveals a markedly dilated main pancreatic duct and amorphous filling defects within the dilated duct. Mucin and papillary mass can contribute to these ectatic changes.

mucus plugging; while IPMN frequently induces an obsturctive pancreatitis. The determination of the exact extent of the tumor by cholangiography or pancreatogaphy is quite difficult in both entities because mucin is also a cause of filling defects on cholangiography or pancreatography, thereby obsecuring the extent of the true tumor.[11,12]

During a cholangioscopic examination of mucin hypersecreting bile duct cancer, the cholangioscopist should be cautious not to overlook a minute mucosal tumor (Fig. 29). The bile duct is usually dilated and the intraductal mucin absorbs some fraction of the light that is emitted from the tip of cholangioscope, which results in a dark visual field . Therefore, it is not easy to detect tiny tumors or determine the extent of

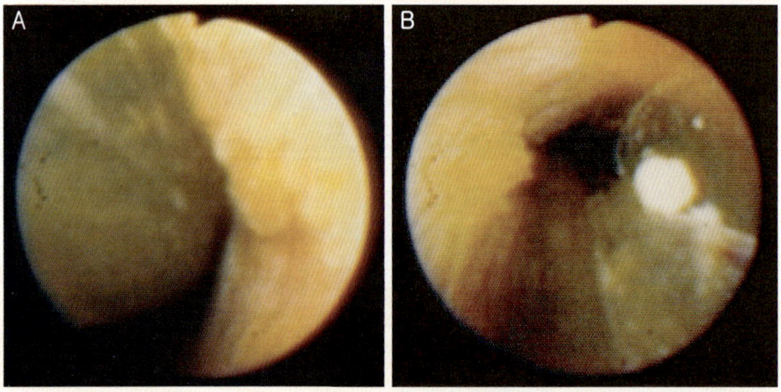

Fig. 29 Cholangioscopic findings of mucin hypersecreting cholangiocarcinoma.

Cholangioscopic examination of a mucin hypersecreting bile duct tumor can reveal various mucosal changes. This patient shows villous mucosal lesions and mucin in the dilated common bile duct.

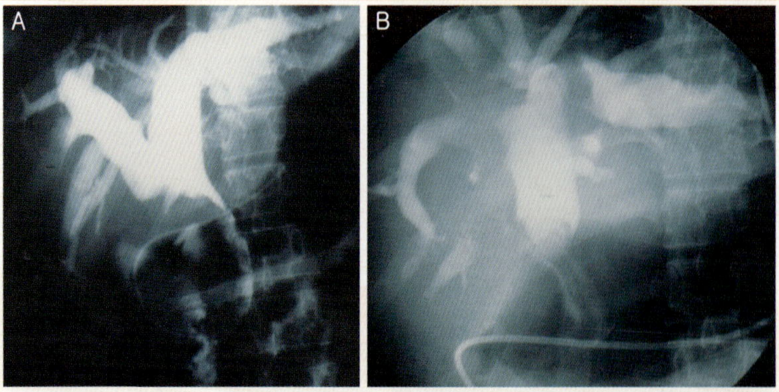

Fig. 30 The viscosity of mucin can be variable.

A: Rather round or elliptical filling defects are visible when the mucin is thick. B: However, when the mucin is thin, thread-like linear filling defects can be seen.

a tumor in the markedly dilated duct full of mucin. Sometimes, even tiny villous or papillary mucosal tumors can produce a massive amount of mucin. Mucin has variable viscosity. Thick mucin tends to cause round filling defects in a cholangiogram; while thin mucin causes thread-like, linear filling defects (Fig. 30). The cholangioscopic finding of mucin hypersecreting bile duct cancer can be either tiny, villous mucosal projections or papillary tumors in the wall of the bile duct. These mucosal lesions are usually highly friable and easily removed by biopsy forceps.

Reference

1. Nimura Y, Kamiya J, Hayakawa N, Shionoya S. Cholangioscopic differentiation of biliary strictures and polyps. Endoscopy 1989;21:351-6.
2. Nimura Y. Staging of biliary carcinoma: cholangiography and cholangioscopy. Endoscopy 1993;25:76-80.
3. Catteli RB, Braasch JW, Kahn F. Polypoid epithelial tumors of the bile ducts. N Engl J Med 1962;266:57-61.
4. Seo DW, Lee SK, Yoo KS, et al. Cholangioscopic findings in bile duct tumors. Gastrointest Endosc. 2000;52:630-4.
5. Seo DW, Kim MH, Lee SK, et al. Usefulness of cholangioscopy in patients with focal stricture of the intrahepatic duct unrelated to intrahepatic stones. Gastrointest Endosc. 1999;49:204-9.
6. Kim HJ, Kim MH, Lee SK, Yoo KS, Seo DW, Min YI. Tumor vessel: valuable cholangioscopic clue of malignant biliary stricture. Gastrointest Endosc. 2000;52:635-8.
7. Seo DW, Lee SK, Kim MH. Biliary papillomatosis. Gastrointest Endosc. 2000;51:67.
8. Kim YS, Myung SJ, Kim SY, et al. Biliary papillomatosis: clinical, cholangiographic and cholangioscopic findings. Endoscopy. 1998;30:763-7.
9. Park HJ, Seo DW, Lee SK, Kim MH. Mucin-hypersecreting cholangiocarcinoma. Gastrointest Endosc. 2000;52:526.
10. Kim HJ, Kim MH, Lee SK, et al. Mucin-hypersecreting bile duct tumor characterized by a striking homology with an intraductal papillary mucinous tumor (IPMT) of the pancreas. Endoscopy. 2000;32:389-93.
11. Sano T, Nimura Y, Hayakawa N, et al. Clinical utility of percutaneous transhepatic cholangioscopy in defining tumor extent: a case of mucin-producing bile duct carcinoma originating in the left caudate lobe. Gastrointest Endosc. 1997;46:455-8.
12. Joo YH, Kim MH, Lee SK, et al. A case of mucin-hypersecreting intrahepatic bile duct tumor associated with pancreatic intraductal papillary mucinous tumor. Gastrointest Endosc. 2000;52:409-12.

4. EUS, EUS-FNA & IDUS

Cholangiocarcinoma is an uncommon malignancy arising from the epithelial cells of the biliary tract. These tumors may arise anywhere along the extrahepatic or intrahepatic biliary tree. Patients with cholangiocarcinoma typically present at advanced stages, and cure rates are low, even with aggressive therapy.

The objectives of the radiologic evaluation of cholangiocarcinoma include the assessment of the level and extent of involvement of the biliary tree, the extent of local invasion including vascular involvement, the identification of hepatic lobe atrophy and hypertrophy, and the detection of local and distant metastasis. These objectives are often accomplished using a combination of complementary diagnostic and imaging modalities.

Endoscopic ultrasonography (EUS) is one of the most recent advances in gastrointestinal endoscopy. Available EUS devices include echoendoscopes, such as radial scanning and linear array echoendoscopes, and catheter ultrasound probes. Endoscopic ultrasonography has various applications, such as staging of gastrointestinal malignancy, evaluation of submucosal tumors, and has grown to be an important modality in evaluating the pancreaticobiliary system. With regard to the biliary system, EUS is useful for the detection and staging of ampullary tumors, detection of microlithiasis and choledocholithiasis and evaluation of benign and malignant bile-duct strictures.[1] EUS may be useful in the evaluation of cholangiocarcinoma and intraductal ultrasound (IDUS) within the bile duct may help differentiate malignant from benign strictures. EUS-guided fine needle aspiration can be helpful in the diagnosis of cholangiocarcinoma, especially in the region of the hilum.

1) Endoscopic Ultrasound

Because EUS reveals the extrahepatic bile ducts in almost all patients, it is the most reliable method for diagnosis of obstructive jaundice. Furthermore, EUS can be used in the differential diagnosis of bile duct masses and strictures.[2] However, the depth of field is limited so that the exploration of the hilum is generally not possible even though imaging has recently improved with the use of a lower frequency of 5 MHz.[3] EUS has proved as a gold standard in the exploration of extrahepatic obstructive jaundice due to its low morbidity and its accuracy.[4,5] Recently, other radiological examinations, such as multi-detector CT (MD-CT) and MRCP, are developed for the diagnosis of the biliary tract diseases. These procedures appear to have advantages because they are non-invasive and able to simultaneously depict the whole biliary tract, pancreatic duct, pancreas, and liver.[3] However, CT and MRCP are limited for the exploration of small lesions.[6,7] Therefore, EUS is still the best procedure for the diagnosis of biliary obstruction, as well as the most accurate when diagnosing extrahepatic obstruction and staging tumors.[2,8]

Although there has been less information published concerning the role of EUS for the detection and staging of cholangiocarcinomas than there has been for other gastrointestinal cancers, such as esophageal, gastric, or pancreatic cancers, it does appear to have a role in identifying and characterizing cholangiocarcinomas, especially for smaller tumors less than 2 cm in diameter.[9] The typical EUS image of a cholangiocarcinoma shows a round or fusiform hypoechoic area arising from or surrounding the bile duct wall (Fig. 1). Although EUS offer a precise diagnosis in the middle and distal segment of biliary tree, more proximal tumors may be difficult to detect due to limited penetration of the echoendoscope transducers. Therefore, MRCP and direct cholangiography, such as ERCP or PTC, are better than EUS in

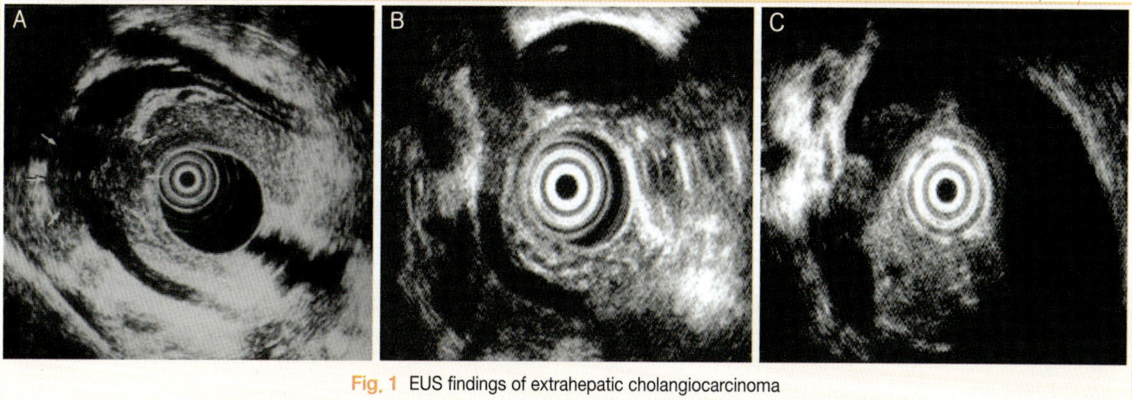

Fig. 1 EUS findings of extrahepatic cholangiocarcinoma

EUS images show round or fusiform hypoechoic area arising from bile duct wall.

the proximal cancers. In a prospective comparative study of ERCP or PTC, MRCP, CT, and EUS, 40 patients with biliary stricture underwent all four imaging tests, the specificity was improved when MRCP was combined with EUS.[10]

EUS staging of cholangiocarcinoma is based on the TNM system. Quilian et al.[11] evaluated the use of EUS for the preoperative assessment of 18 patients with extrahepatic cholangiocarcinomas. The overall accuracy of EUS for T stage was 72% and for N stage was 61%. Tio et al.[12] have conducted the largest volume of work on EUS for staging of proximal bile duct cancers. They found that the overall accuracy of EUS for T stage was 86% and for N stage was 64%. Regarding EUS T staging, overstaging occurs due to inflammation around the CBD and understaging occurs because of microscopic tumor invasion. Although the accuracy of T stage is excellent, the accuracy for lymph nodes is less impressive. The problems with lymph node diagnosis should be largely addressed by EUS-guided fine-needle aspiration biopsy, which has an overall accuracy of about 91%.[13]

2) EUS-guided FNA (fine needle aspiration)

Tissue sampling under EUS guidance should improve the diagnostic rate, depending of the origin of the stenosis. However, there is little information regarding the use of EUS-guided FNA in patients with bile duct massess or strictures.[1]

In a recent retrospective study, the diagnostic yield of EUS was improved by performing EUS-guided FNA, especially in patients with negative brush cytology findings.[14] However, only 3 out of 23 patients had lesions localized in the hilar bile duct. Hilar lesions are often small or diffusely infiltrating, and can therefore be difficult to detect.[1] Hilar cholangiocarcinomas that are unresectable because of anatomic factors and measure less than 3 cm in radial diameter may be amenable to liver transplantation if extrahepatic metastases have been excluded. In a retrospective case series of 47 patients with unresectable hilar cholangiocarcinoma, EUS identified lymph nodes in all patients, and confirmation of malignancy by FNA precluded liver transplantation in 17%.[15] In a single-center, retrospective study, EUS-guided FNA for tissue sampling of proximal biliary strictures after negative or nondiagnostic ERCP brush cytology had a positive predictive value of 100%, but a negative predictive value of 29%.[16] Routine use of EUS-guided FNA for this indication may decrease unnecessary surgical exploration, but the low negative predictive value limits the ability to exclude malignancy. EUS-guided FNA may aid the diagnosis of hilar cholangiocarcinoma when standard methods of tissue diagnosis are inconclusive. Fritscher-Ravens et al.[17] prospectively evaluated 44 patients with stricture at the hepatic hilum. All were suspicious of hilar cholangiocarcinoma but had inconclusive tissue diagnosis. They underwent EUS-guided FNA with linear echoendoscope and 22 gauge needles. Accuracy, sensitivity, and specificity were 91%, 89%, and 100%, respectively. EUS and EUS-guided FNA changed preplanned surgical approach in 27 out of 44 patients. These results suggest that EUS-guided FNA is of value as a new, less-invasive approach for tissue diagnosis of hilar strictures of unknown cause.

EUS-guided FNA is now being used to diagnose and stage cholangiocarcinoma. This procedure is safe, and effective in evaluating proximal biliary strictures. When used in combination with ERCP, it helps distinguish benign from malignant strictures, and facilitates a definitive diagnosis by increasing tissue yield.[18]

3) Intraductal ultrasonography (IDUS)

IDUS with wire-guided, thin caliber, high-frequency probes (Fig. 2) is a feasible and promising imaging modality for the evaluation of a variety of biliary and pancreatic disorders.[19-22] Advantages of these new generation wire-guided probes include ease of biliary cannulation, obviating the need for sphincterotomy in most cases, and the provision of high-resolution, detailed images of ductal and periductal tissues without significantly lengthening the ERCP procedure. Moreover, IDUS can

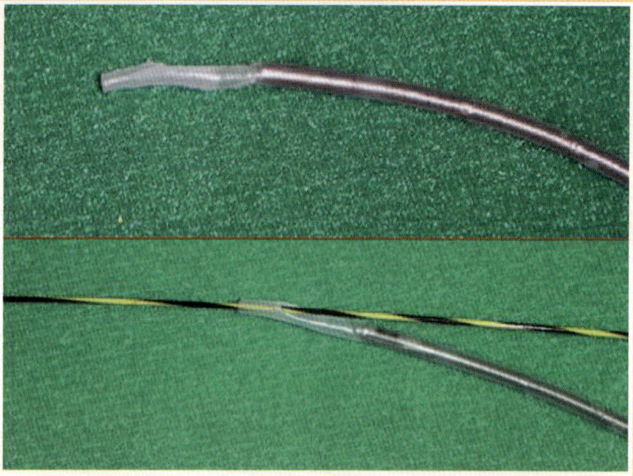

Fig. 2 High-frequency ultrasonic miniature probe. UM-G20-29R probe (Olympus Co., Tokyo, Japan)

provide the local staging required to select patients who would benefit from surgical resection when a malignancy is identified.[23-28] IDUS has consequently emerged as an adjunct to ERCP and percutaneous cholangioscopy (PTC) in the evaluation of biliary strictures.[29-36]

Because their diameter is only about 2 mm, these ultrasonic probes may be passed through the biopsy channel of routinely used duodenoscopes. The small diameter enables IDUS of the biliary tract after transpapillary or transhepatic insertion. The probe tip can be localized fluoroscopically.[21]

IDUS provides an accurate image of bile duct wall and surrounding tissue (Fig. 3). Even when the penetration depth is limited (2 cm), this is sufficient to provide a precise image of an intraductal lesion and possible invasion or compression of adjacent structures. IDUS is faster and easier to learn than conventional EUS.

In the intrapancreatic bile duct, IDUS demonstrates the bile duct wall as a low echoic layer and the pancreatic parenchyma as a fine reticular pattern. In the extrahepatic bile duct, IDUS findings show a two- or three-layer structure; i) an inner

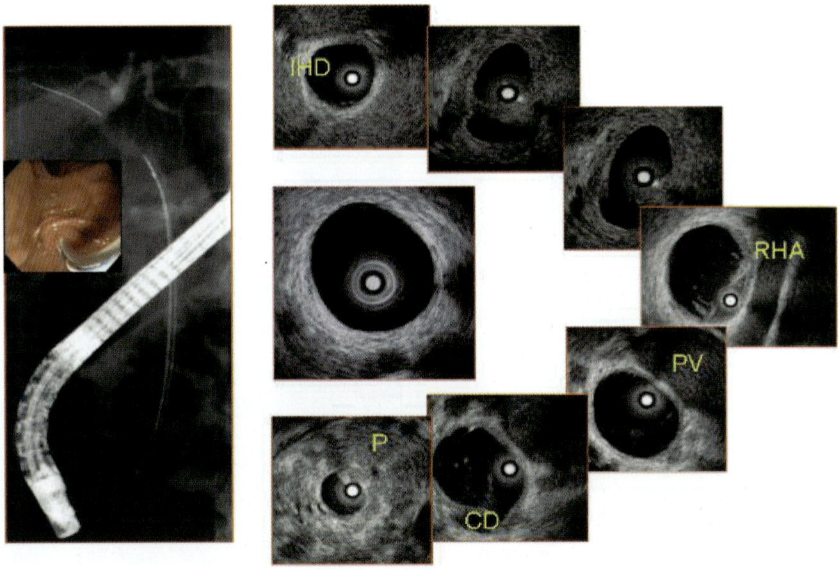

Fig. 3 Normal IDUS findings of biliary tree
IHD, intrahepatic duct; RHA, right hepatic artery; PV, portal vein; CD, cystic duct; P, pancreas.

hypoechoic layer and ii) an outer hyperechoic layer, or the first hyperechoic layer corresponds to the mucosa in addition to a border echo; the second hypoechoic layer is the smooth muscle fibers with fibroelastic tissue; and the third hyperechoic layer is the thin and loose connective tissue with a border echo. During IDUS, portal vein and right hepatic artery are easily seen (Fig. 3).

Cholangiocarcinoma is suspected when IDUS shows hypoechoic masses with irregular margins and inhomogenous echo-poor areas invading surrounding tissues (Fig. 4). Penetration is defined as continuation of the main hypoechoic tumor mass into adjacent structures. On the other hand, homogeneous echo patterns and smoothly defined margins are regarded as benign (Fig. 5).[37] The accuracy of IDUS in differentiating benign from malignant stricture ranges from 76% to 92% in series of patients with various causes of biliary strictures.[30,33,35]

Cholangiocarcinomas are staged according to the following classification, modified from the TNM staging system: T1, limited to the CBD wall; T2, invasion beyound the CBD wall; and T3, invasion of adjacent structures such as the pancreas, duodenum, and portal vein (Fig. 4). The accuracy of IDUS in T-staging was 77.7%.[37] The inner hypoechoic layer of the IDUS images corresponds not olny to the fibromuscular layer but also to a part of the perimuscular connective tissue. Therefore, even though the tumor may be limited to the inner hypoechoic layer, it may be a T2 or T1 tumor.[21] Thus IDUS is not able to differentiate T1 from T2 bile duct cancers.

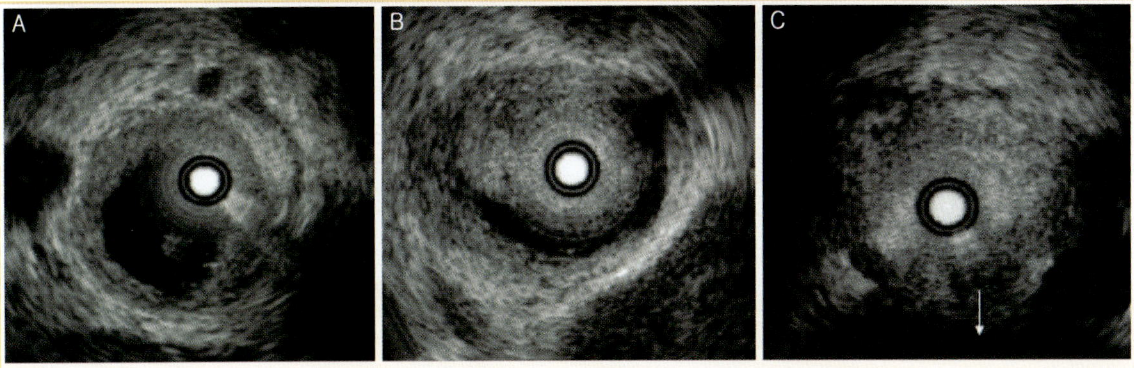

Fig. 4 IDUS findings of T-stage of cholangiocarcinoma

A: T1, Tumor is limited to the bile duct wall and the outer margin of the intramural growth is smooth. B: T2, Tumor invades into the periductal connective tissue and interrupts the outer margin of the bile duct. C: T3, Tumor invades into adjacent blood vessel.

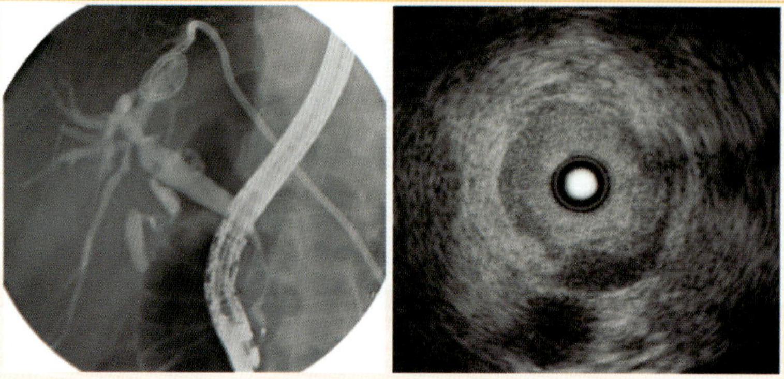

Fig. 5 Benign bile duct stricture

ERC shows long segment narrowing of intrapancreatic distal common bile duct. IDUS finding shows bile duct wall thickening without destruction of wall structure.

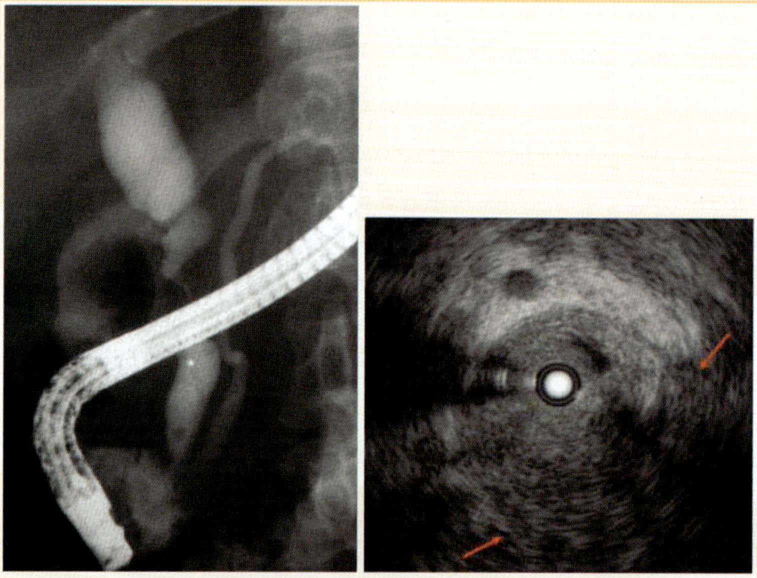

Fig. 6 IDUS finding of pancreatic parenchymal invasion of cholangiocarcinoma

ERCP shows irregular narrowing of mid CBD and dilatation of proximal bile duct and normal appearance of main pancreatic duct. IDUS reveals diffuse irregular destructive thickening of duct wall and interruption of the intrapancreatic bile duct wall, with tumor protrusion into the pancreatic parenchyma (arrows).

Invasion of the adjacent pancreatic parenchyma by a cholangiocarcinoma can be detected by IDUS. Cholangiocarcinoma protruding into the pancreas parenchyma or disruption of the outer bile duct layer are regarded as positive signs of invasion of the pancreatic parenchyma (Fig. 6). Using these criteria, the accuracy of IDUS in assessing tumor invasion to the pancreas was 93~100%.[23]

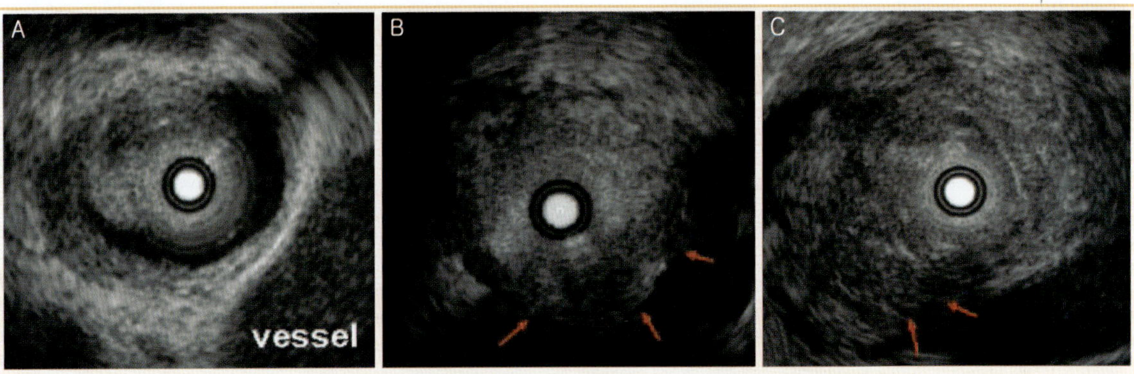

Fig. 7 IDUS findings of vascular invasion of cholangiocarcinoma

A: No invasion of vascular structure. B, C: Invasion of vascular structure. Images show disappearance of the high-echoic layer between the tumor and vessel (arrows).

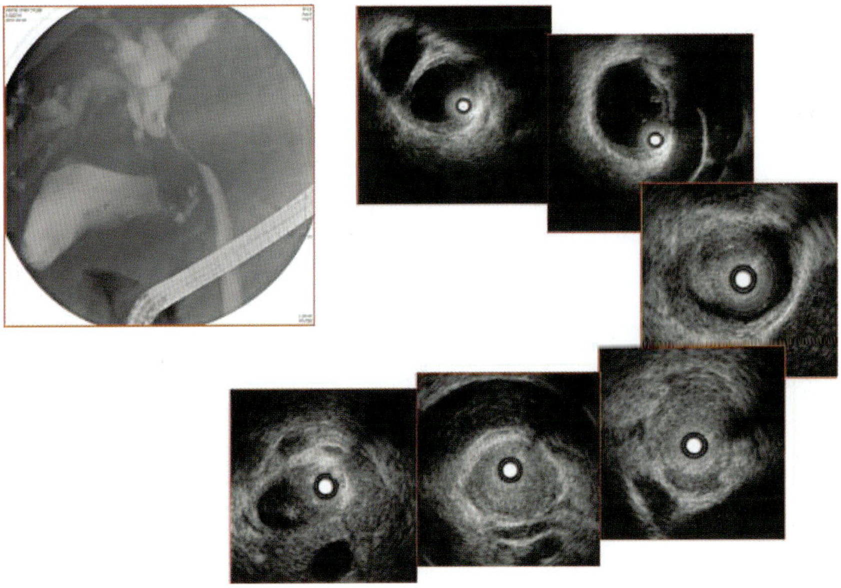

Fig. 8 Assessment of longitudinal tumor extension

IDUS is useful in demonstrating longitudinal extension of bile duct cancer.

IDUS is very accurate (92~100%) in defining portal vein and right hepatic involvement.[9,24,37] Disappearance of the high-echoic layer between the tumor and a vessel is regarded as a positive sign of vascular invasion (Fig. 7). However, left hepatic artery and proper hepatic artery are not easily seen due to anatomical features which cause ultrasound attenuation.

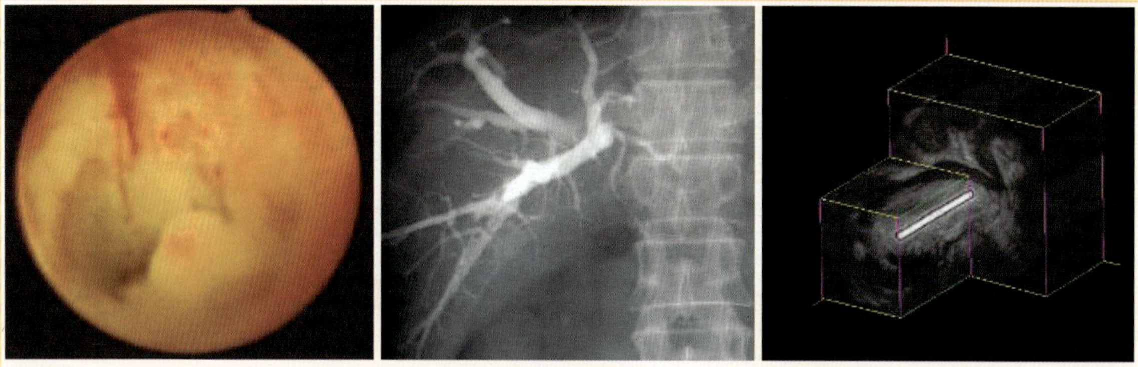

Fig. 9 3D-IDUS finding of cholangiocarcinoma

Cholangioscopy and cholangiogram show stenosis of the bile duct. 3D-IDUS shows the thickening of the bile duct wall. However, the wall structure of bile duct is well preserved.

Intraductal spreading of tumor is known as one of the characteristics of tumor extension of extrahepatic bile duct carcinoma. When irregular thickness of the bile duct is observed consecutively and away from the main lesion, it could be diagnosed that intraductal spreading of cancer existed (Fig. 8).[3] IDUS accuracy in the assessment of longitudinal cancer extension to the hepatic side of the stricture was 72%.[28] This accuracy was increased when asymmetric wall thickness was considered as a criterion of longitudinal tumor spread on both hepatic and duodenal sides, with accuracy of 84% and 86%, respectively.[28]

Because of the limited depth of ultrasonic penetration, IDUS is significantly inferior to conventional EUS with respect to detection of lymph node and distant metastases.[37]

The 3D-IDUS system provides radial and linear real-time images. The 3D-IDUS system consists of an ultrasonic probe that is automatically moved for scanning with an external tube. It carries out linear and radial scanning simultaneously in real-time with on scanning operation (Fig. 9).[1]

Summary

EUS is used to detect and stage biliary malignancies. Endoscopic ultrasound imaging of the biliary system is usually performed with an endosonoscope, but small probes can also be used during ERCP. EUS is used to assist in differentiating between benign and malignant strictures or in the staging of cholangiocarcinoma. Intraductal high frequency ultrasound suggests the presence of malignancy when a hypoechoic infiltration is seen invading through the biliary wall. The findings of a pancreatic mass, irregular bile duct wall, or a bile duct wall of more than 3 mm are suggestive of a malignancy causing biliary obstruction.

Reference

1. Napoleon B, Markoglou C, Lefort C, Durivage G. EUS in bile duct, ampullary, and gallbladder lesions. In: Howes RH, Fokens P. Endosonography. 1st ed. Philadelphia: Saunders, 2006:217-238.
2. Tio TL, Cheng J, Wijers OB, Sars PR, Tytgat GN. Endosonographic TNM staging of extrahepatic bile duct cancer: comparison with pathological staging. Gastroenterology 1991;100:1351-1361.
3. Inui K, Miyoshi H, Yoshino J. Bile duct cancers: what can EUS offer? Intraductal US, 3D-IDUS? FNA-is it possible? Endoscopy 2006;38 (Suppl 1):S47-S49.
4. Amouyal P, Palazzo L, Amouyal G, et al. Endosonography: promising method for diagnosis of extrahepatic cholestasis. Lancet 1989;18:1195-1198.
5. Dancygier H, Nattermann C. The role of endoscopic ultrasonography in biliary tract disease. obstructive jaundice. Endoscopy 1994;26:800-802.
6. Fulcher AS, Turner MA, Capps G, Zfass AM, Baker KM. Half-Fourier RARE MRCP: Experience in 300 subjects. Radiology 1998;207:21-32.
7. Bret PM, Reinhold C. Magnetic Resonance Cholangiopancreatography. Endoscopy 1997;29:472-486.
8. Cannon ME, Carpenter SL, Elta GH, et al. EUS compared with CT, magnetic resonance imaging, and angiography and the influence of biliary stenting on staging accuracy of ampullary neoplasms. Gastrointest Endosc 1999;50:27-33.
9. Stevens PD, Lightdale CJ. Endoscopic ultrasound of the biliary tract. In: Gress FG, Bhattacharya I. Endoscopic ultrasonography. 1st ed. Malden: Blackwell Science, 2001: 103-110.
10. Rösch T, Meining A, Frühmorgen S, et al. A prospective comparison of the diagnostic accuracy of ERCP, MRCP, CT, and EUS in biliary strictures. Gastrointest Endosc 2002; 55:870-876.
11. Qilian Z, Weidong N, Lando Z, Jinyu L. Endoscopic ultrasonography assessment in preoperative staging for carcinoma of ampulla of Vater and extrahepatic bile duct. Chinese Med J 1996;109:622-625.

12. Tio TL, Reeders JW, Sie LH, et al. Endosonography in the clinical staging of Klatskin tumor. Endoscopy 1993;25:81-85.

13. Hoffman BJ, Hawes RH. Endoscopic ultrasonography-guided puncture of the lymph nodes: first experience and clinical consequences. Gastrointest Endosc Clin N Am 1995;5:587-593.

14. Byrne MF, Gerke H, Mitchell RM, et al. Yield of endoscopic ultrasound-guided fine-needle aspiration of bile duct lesions. Endoscopy 2004;36:715-719.

15. Gleeson FC, Rajan E, Levy MJ, et al. EUS-guided FNA of regional lymph nodes in patients with unresectable hilar cholangiocarcinoma. Gastrointest Endosc 2008;67:438-443.

16. DeWitt J, Misra VL, Leblanc JK, McHenry L, Sherman S. EUS-guided FNA of proximal biliary strictures after negative ERCP brush cytology results. Gastrointest Endosc 2006;64: 325-333.

17. Fritscher-Ravens A, Broering DC, Knoefel WT, et al. EUS-guided fine-needle aspiration of suspected hilar cholangiocarcinoma in potentially operable patients with negative brush cytology. Am J Gastroenterol 2004;99:45-51.

18. Chang KJ. State of the art lecture: endoscopic ultrasound (EUS) and FNA in pancreatico-biliary tumors. Endoscopy. 2006;38 (Suppl 1):S56-S60.

19. Stavropoulos S, Larghi A, Verna E, Battezzati P, Stevens P. Intraductal ultrasound for the evaluation of patients with biliary strictures and no abdominal mass on computed tomography. Endoscopy 2005;37:715-721.

20. Menzel J, Domschke W. Intraductal ultrasonography (IDUS) of the pancreato-biliary duct system: personal experience and review of literature. Eur J Ultrasound 1999;10:105-115.

21. Tamada K, Inui K, Menzel J. Intraductal ultrasonography of the bile duct system. Endoscopy 2001;33:878-885.

22. Levy MJ, Vazquez-Sequeiros E, Wiersema MJ. Evaluation of the pancreaticobiliary ductal systems by intraductal US. Gastrointest Endosc 2002;55:397-408.

23. Tamada K, Ido K, Ueno N, et al. Preoperative staging of extrahepatic bile duct cancer with intraductal ultrasonography. Am J Gastroenterol 1995;90:239-246.

24. Tamada K, Ido K, Ueno N, et al. Assessment of portal vein invasion by bile duct cancer using intraductal ultrasonography. Endoscopy 1995;27:573-578.

25. Tamada K, Ido K, Ueno N, et al. Assessment of hepatic artery invasion by bile duct cancer using intraductal ultrasonography. Endoscopy 1995;27:579-583.

26. Tamada K, Ido K, Ueno N, et al. Assessment of the course and variations of the hepatic artery in bile duct cancer by intraductal ultrasonography. Gastrointest Endosc 1996;44: 249-256.

27. Tamada K, Ueno N, Ichiyama M, et al. Assessment of pancreatic parenchymal invasion by bile duct cancer using intraductal ultrasonography. Endoscopy 1996;28:492-496.

28. Tamada K, Nagai H, Yasuda Y, et al. Transpapillary intraductal US prior to biliary drainage in the assessment of longitudinal spread of extrahepatic bile duct carcinoma. Gastrointest Endosc 2001;53:300-307.
29. Gress F, Chen YK, Sherman S, et al. Experience with a catheter-based ultrasound probe in the bile duct and pancreas. Endoscopy 1995;27:178-184.
30. Tamada K, Ueno N, Tomiyama T, et al. Characterization of biliary strictures using intraductal ultrasonography: comparison with percutaneous cholangioscopic biopsy. Gastrointest Endosc 1998;47:341-349.
31. Riemann B, Menzel J, Schiemann U, et al. Ultrasound-guided biopsies of abdominal organs with an automatic biopsy system: a retrospective analysis of the quality of biopsies and of hemorrhagic complications. Scand J Gastroenterol 2000;35:102-107.
32. Chak A, Isenberg G, Kobayashi K, et al. Prospective evaluation of an over-the-wire catheter US probe. Gastrointest Endosc 2000;51:202-205.
33. Vazquez-Sequeiros E, Baron TH, Clain JE, et al. Evaluation of indeterminate bile duct strictures by intraductal US. Gastrointest Endosc 2002;56:372-379.
34. Farrell RJ, Agarwal B, Brandwein SL, et al. Intraductal US is a useful adjunct to ERCP for distinguishing malignant from benign biliary strictures. Gastrointest Endosc 2002;56: 681-687.
35. Tamada K, Tomiyama T, Wada S, et al. Endoscopic transpapillary bile duct biopsy with the combination of intraductal ultrasonography in the diagnosis of biliary strictures. Gut 2002; 50:326-331.
36. Domagk D, Poremba C, Dietl KH, et al. Endoscopic transpapillary biopsies and intraductal ultrasonography in the diagnostics of bile duct strictures: a prospective study. Gut 2002;51: 240-244.
37. Menzel J, Poremba C, Dietl KH, Domschke W. Preoperative diagnosis of bile duct strictures-comparison of intraductal ultrasonography with conventional endosonography. Scand J Gastroenterol 2000;35:77-82.

VIII・IV

The Role of ^{18}F-Fluorodeoxyglucose PET(Positron Emission Tomography) in Cholangiocarcinoma

Introduction

Cholangiocarcinoma is a serious malignancy because most patients present with advanced disease. Only 20% are resectable at the time of diagnosis. In addition, surgical resection offers the only possibility for cure, and systemic chemotherapy and radiation therapy have been largely ineffective in patients with inoperable cancer. A lack of imaging modalities for early detection, advanced age at presentation, and the significant morbidity of radical surgery are also related to the poor prognosis of cholangiocarcinoma.[1-4]

Current imaging modalities of cholangiocarcinoma include ultrasound (US), computed tomography (CT), or magnetic resonance imaging (MRI).[5] They provide information on tumor extension, dilation of bile ducts, and enlargement of regional lymph nodes.[2,3] However, they cannot differentiate between malignant and benign lesions and invasive procedures are needed to obtain pathologic confirmation and conclusive diagnosis.[6] Brush cytology and biopsy during endoscopic retrograde cholangio-pancreatography (ERCP) is helpful for differentiating between benign and malignant strictures. These techniques may prove the presence of malignancies in up to 70~90% of cases,[7-9] but a benign result does not reliably exclude a malignant tumor. Thus, new technology must be evaluated and applied in the appropriate clinical situations.

Positron emission tomography (PET) scanning, particularly using [^{18}F] fluoro-2-deoxy-D-glucose (^{18}FDG), has recently emerged as a powerful functional imaging tool for detection and staging of various malignancies. [18]FDG-PET enables the creation of metabolic images through an increased rate of glucose metabolism, one of the characteristics of malignant cells.[10-13] Cellular [18]FDG uptake is predominantly related to expression of the protein glucose uptake transport 1(GLUT 1). GLUT 1 is expressed in almost all cell types, but it is frequently overexpressed in malignant tissue and can lead to intracellular accumulation of [18]FDG, which then can be visualized by PET. [18]FDG is transported intracellularly by GLUT 1 and phosphorylated by hexokinase to FDG-6-phosphate through the same membrane transport pathway as glucose. However, unlike glucose, FDG-6-phosphate is trapped intracellularly due to lack of further metabolism because of insufficient amounts of glucose phosphatase. In cholangiocarcinoma, [18]FDG accumulation seems to be primarily correlated to increased expression of GLUT 1, but is unrelated to upregulation of type II hexokinase.[14-18]

[18]FDG-PET, which assesses the metabolic and functional features of malignancies, has proven to be useful in the diagnosis and management of patients with various types of cancers. [18]FDG-PET is used for many cancers, mainly for staging, follow-up, and monitoring responses during therapy. Specifically, it is useful to detect recurrent tumors after surgery or radiation therapy that may be obscured by scarring and necrosis.[19,20] There are many studies reporting the value of this method for the assessment of various cancers, most notably malignant lymphoma, melanoma, breast cancer, lung cancer, esophageal cancer, colorectal cancer, and gastric cancer.[20] In malignant lymphoma, [18]FDG-PET is roughly 10% more sensitive than conventional techniques and provides a therapeutically relevant change in disease staging in about 10% of patients.[21] In addition, it is very useful for restaging, as it determines the true extent of lymphoma recurrence and evaluates patients' responses after chemotherapy or immunotherapy.[22] Recently, many investigators have reported on the efficacy of [18]FDG-PET in cholangiocarcinoma.

1. Diagnosis of Primary Tumors

One of the important roles of [18]FDG-PET is differentiation of benign from malignant tumors, such as solitary pulmonary nodules or other gastrointestinal malignancies.[20] In a meta-analysis of 1,474 focal pulmonary lesions, Gould et al.[23] reported that ^{18}FDG-PET had a sensitivity of 96.8% and specificity of 77.8%, and they suggested that PET scanning had high accuracy for detecting malignancy. PET also has high sensitivity (90~100%) for the detection of primary esophageal cancer, this sensitivity is higher than that of CT.[24-29] In the detection of primary carcinomas and premalignant lesions of the large bowel, the sensitivity of PET is 76% in high-grade lesions and 89% in carcinomas if the tumor is larger than 1 cm.[30]

Several study groups have reported that ^{18}FDG-PET has a 90% or greater sensitivity for primary cholangiocarcinoma.[31-33] Kluge et al.[31] reported that visual analysis of PET resulted in a sensitivity of 92.3% and a specificity of 92.9% for the diagnosis of perihilar cholangiocarcinoma(Table 1). However, other investigators demonstrated that ^{18}FDG-PET revealed increased ^{18}FDG uptake in the biliary tract, which was regarded as a positive finding, in only 18 (60%) of the 30 patients with extrahepatic bile duct cancer.[34] In a study by Moon et al.,[35] the overall sensitivity and specificity of ^{18}FDG-PET were 89.1% and 87.5% for primary cholangiocarcinoma, respectively, but the sensitivity of ^{18}FDG-PET in perihilar cholangiocarcinoma was lower than the value of intrahepatic and common bile duct cancers (83.3 % vs. 91.3%, 90.9%, respectively)(Table 1). These results are possibly caused by the fact that perihilar carcinomas are frequently accompanied by obstructive jaundice with or without cholangitis. Thus the sensitivity and accuracy of PET varies according to different anatomic locations i.e. when the primary lesions are divided into intrahepatic, perihilar, and extrahepatic bile duct levels. The different accuracies of

Table 1. Summary of diagnostic accuracy of ^{18}FDG-PET in primary cholangiocarcinoma

Investigator	Year	Anatomic locations	Sensitivity (%)	Specificity (%)
Kluge et al.[31]	2001	Perihilar bile duct lesions (n=54)	24/26 (92.3)	26/28 (92.9)
Kato et al.[32]	2002	Extrahepatic bile duct lesions (n=30)	18/30 (60.0)	
Anderson et al.[36]	2004	Perihilar and common bile duct lesions (n=36)	19/31 (61.3)	4/5 (80.0)
Moon et al.[35]	2007	Overall (n=54)	41/46 (89.1)	7/8 (87.5)
		Intrahepatic bile duct lesions (n=28)	21/23 (91.3)	4/5 (80.0)
		Perihilar bile duct lesions (n=13)	10/12 (83.3)	1/1 (100)
		Common bile duct lesions (n=13)	10/11 (90.9)	2/2 (100)

Table 2. Summary of diagnostic accuracy of ^{18}FDG-PET according to the growth patterns of suspicious cholangiocarcinoma

Investigator	Year	Nodular type (mass ≥1 cm)		Infiltrative type	
		Sensitivity (%)	Specificity (%)	Sensitivity (%)	Specificity (%)
Anderson et al.[36]	2004	17/20 (85.0)	1/2 (50.0)	2/11 (18.2)	3/3 (100)
Moon et al.[35]	2007	27/30 (90.0)	4/4 (100)	14/16 (87.5)	3/4 (75.0)

PET scans appear to be related to the different characteristics of the study populations. For example, the patients in the study of Kato et al.[34] had early-stage bile duct cancer and had more frequent primary tumors showing no tumoral mass on CT as compared to those in the other studies.[31,35]

The diagnostic outcomes of ^{18}FDG-PET in cholangiocarcinoma are also related to the growth patterns and histopathologic subtypes of these malignancies. Anderson et al.[36] reported that the rate of detection of tumors is higher for the nodular type than for the infiltrating type; the sensitivity was 85% for the nodular morphology, whereas it was only 18% for infiltrating morphology (Table 2).

^{18}FDG-PET generally does not seem to detect lesions 0.8 cm in size or less and will thus often fail to detect the more frequently occurring ductal infiltrating type of cholangiocarcinoma.[37] In one study,[38] while all true positive cases were of the tubular type of cholangiocarcinoma with a high amount of tumor cells and low production of mucin, all false negative cases were mucinous adenocarcinomas. As mucin cannot take up glucose over a short period, the residual tumor cell volume that has a high glucose metabolism may be too small to show a significant PET signal. In addition, ^{18}FDG-PET must be carefully interpreted in patients with specific benign conditions, such as primary sclerosing cholangitis, biliary stents, granulomatous diseases, or other conditions that present with high FDG uptake. However, several investigators have reported high sensitivity in the detection of cholangiocarcinomas in patients with primary sclerosing cholangitis.[31,32,36] In a study of seven patients with underlying primary sclerosing cholangitis, the overall sensitivity and specificity was 100% (2/2) and 80% (4/5), respectively.[36] Other investigators have reported that no false positive results were observed in patients that had only primary sclerosing cholangitis.[31] In the study by Keiding et al.,[32] a positive PET scan was obtained in six patients with primary sclerosing cholangitis and known cholangiocarcinoma, and in none of 15 controls. Comparative analysis of ^{18}FDG-PET with CT scans indicates that the limited accuracy of ^{18}FDG-PET precludes its replacement of conventional CT in the discrimination of malignant versus benign diseases in the bile duct (Fig. 1 and Fig. 2). In the study by Kato et al.,[34] the sensitivity of ^{18}FDG-PET for primary cholangiocarcinoma was lower than that of CT (60% vs. 80%) even though PET scan could detect the primary tumors in three of six patients (50%) not found to have malignant tumors on CT (Fig. 3). However, another study demonstrated that the overall accuracy of ^{18}FDG-PET for discriminating malignant diseases from benign conditions was slightly higher than that of CT scan (88.9% vs. 81.5%).[35]

2. Evaluation of Locoregional and Distant Metastasis

The resectability of the tumor depends on its locoregional and distant spread. With regards to use of a PET scan in detection of locoregional lymph node metastasis (Table 3), several studies have reported that PET scans showed a higher specificity with lower sensitivity in various gastrointestinal malignancies.[39-45] In a prospective study of 26 patients with bile duct cancer, low sensitivity (13%) of ^{18}FDG PET was reported for regional lymph node metastases,[31] and another study similarly demonstrated a lower sensitivity (38%) and higher specificity (100%) of PET compared to CT (sensitivity 54%, specificity 59%).[34] The reason for this poor result is assumed to arise from the difficulty of discriminating between extrahepatic parts of the tumor itself and FDG-accumulating lymph nodes in the perihilar region. However, Moon et al.[35] reported ^{18}FDG-PET could detect lymph node metastasis

Table 3. Summary of diagnostic accuracy of ^{18}FDG-PET in locoregional metastases of cholangiocarcinoma compared with CT

Investigator	Year	CT scan		^{18}FDG-PET scan	
		Sensitivity (%)	Specificity (%)	Sensitivity (%)	Specificity (%)
Kluge et al.[31]				2/15 (13.3)	
Kato et al.[32]	2002	7/13 (53.8)	10/17 (58.8)	5/13 (38.5)	17/17 (100)
Moon et al.[35]	2007	4/13 (30.8)		10/13 (76.9)	

undetected by CT (Fig. 4), and changed treatment plans in a significant number of cases even though the sensitivity of PET was only 50%. Thus, for a preoperative diagnosis of regional lymph node metastasis, ^{18}FDG-PET can provide additional information about staging and is complementary to CT scanning.

On the contrary, ^{18}FDG-PET shows promise for the detection of distant metastasis. Previous investigators have demonstrated that ^{18}FDG-ET has high accuracy for the detection of unsuspected distant metastases of cholangio-carcinoma.[31,32,35,36] PET scanning detected 7 of 10 distant metastases in a population of 26 patients with perihilar carcinomas.[31] In another study, even though the sensitivity for detecting distant metastases was only 65%, all the lesions visible on PET went undetected by other methods, and their discovery led to a change in management in 30% of patients for cholangiocarcinoma.[36] Another study reported nine distant metastatic lesions detected with PET that were not detected using other imaging modalities.[35] An ^{18}FDG-PET scan, due to detection of hidden metastatic foci, also allowed exclusion of two patients for whom a laparatomy had been planned thus avoiding unnecessary operations.

3. Monitoring of Response

^{18}FDG-PET appears to have a great potential in malignant lymphoma and gastrointestinal malignancies such as colorectal cancer and esophageal cancer for assessing treatment response or prognosis.[46,47] It has been reported that a PET scan is the most sensitive and specific tool for end-of-treatment evaluation and superior to conventional imaging modalities in Hodgkin's lymphoma. ^{18}FDG-PET can predict outcome more accurately than classic risk evaluation by pretreatment prognostic score systems.[46] In colorectal cancer, it has been reported that a PET scan can predict histopathologic response to neoadjuvant therapy and monitor the success of radiofrequency ablation, owing to its ability to differentiate scar tissue from recurrent tumor.[47] However, there have been few reports available on the utility of ^{18}FDG-PET in assessing treatment response in patients with cholangiocarcinoma. One recent study investigated the feasibility of ^{18}FDG-PET as a follow-up screening method in patients with nonresectable hilar cholangiocarcinoma who underwent photodynamic therapy.[48] Patients were examined by PET scan before and 4~6 weeks after therapy. Interestingly, photodynamic therapy did not effectively reduce tumor volume in hilar cholangiocarcinoma, despite significant reduction of cholestasis. PET imaging also did not show a significant change after treatment. In cholangiocarcinoma, further studies need to be carried out on a larger number of patients.

Nevertheless, ^{18}FDG-PET scans are limited by poor resolution and poor anatomic localization of positive PET lesions. In particular, the abdominal and pelvic areas are often difficult to interpret on a PET scan due to various patterns of bowel and urinary activity.[49] To overcome the poor image quality of PET scans, a combined PET and CT system was developed and has become widely used in clinical oncology. PET-CT has been shown to improve diagnostic accuracy and confidence by providing metabolic and morphologic imaging in a single session.[50] It has recently been confirmed that PET-CT has better diagnostic accuracy in lung cancer, pancreatic cancer, colorectal cancer, and cholangiocarcinoma.[51-55] However, future studies should evaluate the cost benefit of PET-CT before its routine use for cholangio-carcinoma.

Conclusion

^{18}FDG-PET seems to be additive rather than confirmative for diagnosis of primary cholangiocarcinoma and regional lymph node metastases. However, it has been proven that ^{18}FDG-PET is highly valuable for detecting unsuspected distant metastases. In cholangiocarcinoma, accurate diagnosis of distant metastases with PET scan impacts patient management decisions. As such, ^{18}FDG-PET should be considered an essential tool in patients for whom local curative surgery or receive local chemoradiation therapy for the primary tumor is planned.

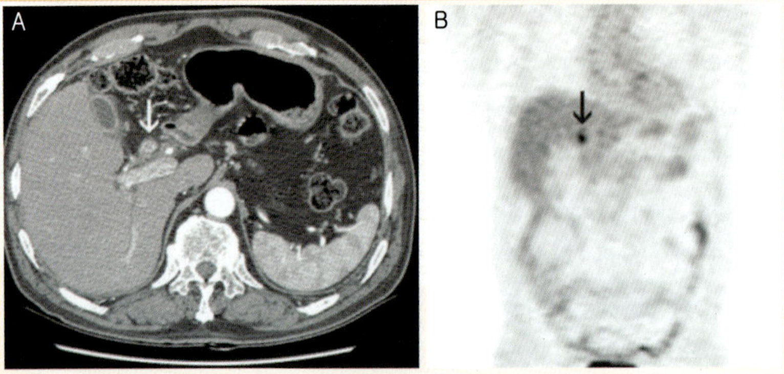

Fig. 1 Computed tomography (CT) scan and ^{18}F-fluoro-2-deoxy-D-glucose positron emission tomography (^{18}FDG-PET) of a patient with perihilar bile duct cancer.

(A) A contrast-enhanced lesion detected with CT scan (indicated with white arrow) also showed increased glucose uptake with (B) ^{18}FDG-PET (indicated with black arrow).[35]

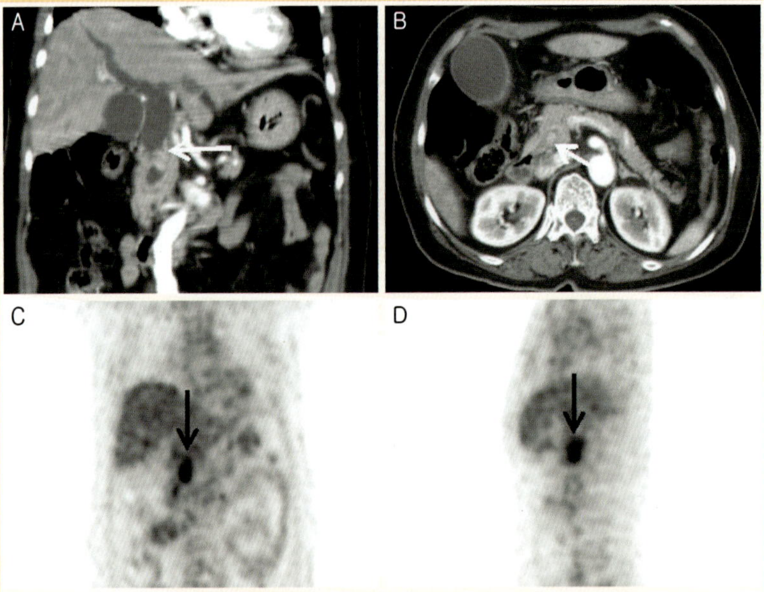

Fig. 2 Computed tomography (CT) scan and ^{18}F-fluoro-2-deoxy-D-glucose positron emission tomography (^{18}FDG-PET) of a patient with common bile duct cancer.

(A, B) CT scan found a lesion suspicious for cholangiocarcinoma (indicated with white arrow), and (C, D) 18FDG-PET detected a focus of intense uptake that was confirmed as adenocarcinoma of common bile duct cancer (indicated with black arrow).

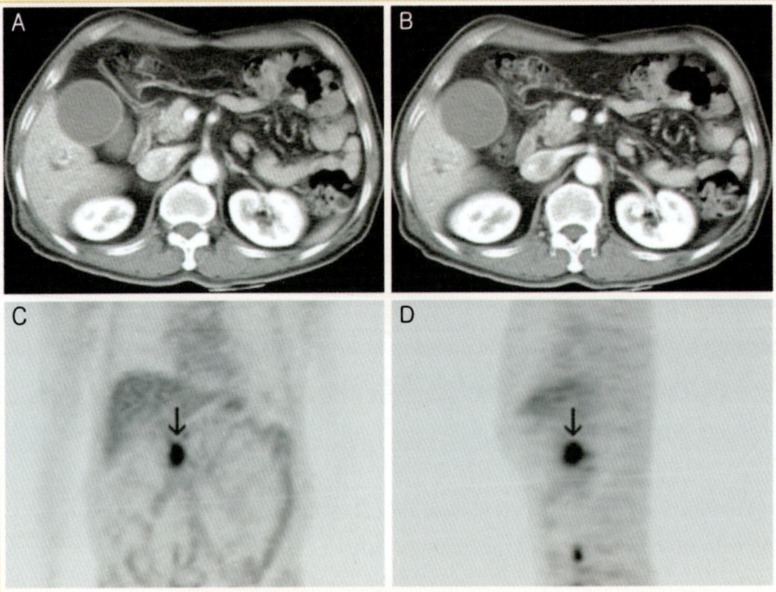

Fig. 3 Computed tomography (CT) scan and ^{18}F-fluoro-2-deoxy-D-glucose positron emission tomography (^{18}FDG-PET) of a patient with common bile duct cancer.

(A, B) CT scan could not find a definite lesion, but (C, D) ^{18}FDG-PET detected a focus of intense uptake that was later confirmed as adenocarcinoma of common bile duct cancer (indicated with black arrow).[35]

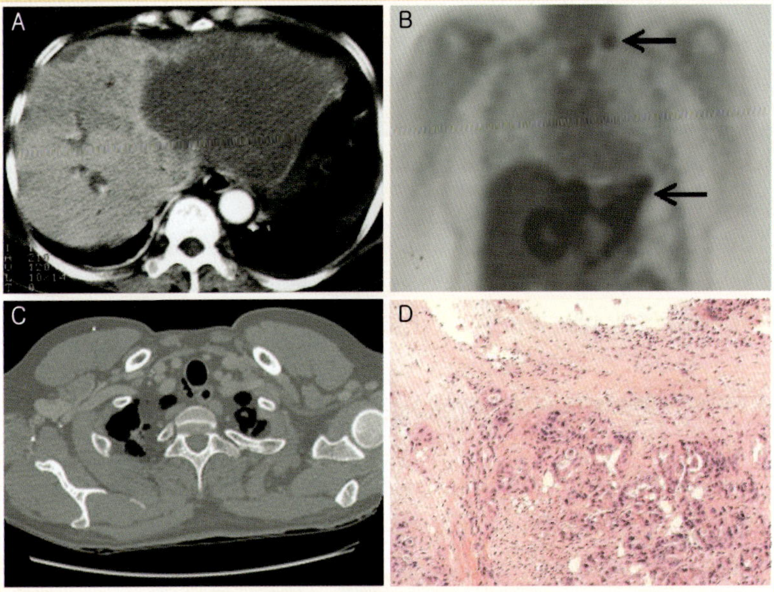

Fig. 4 Computed tomography (CT) scan and ^{18}F-fluoro-2-deoxy-D-glucose positron emission tomography (^{18}FDG-PET) of a patient with intrahepatic bile duct cancer.

(A) CT scan found a huge suspicious lesion for intrahepatic bile duct cancer and (B) 18FDG-PET detected two lesions of increased glucose uptake (indicated with black arrow). One was later confirmed as primary intrahepatic bile duct cancer, and the other was a biopsy-proven metastatic adenocarcinoma at the left supraclavicular lymph node (D). CT scan could not find a definite lesion at the left supraclavicular lymph node (C).

Reference

1. Khan SA, Davidson BR, Goldin R, et al. Guidelines for the diagnosis and treatment of cholangiocarcinoma: consensus document. Gut 2002;51(suppl 6):VI 1-9.
2. De Groen PC, Gores GJ, LaRusso NF, et al. Biliary tract cancers. N Engl J med 1999; 341: 1368-1379.
3. Gores GJ. Early detection and treatment of cholangiocarcinoma. Liver Transpl 2000;6: S30-34.
4. Singh P, Patel T. Advances in the diagnosis, evaluation and management of cholangio-carcinoma. Curr Opin Gastroenterol. 2006;22:294-299.
5. Zech CJ, Shoenberg SO, Reiser M, et al. Cross-sectional imaging of biliary tumors: current clinical status and future developments. Eur Radiol. 2004;14:1174-1187.
6. Feydy A, Vilgrain V, Denys A, et al. Helical CT assessment in hilar cholangiocarcinoma: correlation with surgical and pathologic findings. AJR 1999;172:73-77.
7. Pugliese V, Conio M, Nicolo G, et al. Endoscopic retrograde forceps biopsy and brush cytology of biliary strictures : a prospective study. Gastrointest Endosc 1995;42:520-526.
8. Schoefl R, Haefner M, Wrba F, et al. Forceps biopsy and brush cytology during endoscopic retrograde cholangiopancreatography for the diagnosis of biliary stenoses. Scand J Gastoenterol 1997;32:363-368.
9. Glasbrenner B, Ardan M, Boeck W, et al. Prospective evaluation of brush cytology strictures during endoscopic retrograde cholangiopancreatography. Endoscopy 1999; 31: 712-717.
10. Filer JS, Muecker MM, Usher P, Lodish HF. Elevated levels of glucose transport and transporter messanger RNA are induced by ras or src oncogenes. Science 1987;235:1492-1495.
11. Diederichs CG, Staib L, Vogel J, et al. Values and limitations of ^{18}F-fluorodeoxyglucose-positron emission tomography with preoperative evaluation of patients with pancreatic masses. Pancreas 2000;20:109-116.
12. Schiepers C, Penninckx F, deVadder N. Contribution of PET in the diagnosis of recurrent colorectal cancer: comparison with conventional imaging. Eur J Surg Oncol 1995;21:517-522.
13. Lowe VJ, Fletcher JW, Gobar L. Prospective investigation of positron emission tomography in lung nodules. J Clin Oncol 1998;16:1075-1084.
14. Shiomi S, Nishiguchi S, Ishizu H, et al. Usefulness of positron emission tomography with fluorine-18 fluorodeoxyglucose for predicting outcome in patients with hepatocellular carcinoma. Am J Gastroenterol 2001;96:1877-1880.

15. Higashi T, Tamaki N, Honda T, et al. Expression of glucose transporters in human pancreatic tumors compared with increased FDG accumulation in PET study. J Nucl Med 1997;38:1337-1344.

16. Scheck N, Hall BL, Finn OJ. Increased glyceraldehydes-3-phosphate dehydrogenase gene expression in human pancreatic adenocarcinoma. Cancer Res 1988;48:6354-6359.

17. Higashi K, Clavo AC, Wahl RL. Does FDG uptake measure proliferative activity of human cancer cells? In vivo comparison with DNA flow cytometry and tritiated thymidine uptake. J Nucl Med 1993;34:414-419.

18. Lee JD, Yang WI, Park YN, et al. Different glucose uptake and glycolytic mechanisms between hepatocellular carcinoma and intrahepatic mass-forming cholangiocarcinoma with increased (^{18})F FDG uptake. J Nucl Med. 2005;46:1753-1759.

19. Kostakoglu L, Agress HJ, Goldsmith SJ. Clinical role of FDG-PET in evaluation of cancer patients. Radiographics 2003;23:315-340.

20. Keigo Endo, Noburo Oriuchi, Tetsuya Higuchi et al. PET and PET/CT using ^{18}F-FDG in the diagnosis and management of cancer patients. Int J Clin Oncol 2006;11:286-296.

21. Reske SN, Kotzerke J. FDG-PET for clinical use Results of the 3rd German Interdisciplinary Consensus Conference, "Onko-PET III", 21 July and 19 September 2000. Eur J Nucl Med 2001;28:1707-1723.

22. Juweid ME, Cheson BD. Role of positron emission tomography in lymphoma. J Clin Oncol 2005;23:4577-4580.

23. Gould MK, Maclean CC, Kuschner WG, et al. Accuracy of positron emission tomography for diagnosis of pulmonary nodules and mass lesions. JAMA 2001;285:914-924.

24. Flamen P, Lerut A, Van Cutsem E, et al. Utility of positron emission tomography for the staging of patients with potentially operable esophageal carcinoma. J Clin Oncol 2000; 18: 3202-3210.

25. Yoon YC, Lee KS, Shim YM, et al. Metastasis to regional lymph nodes in patients with esophageal squamous cell carcinoma: CT versus FDG PET for presurgical detection prospective study. Radiology 2003;227:764-770.

26. Gambhir SS, Czernin J, Schwimmer J, et al. A tabulated summary of the FDG PET literature. J Nucl Med 2001;42:1S-93S.

27. Skehan SJ, Brown AL, Thompson M, et al. Imaging features of primary and recurrent esophageal cancer at FDG-PET. Radiographics 2000;20:713-723.

28. Fukunaga T, Okazumi S, Koide Y, et al. Evaluation of esophageal cancers using fluorine-18-fluorodeoxyglucose PET. J Nucl Med 1998;39:1002-1007.

29. Block MI, Patterson GA, Sundaresan RS, et al. Improvement in staging of esophageal cancer with the addition of positron emission tomography. Ann Thorac Surg 1997;64: 770-776.

30. van Kouwen MC, Nagengast FM, Jansen JB, et al. 2-(18F)-fluoro-2-deoxy-D-glucose positron emission tomography detects clinical relevant adenomas of the colon: a prospective study. J Clin Oncol 2005;023: 3713-3717.

31. Kluge R, Schmidt F, Caca K, et al. Positron emission tomography with [^{18}F]fluoro-2-deoxy-D-glucose for diagnosis and staging of bile duct cancer. Hepatology 2001;33:1029-1035.

32. Keiding S, Hansen SB, Rasmussen HH, et al. Detection of cholangiocarcinoma in primary sclerosing cholangitis by positron emission tomography. Hepatology 1998;28:700-706.

33. Widjaja A, Mix H, Wagner S, et al. Positron emission tomography and cholangiocarcinoma in primary sclerosing cholangitis. Z Gastroenterol 1999;37:731-733.

34. Kato T, Tsukamoto E, Kuge Y, Katoh C, Nambu T, Nobuta A, Kondo S, Asaka M, Tamaki N. Clinical role of ^{18}F-FDG PET for initial staging of patients with extrahepatic bile duct cancer. Eur J Nucl Med 2002;29:1047-1054.

35. Moon CM, Bang S, Chung JB, et al. Usefulness of ^{18}F-fluorodeoxyglucose positron emission tomography in differential diagnosis and staging of cholangiocarcinomas. J Gastroenterol Hepatol. 2008;23:759-765.

36. Anderson CD, Rice MH, Pinson CW, et al. Fluorodeoxyglucose PET imaging in the evaluation of Gallbladder Carcinoma and Cholangiocarcinoma. J Gastrointest Surg 2004; 8: 90-97.

37. Gores GJ. Cholangiocarcinoma: current concepts and insights. Hepatology 2003;37: 961-969.

38. Fritscher-Ravens A, Bohuslavizki KH, Broering DC, et al. FDG PET in the diagnosis of hilar cholangiocarcinoma. Nucl Med Commun. 2001;22:1277-1285.

39. Flanagan FL, Dehdashti F, Siegel BA, et al. Staging of esophageal cancer with ^{18}F-fluorodeoxyglucose positron emission tomography. Am J Roentgenol. 1997;168:417-424.

40. Meltzer CC, Luketich JD, Friedman D, et al. Whole-body FDG positron emission tomographic imaging for staging esophageal cancer comparison with computed tomography. Clin Nucl Med. 2000;25:882-887.

41. McAteer D, Wallis F, Couper G, et al. Evaluation of ^{18}F-FDG positron emission tomography in gastric and oesophageal carcinoma. Br J Radiol. 1999;72:525-529.

42. Kalady MF, Clary BM, Gottfried M, et al. Clinical utility of positron emission tomography in the diagnosis and management of periampullary neoplasms. Ann Surg Oncol 2002;9: 237-242.

43. Valinas R, Barrier A, Montravers F, et al. 18F-fluorodeoxyglucose positron emission tomography for characterization and initial staging of pancreatic cancer. Gastroenterol Clin Biol 2002;9:799-806.

44. Bares R, Dohmen BM, Cremerius U, et al. Results of positron emission tomography with fluorine-18 labelled fluorodeoxyglucose in differential diagnosis and staging of pancreatic carcinoma. Radiology 1996;36:435-440.

45. Abdel-Nabi H, Doerr RJ, Lamonica DM, et al. Staging of primary colorectal carcinomas with fluorine-18 fluorodeoxyglucose whole-body PET: correlation with histopathologic and CT findings. Radiology 1998;206:755-760.

46. Brepoels L, Stroobants S. Is [18F]fluorodeoxyglucose positron emission tomography the ultimate tool for response and prognosis assessment? Hematol Oncol Clin North Am 2007; 21:855-869.

47. Esteves FP, Schuster DM, Halkar RK, et al. Gastrointestinal tract malignancies and positron emission tomography: An overview. Semin Nucl Med 2006;36:169-181.

48. Muller D, Weidmann M, Kluge R, et al. Is 18F-FDG-PET suitable for therapy monitoring after palliative photodynamic therapy of non-resectable hilar cholangiocarcinoma? J Gastroenterol 2005; 43:439-443.

49. Hustinx R, Dolin RJ, Benard F, et al. Impact of attenuation correction on the accuracy of FDG-PET in patients with abdominal tumors: a free-response ROC analysis. Eur J Nucl Med 2000;27:1365-1371.

50. Townsend DW. From 3-D positron emission tomography to 3-D positron emission tomography computed tomography: what did we learn? Mol Imaging Biol. 2004;6:275-290.

51. Lardinois D, Weder W, Hany TF et al. Staging of non-small-cell lung cancer with integrated positron-emission tomography and computed tomography. N Engl J Med 2003; 348:2500-2507.

52. Selzner M, Hany TF, Wildbrett P, et al. Does the novel PET/CT imaging modality impact on the treatment of patients with metastatic colorectal cancer of the liver? Ann Surg 2004; 240:1027-1034.

53. Heinrich S, Goerres GW, Schafer M, et al. Positron emission tomography/computed tomography influences on the management of resectable pancreatic cancer and its cost-effectiveness. Ann Surg 2005;242:235-243.

54. Reinhardt MJ, Strunk H, Gerhardt T, et al. Detection of Klatskin's tumor in extrahepatic bile duct strictures using delayed 18F-FDG PET/CT: preliminary results for 22 patient studies. J Nucl Med 2005;46:1158-1163.

55. Petrowsky H, Wildbrett P, Husarik DB, et al. Impact of integrated positron emission tomography and computed tomography on staging and management of gallbladder cancer and cholangiocarcinoma. J Hepatol 2006;45:43-50.

IX. Preoperative Assessment for Resectability

IX Preoperative Assessment for Resectability

Sun-Whe Kim, M.D.

IX
Preoperative Assessment for Resectability

This chapter focuses on the determination of resectability for extrahepatic bile duct carcinoma, including hilar cholangiocarcinoma (Klatskin tumor). Radicality and safety are two essential conditions for curative surgical resection as local control of a surgical disease. Because the two conditions are sometimes in opposition, there is considerable controversy in resectability criteria. Reported resectability varies widely from 20% to>80%, based on the location of the tumor and the surgeon's attitude.[1]

In order to determine resectability, the following are required; (1) an understanding of the anatomy of the biliary tract system and adjacent structures; (2) the mode of tumor spread; (3) adequate preoperative diagnostic tools for staging workup; and (4) reasonable criteria of resectability.

1. Anatomy of the Biliary Tract System and Adjacent Structures

The extent of local invasion into the adjacent tissues, including major vessels, is the most critical factor in determining the type of management. A significant portion of the hilar bile duct is located in the liver parenchyma and the distal common bile duct is surrounded by the pancreatic parenchyma. Therefore, tumors in this location easily infiltrate into the liver or pancreas, which need to be removed to some extent. The common hepatic duct (CHD) and the proximal common bile duct (CBD) course along the hepatoduodenal ligament, together with the hepatic artery and portal vein.

The relative location between the bile duct and the vessels is important in understanding the vascular invasion of a tumor. At the level of the intrapancreatic CBD, there is some distance between the duct and vessels (the superior mesenteric/portal vein and common hepatic artery). As the common duct approaches the liver hilum, the portal vein and proper hepatic artery run very close to the bile duct, and finally they become a single unit, the Glissonian unit, at the level of the hilum. The portal vein runs from the left posterior side to the posterior side of the CHD, the hepatic artery runs on the left side of the duct, and the right hepatic artery usually crosses the bile duct posteriorly at the level of the CHD.

There are a number of anatomical variations in the bile duct and vessels. Considering that the most common type accounts for<50%, it becomes very difficult to apply the same consistent principle of resectability criteria to all cases.

2. Mode of Local Spread of the Tumor

Bile duct cancer is known to be a slow-growing tumor. The tumor often spreads locally over a long period of time, and distant metastasis is rare. Loco-regional spread, including direct invasion, neural and perineural infiltration, and lymphatic metastasis are important modes of spread.

1) Direct local invasion

(1) Extra-bile duct wall invasion (depth of invasion)

Most bile duct cancers present after they have already invaded the fibromuscular layer and adjacent soft tissues. According to the location, the tumor invades the liver parenchyma, soft tissue in the hepatoduodenal ligament, pancreas, portal vein, and hepatic artery. Vascular invasion is more common in proximal bile duct cancers. Tumors involving the CHD easily invade the right hepatic artery because of its course. The right hepatic artery or sectional branch, that originates from the superior mesenteric artery, usually courses posterior to the CBD, and is thus easily infiltrated. The main portal vein and its main branches are common sites of direct tumor infiltration, especially in proximal bile duct cancer. In some cases, contralateral arterial invasion develops, as Bismuth type IIIb is sometimes seen with left portal invasion and right arterial invasion.

(2) Intramural invasion

Bile duct cancer spreads longitudinally (proximally and distally) along the bile duct wall. Diffuse involvement is not rare. Bile duct cancer can spread along the mucosal layer, but in most cases it spreads along the periductal fibrous tissues and the Glissonian sheath in the proximal duct. In sclerosing-type tumors, tumor spread more than 1~2 cm beyond the gross tumor margin is seen quite often and in the mucosal spread-type papillary tumor, proximal spread over 4~5 cm is common.[2] This pattern of tumor spread is the rationale for pancreatoduodenectomy for proximal common bile duct cancer or liver resection, including caudate lobectomy for the Klatskin tumor.[3]

2) Lymph node metastasis

Lymph node metastasis is detected in 20~40% of resected cases.[1] Usually, the order of lymphatic spread is as follows: pericholedochal nodes (12h, 12c); hepatoduodenal ligament nodes (12b, 12a); posterior pancreatic head (13a,b); common hepatic artery nodes (8); and lymph nodes around the superior mesenteric artery (14)/celiac artery (9). Lymphatic spread to the para-aortic lymph nodes (16a,b) is no longer regional and is considered as distant metastasis site. Skipped metastases rarely develop.

3) Perineural invasion

Perineural invasion is one of the most important prognostic factors and is considered an important cause of local treatment failure. Therefore, it is very important to remove all the soft tissues, including the nerve plexus in the hepatoduodenal ligament and the hepatic artery, which is referred to as 'skeletonization of vessels.' However, in cases with overt peri-vascular neural and perineural infiltration, which is sometimes observed as a 'frozen hepatoduodenal ligament,' R0 resection is nearly impossible.

3. Diagnostic Modalities to Determine Resectability

Radical surgeries for bile duct cancer (hepatobiliary resection and pancreato-duodenectomy) have become relatively safe surgical procedures. However, they are still associated with high morbidity and mortality that place an enormous burden on the patients and surgeons, both physically and mentally. Therefore, a patient's general condition (host factor) as well as the disease factor should be considered to determine the treatment modality and type/extent of surgery.

The diagnostic modalities for the preoperative work-up are listed below. The details of each procedure are covered in other chapters.

1) Ultrasonography

Abdominal ultrasonography should be a first-line screening test to confirm obstructive jaundice. The value of abdominal ultrasonography as a tool to determine resectability is limited. Abdominal ultrasonography can be helpful by detecting distant metastasis, including liver metastasis and ascites.

2) Computed tomography (CT)

Abdominal CT is a gold standard to determine resectability. The extent of local invasion into the adjacent organs and major vessels, lymph node metastasis, and distant metastasis (including liver metastasis) can be evaluated by CT. Advanced CT techniques, such as MD-CT, CT angiography, and 3-D CT give more precise information on the extent of tumor and anatomical variation.[4,5]

3) ERCP

Because most patients have obstructing lesions, ERCP is helpful only to look at the distal margin of the tumor. Therefore, it is not a critical tool for resectability.

4) PTC

PTBD with PTC is a standard tool for evaluation of the proximal extent of the tumor. It is an essential procedure in most of the Klatskin tumor cases.

5) MRI /MR cholangiography

Although it is a non-invasive procedure, it costs more and the quality of cholangiography is inferior to PTC. It is a good alternative when the bile duct is not sufficiently dilated. MRI is considered superior to CT to confirm liver metastasis.

6) Percutaneous transhepatic cholangioscope (PTCS)

In the papillary tumor with a mucosal spreading pattern, it is difficult to determine the extent of tumor by CT and cholangiography. PTCS and biopsy is necessary for accurate mapping the proximal extent of the tumor.

7) Miscellaneous tools

Endoscopic ultrasonography (EUS), pre-exploratory staging laparoscopy with laparoscopic ultrasonography, and positron emission tomography (PET) can be used to detect hidden distant metastases and to confirm suspicious metastases.

4. Resectability Criteria

The diagnosis of bile duct cancer is not so difficult, but it is sometimes very difficult to determine resectability; the reasons are as follows: (1) there are a number of anatomical variations of the bile duct, hepatic artery, and portal vein; (2) the preoperative determination of the extent of the tumor is sometimes very difficult; (3) radical surgery is technically complicated and time-consuming and is associated with high morbidity and mortality; and (4) the criteria of resectability is not well-established. In general, the following are regarded as criteria of non-resectability: (1) bilateral extensive involvement of the intra-hepatic duct (Bismuth IV); (2) extensive lymph node metastasis, especially para-aortic lymph node metastasis; (3) main portal vein or proper hepatic artery involvement or contralateral (to the side of the extensive involvement of bile duct) hepatic or portal vein involvement that is not removable; (4) distant metastasis (liver metastasis and peritoneal metastasis); (5) poor hepatic reserve function or insufficient volume of residual liver; and (6) high operative risk patients due to systemic problems.

1) Extent of bile duct invasion

Resectability should be determined preoperatively. Intraoperative determination is very difficult and sometimes impossible. The proximal extent of the tumor can be determined by cholangiography (PTC through a PTBD tube or MRCP, PTCS with biopsy if needed, or CT). At least 0.5~1 cm proximal and distal normal-appearing bile duct should be removed.

Bismuth type IV is generally considered non-resectable. Although most surgeons are using Bismuth classification to determine resectability, it cannot be a strict criteria because many patients have anatomical variations of the bile duct and resectability criteria differs according to the centers. If a trisectionectomy is regarded as curative surgery, the tumor involvement of the confluence of sectional ducts is not a contraindication. However, trisectionectomy is associated with a high risk of hepatic failure and dissection of branches of hepatic and portal vasculature from the bile duct in the Glissonian sheath can be considered oncologically-unacceptable.

The Bismuth type is sometimes related to the intrahepatic extent of the tumor. Bismuth type IV can sometimes be resectable, depending on the bile duct anatomical variation, the location of the hilum, or the distance from the main confluence to the second order confluence. If the hilum has a trifurcation variation, the extent of tumor to the right side hepatic duct can lead to overinterpretation. If the confluence of the left medial and lateral sectional ducts is close to the hilum, left lateral section or sometimes left lobe of liver can be preserved even in Bismuth type IV. If a trisectionectomy is adapted and the confluence of left lateral segmental ducts (B2 and B3) or the confluence of right posterior segmental ducts (B6 and B7) is preserved, Bismuth type IV is no longer a contraindication. In such cases, residual liver function or involvement of a vascular pedicle is more often critical.

2) Extent of vascular invasion

Vascular invasion and anatomic variation are important factors for determination of resectability and type of surgery. Conventional angiography is no longer used because of its invasiveness. CT and MRI with their reconstruction technique are the methods of choice. Different extents of vascular encasement, luminal change, and development of collateral vessels are positive findings. Because a desmoplastic reaction around the tumor is seen like a vascular encasement, equivocal cases should be explored.

The proper hepatic artery and the right or left hepatic artery can be invaded according to the location of the tumor. The proper hepatic artery can be invaded in cases with extensive hepatoduodenal ligament infiltration that is mostly non-resectable. Ipsilateral hepatic artery invasion in Bismuth IIIa or IIIb is not a contraindication. The right hepatic artery is easily involved in all the types of proximal cancer, including Bismuth IIIb because it crosses the bile duct just behind the CHD. Contralateral involvement, for instance Bismuth type IIIb and right hepatic artery involvement, is usually considered non-resectable. A short involved segment of the hepatic artery can be removed and reconstructed, but the benefit of the technique has not been documented yet. The right hepatic artery originated from superior mesenteric artery is also easily involved because it runs posterior to the common duct through the pericholedochal soft tissue including the lymph nodes. The right hepatic artery from the superior mesenteric artery, the left hepatic artery from the left gastric artery, and some variable courses of artery sometimes make resection easier or difficult according to the location of the tumor.

Curative (R0) resection of the tumor with arterial involvement is almost impossible because arterial invasion means infiltration into periarterial soft tissues, including the periarterial nerve plexus. Arterial resection and reconstruction are technically difficult and complications of this site easily lead to hepatic failure and mortality. Pancreatic leakage easily leads to complications of arterial anastomosis. Therefore, arterial resection and reconstruction should be carefully performed in selected cases with very short segmental involvement in good risk patients by experienced vascular surgeons.

Main portal veins are rarely involved in distal bile duct cancer. The main portal vein and its branch near the bifurcation area are frequently involved by proximal bile duct cancer. Peripheral ipsilateral portal vein involvement can be removed with ipsilatral hepatectomy, but involvement of the bifurcation area or the contralateral vein invasion needs to be individualized to determine resectability. Because the portal vein has a large lumen and some redundancy and no tightly attached nerve plexus, portal vein surgery, including wedge resection and segmental resection and reconstruction with or without graft is applied more frequently. If the bifurcation area of the portal vein is histologically-involved, long-term survival is extremely rare. Involvement of the long segment that might need a graft has not shown any convincing data for benefit of resection. However, radiologic and sometimes gross findings are not always consistent with pathologic findings. So exploration should be performed for cases with equivocal findings.

3) Lymph node metastasis

Definitive para-aortic lymph node metastasis or extensive conglomerated metastasis of regional lymph node indicates non-resectability. If these findings are suggested on CT, PET can be performed to confirm. CT has a limited value for metastasis of individual lymph nodes, so a few positive nodes, even in the para-aortic area, is not a contraindication for surgery.

4) Residual liver function and volume

In the patients who need major liver resection, biliary drainage (preferably PTBD) is needed to relieve jaundice and evaluate residual liver function. Expected function and volume of the residual liver are critical for postoperative recovery.[6] It is especially important when the patients have chronic liver disease or trisectionectomy should be performed, otherwise R0 resection is impossible. If the right and left hepatic ducts are separated, the remaining liver should be drained to improve function. If jaundice is not relieved with 2~3 weeks of adequate biliary drainage, liver resection would be risky. It would be ideal if the bilirubin level is normalized, but most surgeons agree that 3~5 mg% is sufficient. The rate of decreasing jaundice is also significant. After jaundice is relieved, an ICG test and oral glucose tolerance test can be done to estimate residual liver function. Residual liver volume can be measured using CT volumetry. In general, at least 30% of liver volume should remain.

If the expected residual liver volume is too small, percutanous trans-hepatic portal vein embolization (PTPE) can be performed.[7] PTPE induces hypertrophy of the remaining liver by blocking portal blood inflow to the liver to be removed. It can be indicated in proximal bile duct cancer in those patients who need hepatectomy if the remaining liver volume is expected to be<30% of the total liver volume or trisectionectomy is needed, in patients who have chronic liver disease and need major liver resection, and in patients who need combined pancreatoduodenectomy. However, the effectiveness of PTPE to prevent postoperative liver failure has not been clearly documented and evidence is not sufficient. If PTPE is not working, other modalities should be considered.

5) Other challenging trials to increase resectability

Active application of vascular surgery increases resectability of bile duct cancer. It needs to be investigated whether the procedures have a significant benefit of better long-term outcome without a significant increase of early morbidity and mortality. Hepatoligamentopancreatoduodenectomy is the extreme of extensive resection that has been reported, but it has not popularized because of high operative mortality.

Liver transplantation can be tried for a non-resectable Klatskin tumor.[8] The candidate should be selected strictly to the cases without dissemination, lymph node metastasis or distant metastasis. High recurrence rate, high operative morbidity and mortality, and donor shortage are the problems of liver transplantation for cholangiocarcinoma to overcome.

Conclusion

Resectability rates vary widely according to the different institutes. Different view point on the tumor characteristics and natural course make surgeons have different criteria of resectability. For the last couple of decades, thanks to the development of perioperative care and diagnostic tools, the extent of surgery has been expanded gradually. However, it is time to reconsider the trend of extensive surgery in a viewpoint of evidence-based surgery.

Reference

1. Jang JY, Kim SW, Park DJ, Ahn YJ, Yoon YS, Choi MK, Suh KS, Lee KU, Park YH. Actual long-term outcome of extrahepatic bile duct cancer after surgical resection. Ann Surg 2005; 241(1):77-84.
2. Ogura Y, Takahashi K, Tabata M, Mizumoto R. Clinico-pathological study on carcinoma of the extrahepatic bile duct with special focus on cancer invasion on the surgical margins. World J Surg 1994;18:778-784.
3. Mizumoto R, Suzuki H. Surgical anatomy of the hepatic hilum with special reference to the caudate lobe. World J Surg 1988;12:2-10.
4. Chen HW, Pan AZ, Zhen ZJ, Su SY, Wang JH, Yu SC, et al. Preoperative evaluation of Resectability of Klatskin tumor with 16-MDCT angiography and cholangiography. Am J Roentgenol 2006;186:1580-1586.
5. Cha JH, Han JK, Kim TK. Preoperative evaluation of Klatskin tumor; Accuracy of spiral CT in determining vascular invasion as a sign of unresectability. Abdom Imaging 2000; 25:500-507.
6. Nagino M, Nimura Y, Hayakawa N, Kamiya J, Kondo S, Sasaki R, Hamajima N. Logistic regression and discri-minant analyses of hepatic failure after liver resection for carcinoma of the biliary tract. World J Surg 1993;17:250-255.
7. Nagino M, Kamiya J, Nishio H, Ebata T, Arai T, Nimura Y. Two hundred forty consecutive portal vein embolizations before Extended hepatectomy for biliary cancer: Surgical outcome and long-term outcome. Ann Surg 2006;243:364-372.
8. Rea DJ, Heimbach JK, Rosen CB, Haddock MG, Alberts SR, Kremers WK, et al. Liver transplantation with neoadjuvant chemoradiation is more effective than resetion for hilar cholangiocarcinoma. Ann Surg 2005;242:451-458.

X • Treatment

X·I

Surgical Treatment for Cholangiocarcinoma

Surgical resection is a potentially curative treatment modality for both intrahepatic and extrahepatic cholangiocarcinoma. Nevertheless, for all intrahepatic and most extrahepatic cholangiocarcinomas, complete surgical removal of the malignancy necessitates major hepatectomy. For this reason, many patients do not qualify for surgery because of the existence of other comorbidities. Unfortunately, more than half of cholangiocarcinoma patients present with advanced unresectable disease. In such cases, palliative therapies, such as biliary stenting and/or photodynamic therapy, can provide symptom relief and possibly have a positive effect on survival.[1,2]

The type and extent of the surgery depends on the location of the cancer within the liver or the bile duct. Surgical treatment of intrahepatic cholangiocarcinoma consists of a partial hepatectomy with regional lymphnodes dissection.[3] For extrahepatic cholangiocarcinoma affecting the common bile duct, the biliary tree and hilar lymphatics are resected. Most patients with extrahepatic tumors where the confluence of the bile ducts is also affected, will additionally require a partial hepatectomy with caudate lobectomy to adequately resect the cancer.[4] Distal cholangiocarcinomas are managed by pancreato-duodenectomy, as with ampullary or pancreatic head cancers, with the aim of a margin-negative resection.[2]

To date, chemo- and/or radiation therapy for cholangiocarcinomas have not been evaluated in randomized controlled trials, including adjuvant treatment after surgical resection to diminish the risk of cholangiocarcinoma recurrence.[2] Recently, selected patients with intrahepatic or hilar cholangiocarcinoma have undergone liver transplantation with curative intent at some liver transplantation centers.[5,6]

Given that the type and extent of surgery is markedly different according to the location of the tumor, this chapter will be divided first intrahepatic and extrahepatic cholangiocarcinomas. Extrahepatic cholangiocarcinoma will further be subdivided into proximal cholangiocarcinoma, distal cholangiocarcinoma, diffuse cholangiocarcinoma, and extrahepatic cholangiocarcinoma with vascular invasion. We will also describe the surgical treatment for respective groups and discuss the role of liver transplantation in patients with cholangiocarcinoma.

1. Intrahepatic Cholangiocarcinoma

Intrahepatic cholangiocarcinoma is the second common primary liver cancer after hepatocellular carcinoma. It accounts for about 10% of primary liver malignancies and has been reported to occur with increasing incidence in recent years.[7-8] Due to its intrahepatic localization, early symptoms are rare, and the majority of patients presents with advanced and often already existing extrahepatic tumors. The prognosis for this type of lesion has been shown to be generally poor, and the reported median survival is usually below 6 to 9 months in the majority of patients after diagnosis.[9-11]

The Korean Society of Liver Surgeons conducted a survey on the status of the surgical management of primary liver cancers in Korea. The study was based on the clinical data of resected cases from 16 major medical centers throughout the country, including 14 university hospitals. A total of 223 patients with intrahepatic cholangiocarcinoma underwent liver resection over a period of 12 years (January 1985-December 1996). There were 146 males and 77 females with a ratio of 1.9:1. Associated hepatobiliary diseases included intrahepatic stones (27.6%), clonorchiasis (19.2%), and cirrhosis (9.2%). Three quarters of the tumors presented with mass-forming and expanding growth pathology. CA19-9 was the most frequently elevated tumor marker. Forty percent of the patients had lymph node metastasis detected by postoperative pathology. The operative mortality rate was 2.7%, while the actuarial survival rates at 1, 3, 5, and 10 years were 61.5%, 31.7%, 22.6%, and 15%, respectively. The median survival time for the above patients was 17 months. The most significant prognostic factor was lymph node metastasis at the time of surgery.[12]

There are two principles of surgery for intrahepatic cholangiocarcinomas that differ from surgery for hepatocellular carcinoma: attainment of sufficient resection margin of the liver parenchyma, and adequate dissection of lymph nodes.[13-18] As the spread of an intrahepatic cholangiocarcinoma is characterized by the growth pattern of the tumor which is along the bile duct, it is advisable to resect the tumor with more sufficient free resection margins, which should be confirmed by intraoperative frozen section of the resected bile duct. The incidence of accompanying liver cirrhosis of intrahepatic cholangiocarcinoma compared with hepatocellular carcinoma, is a significantly lower 10%,[19-22] and therefore a major hepatectomy, other than a lobectomy, is strongly recommended. Approximately half of all intrahepatic cholangiocarcinomas are associated with lymph node metastasis. It has therefore been strongly advised that lymph node dissection be performed in all such patients.[13-16,23,24] Lymph node metastasis occurs most frequently in the lymph nodes located around the hepatoduodenal ligament, regardless of the site of the primary tumor, followed by metastasis of the periaortic lymph nodes, retropancreatic lymph nodes, and common hepatic artery lymph nodes. Likewise, Yamamoto et al[23] has suggested that the hepatoduodenal ligament lymph nodes act as sentinel lymph nodes in patients with intrahepatic cholangiocarcinoma. Also, in patients with intrahepatic cholangiocarcinoma that is located in the left lobe of the liver, cancer tend to metastasize to the left gastric artery lymph nodes and lesser curvature of the stomach lymph nodes. It has therefore been proposed by Tsuji et al[24] that extended lymph node dissection including lymph nodes along the lesser curvature of the stomach should accompany the hepatectomy of such patients.

The pattern of spread of intrahepatic cholangiocarcinoma differs according to the gross appearance of the tumor. The periductal infiltrative type progresses around the bile ducts along the Glisson's capsule, and therefore lymph node metastasis of the hilum of the liver is a common finding. In advanced cases, it is necessary to perform caudate lobectomy, resection of the extrahepatic bile duct and adequate lymph node dissection, as well as ipsilateral hemihepatectomy.[18,24,25] In the early stage of mass-forming type, the tumor commonly metastasizes along the portal vein and forms satellite nodules in the liver, demonstrating similar tumor growth patterns to

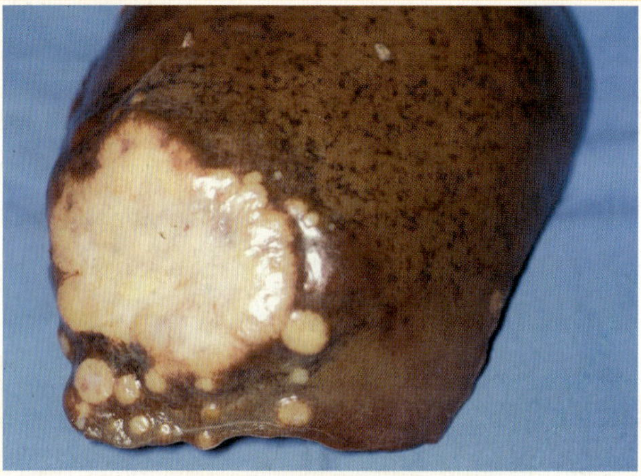

Fig. 1 Operative specimen after extended right hemihepatectomy showing intrahepatic cholangiocarcinoma with multiple satellite nodules

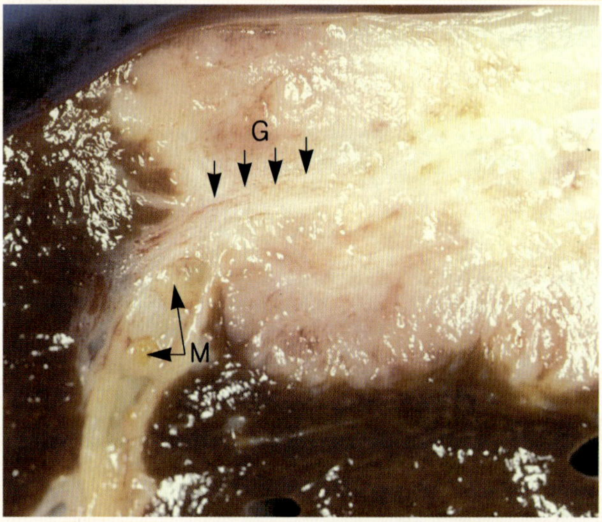

Fig. 2 Operative specimen of advanced intrahepatic cholangiocarcinoma
G: Invasion of Glisson sheath, M: mucosal spread of intrahepatic bile duct.

hepatocellular carcinomas. It is therefore important to obtain sufficient surgical margins (Fig. 1).[18,25] Shimada et al compared the 5-year survival rates of patients with mass-forming type of intrahepatic cholangiocarcinoma without lymph node metastasis according to the surgical margin status, the obtained results were 65% and 17% for surgical margin negative and positive patients, respectively.[26] While lymph node dissection may not be of major significance in patients with small sized tumors, careful attention should be given to surgical margin status, as in surgery for cholangiocarcinoma, for tumors that spread by the invasion of the Glisson's capsule. Lymph node dissection has also been noted to assist in improving survival (Fig. 2).[13,18,25]

Given that intraductal growth type of intrahepatic cholangiocarcinoma has only been recently described in the literature, elaborate studies regarding the mode of therapy are consequently relatively sparse. It is based on this that this condition is associated generally with favorable prognosis compared to other gross types of intrahepatic cholangiocarcinomas.[27] A study by Suh et al,[13,28] which reported no cases with lymph node metastasis among 16 patients who received hepatectomy surgery for intraductal growth type further highlight this view. Nevertheless, as the intraductal growth type has a tendency for intraductal mucosal spreading, careful consideration should be given to the status of the surgical margins,[27] and since this type is basically a form of cholangiocarcinoma, it is suggested that it would be safer to perform lymph node dissection during surgery as in other cases of invasive cholangiocarcinoma.[13]

2. Extrahepatic Cholangiocarcinoma

Infiltration by extrahepatic cholangiocarcinoma includes longitudinal extension and vertical invasion. Microscopic extension of cholangiocarcinoma beyond the border visualized by cholangiography or the margin observed macroscopically is often detected, and is diagnosed as a microscopically positive margin (R1). Longitudinal extension consists of superficial and submucosal infiltration and sometimes includes direct, lymphatic, or perineural invasion.[29-33] Sakamoto et al[32] pointed out a correlation between the gross type of the tumor and the pattern of spread beyond the macroscopic margin at the proximal border. The submucosal spread was predominant in infiltrating types, and the mean length was 6 mm. The superficial extension was predominant in the papillary and nodular types, and the mean length was 20 mm. Ebata et al[33] investigated 80 resected specimens with microscopically positive margins, and observed invasive (submucosal) extent within 10 mm in all cases, and non-invasive (superficial) spread within 20 mm in 90% of cases. Considering these results, free surgical margins from the gross edge should exceed 10 mm in the invasive type and over 20 mm in the papillary and nodular types. Intraoperative pathologic examination by frozen sections is also advocated to confirm the margin of the cut end of the bile duct. When the margin is positive for cancer, additional resection is necessary to obtain R0 resection whenever possible.[29]

Extrahepatic cholangiocarcinoma vertically infiltrates into the hepatoduodenal ligament, in which the hepatic artery and the portal vein are located adjacent to the bile duct. Therefore, the skeletonization of vessels in the hepatoduodenal ligament and the clearance of all perivascular connective tissue is the standard surgical procedure.[29,34,35] Hilar cholangiocarcinoma easily invades the right hepatic artery, which usually lies behind the common bile duct, and involves the portal vein. If the tumor shows signs of invasion of the perivascular connective tissue, en-bloc resection of the right hepatic artery is advocated to obtain a negative surgical margin; therefore, right hemihepatectomy is recommended. If the tumor invades the portal vein, combined resection and reconstruction of the portal vein are the treatment of choice to obtain a negative surgical margin.[29,36,37]

With these general principles in mind, to attain the margins free R0 resection status, which directly correlates with tumor prognosis, major hepatectomy may be occasionally required and sometimes additional pancreatoduodenectomy may also be needed.

1) Proximal cholangiocarcinoma

Entering into the 1990's, while extended hepatectomy including the caudate lobectomy and bile duct resection has improved the hilar cholangiocarcinoma R0 resection rate to above 50%, the mortality rate has also increased to more than 10% due to this extended surgical procedure. The 5-year survival rates after hepatectomy for hilar cholangiocarcinoma reported in literature published in the 1990's ranged from 20~40%.[38] Recent advances in precision preoperative intervention techniques such as preoperative percutaneous biliary drainage and preoperative portal vein embolization tend to be more effective in preventing hepatic failure after extended hepatectomy. Extended hemihepatectomy has therefore recently been recognized as the standard curative treatment for hilar cholangiocarcinoma with acceptable mortality.[39-41]

(1) Preoperative treatments

a. Percutaneous transhepatic biliary drainage (PTBD)

The aims of preoperative biliary drainage are the restoration of hepatic function and decreased postoperative morbidity and mortality after extended hepatectomy.[42-44] There are two types in the biliary drainage procedures: endoscopic technique and PTBD. Generally, as there is a higher risk of bile contamination and difficulty in obtaining intrahepatic bile duct imaging in endoscopic biliary drainage, the majority of institutions prefer PTBD as the preoperative biliary drainage procedure. However, in addition to recent reports claiming that preoperative PTBD only minimally affects postoperative course, other studies have demonstrated that preoperative PTBD causes bile contamination, which may lead to cholangitis and sepsis, as well as the possibility of catheter tract seeding of the tumor.[42-47]

To further clarify this question, Seyama et al extensively reviewed previous literature pertaining to opinions against preoperative PTBD, and found that since the curative resection rate was too low (around 15%), and that the majority of the curative resection procedures did not include hepatectomy, the analyzed data available to date did not conclusively evaluate the effectiveness of preoperative PTBD in curative resection including hepatectomy. It was also pointed out in the same study that if the total bilirubin fell to 10mg/dL 10~14 days after preoperative PTBD, surgery was conducted under conditions whereby hepatic function recuperation was inadequate. In contrast, several studies from Japanese colleagues have shown that in patients who received surgery after preoperative PTBD and full normalization of hepatic function as confirmed by a total bilirubin of less than 2.0 mg/dL, postoperative hepatic dysfunction was significantly reduced, which was stated to take approximately 4~6 weeks.[29,39,40]

It is not uncommon for preoperative PTBD to be accompanied by suppurative cholangitis, and postoperative bile contamination increases infectious complications and mortality. The mechanisms of cholangitis development are contaminated bile filling of the undrained area during cholangiography and inadequate bile drainage of the tube. In order to prevent or minimize cholangitis after PTBD, it is recommended that cholangiography should be limited to during PTBD catheter insertion on the afternoon of the day before surgery. The reason for this recommendation is that bile juice contamination usually occurs within 3 days of the procedure. However, irrespective of the cause, if and when cholangitis develops, the obstructed PTBD catheter should be made patent with antibiotic irrigation or a newly inserted tube. If an undrained duct is present, a new tube should be inserted via a percutaneous transhepatic route to drain the contaminated bile. Bacterial culture studies and antibiotic sensitivity tests of the drained bile have also been recommended.[29]

It has been reported by various investigators that catheter tract seeding of cholangiocarcinoma occurs in 5~10% of patients after PTBD,[39,48] and that since the majority were patients already with a far-advanced primary tumor disease, who later developed multiple recurrent disease, the tract seeding does not seem to significantly affect prognosis.[29] In a study by Sakata et al[48] it was reported that excision of the isolated metastasis along the catheter tract improved survival, and that while catheter seeding is not an uncommon complication of biliary malignancy, the overall incidence is generally acceptable. The above study also suggested that in selected cases, wide excision will afford long term survival.

b. Portal Vein Embolization (PVE)

In 1982, Makuuchi et al[49,50] performed PVE for the first time to prevent liver failure after extended hemihepatectomy in patients with hilar cholangiocarcinoma. Major hepatectomy leads to acute decrease in liver volume and sudden increase in the portal pressure. If preoperative PVE is performed, the degree of portal pressure increase and decrease in liver volume is lessened according to the atrophy-hypertrophy complex theory, thus reducing the risk of hepatic dysfunction after major hepatectomy.[29] Kubota et al[51] also suggested a PVE indication guideline utilizing the volume of a liver that is expected to be removed as calculated by CT volumetry, and ICG R15. Recent published data have shown that 2 weeks after PVE for patients with jaundice associated with hilar cholangiocarcinoma the remnant expected liver volume increase rate ranges from 8~12%, and that major hepatectomy is a safe procedure for such patients.[29,39,40,52-54]

c. Safe strategy for major hepatectomy in hilar cholangiocarcinoma

Seyama et al[29,40] have suggested a safe strategy for major hepatectomy with preoperative PTBD and PVE in hilar cholangiocarcinoma. A flow chart for preoperative treatment is shown in Fig. 3. If a patient shows evidence of

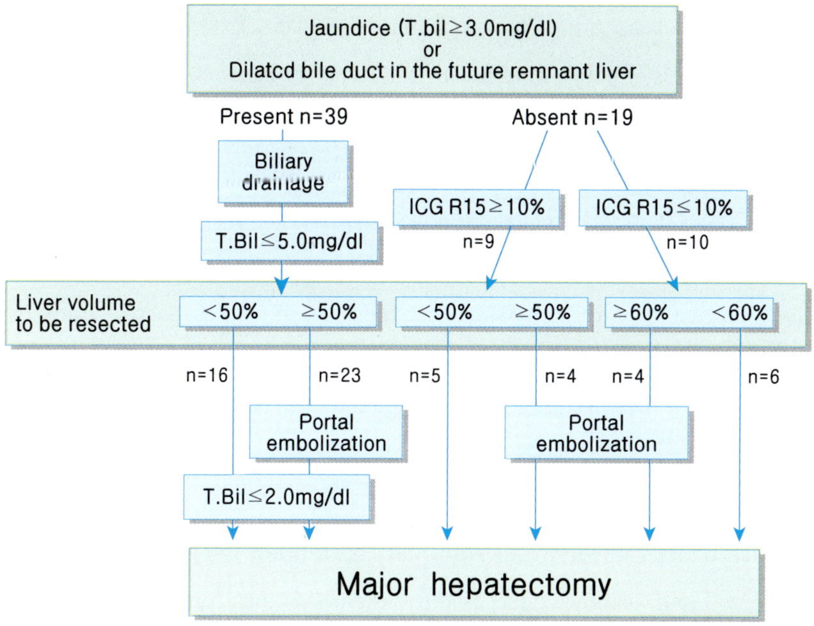

Fig. 3 Flow chart for preoperative treatment

T. Bil, serum total bilirubin concentration; ICG R15, indocyanine green retention rate at 15 minutes.[29,40]

jaundice or if there are dilated bile ducts in the future remnant liver, PTBD should be performed. Whether PVE is indicated depends on liver function and the volume of the future remnant liver, which is calculated by CT volumetry. In patients with normal liver function, i.e. an ICG R15 value under 10%, PVE is indicated when the future remnant liver volume is less than 40%. In patients with jaundice or an ICG R15 value over 10%, PVE is indicated if the future remnant hemiliver volume is less than 50%. As the standard operative procedure for hilar cholangiocarcinoma consists of extended hemihepatectomy including the caudate lobe, the remaining hemiliver volume should have a margin from the safety zone. After reevaluation of the liver volume to be resected, hepatectomy should be performed if the patient fulfilled the criteria.[29]

(2) Surgical treatment for hilar cholangiocarcinoma

To achieve radical resection of hilar cholangiocarcinomas, two important factors should be taken into consideration: The first is removal of the liver parenchyme adjacent to the hepatic hilum as well as the hilar plate. Extended right or left hemihepatectomy is effective in removing the tumor invasion of the right and left bile duct. The second is resection of the caudate lobe and the inferior area of segment IV in order to remove the cancer infiltration to the fine bile ducts around the hilum.[29] After being firstly suggested by Nimura et al, many Japanese authors have described the necessity of resecting the caudate lobe.[55-57] The clinical significance of caudate resection was first reported in a retrospective study by Sugiura et al[58], that showed that the 5-year survival rate was 46% in patients who received caudate lobectomy as opposed to 12% in those who did not.

a. Extended hemihepatectomy

Because of its radicalty and simplicity, extended hemihepatectomy is recognized and acknowledged as the standard surgical procedure for hilar cholangiocarcinoma.[29,39,40,52] Extended right hemihepatectomy comprises resection of the right liver, the inferior part of Couinaud's segment IV, and the entire caudate lobe, while extended left hemihepatectomy comprises resection

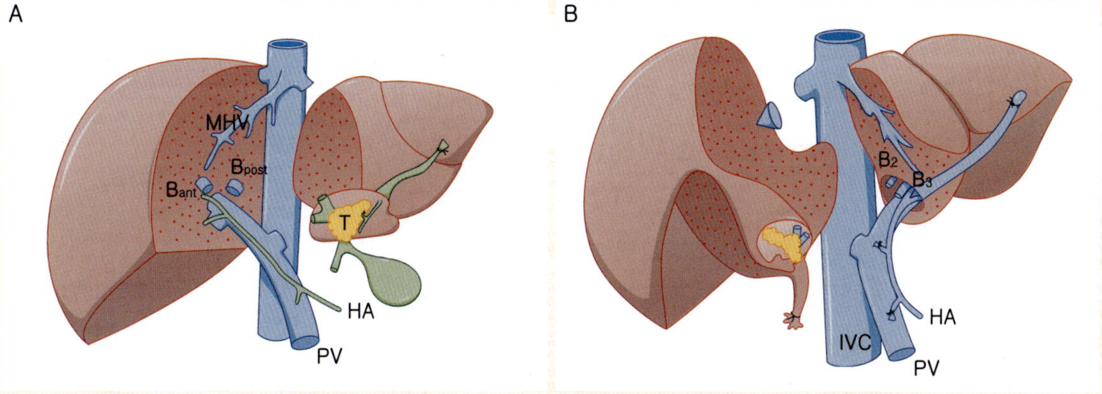

Fig. 4 Standard surgery for hilar cholangiocarcinoma

A: Extended left hemihepatectomy with caudate lobectomy and extrahepatic bile duct resection; B: Extended Right hemihepatectomy with caudate lobectomy and extrahepatic bile duct resection, Green area, resected organ and tissues; HA, hepatic artery; PV, portal Vein; MHV, middle hepatic vein; Bant, anterior branch of intrahepatic bile duct; Bpost, posterior branch of intrahepatic bile duct; T, tumor.

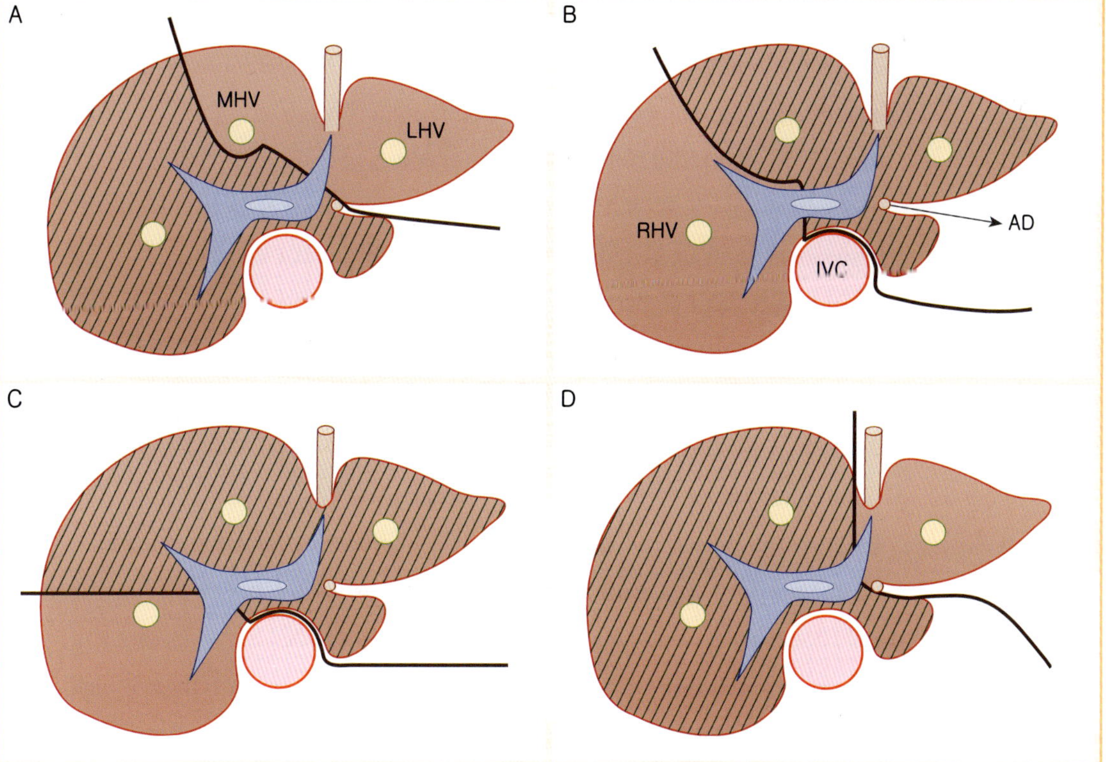

Fig. 5 Resection lines in various types of hepatectomy with caudate lobectomy for hilar cholangiocarcinoma

A: Extended right hemihepatectomy; B: Extended left hemihepatectomy; C: Left trisectionectomy; D: Right trisectionectomy. Red lines, resection lines; Green area, resected liver parenchyme; Brown area, resected branches of portal veins. RHV, right hepatic vein; MHV, middle hepatic vein; LHV, left hepatic vein; AD, Arantius duct.

of the left liver, the ventral part of the anterior segment, and most of the caudate lobe (Fig. 4) (Fig. 5). Even in patients with Bismuth type I or type II lesions, extended hemihepatectomy may be necessary to achieve successful curative resection according to the mode of tumor extension.[29,39,40,52]

b. Right or left trisectionectomy

Trisectionectomy is sometimes required for curative resection in hilar cholangiocarcinoma that widely spreads into the hepatic hilum (Fig. 5). Right or left trisectionectomy is advantageous in obtaining a cancer-free-margin of the hepatic duct. Previous studies[29,59,60] have reported that negative proximal margins were observed after left trisectionectomy in 75% of patients, and in 87.5% of patients after right trisectionectomy, and these figures are significantly higher than that for extended hemihepatectomy procedures. However, since the operative risk after trisectionectomy is greater than that of extended hemihepatectomy, preoperative PTBD and PVE are strongly advised. Despite preoperative PVE, Nagino et al[60] reported a 7.1% mortality rate. However, Shimada et al[59] observed a zero mortality among 12 consecutive patients with hilar cholangiocarcinoma who received left trisectionectomy after routine preoperative PTBD and PVE. Therefore, for patients with hilar cholangiocarcinoma who are planning to undergo radical high-risk surgery such as trisectionectomy, proper patient selection and adequate preoperative treatment is required.

c. Limited resections for hilar cholangiocarcinoma

Parenchyma preserving hepatectomy is a less invasive procedure for hilar cholangiocarcinoma patients, which comprises various forms of hepatic resection, such as segmental (S4 or S1), S4+S1 or S4a+S5+S1. A drawback of this procedure is that since the tumor spreads along the bile duct, there is high incidence of tumor involvement of the resection margin.[29,61,62] Another problem is the complexity of the surgical procedure which entails lengthy operation time, significant intraoperative bleeding, and difficult biliary reconstruction. Consequently, parenchyma preserving hepatectomy for hilar cholangiocarcinoma should be reserved as an alternative procedure for patients with poor general condition or those with high-risk factors.

Bile duct resection without hepatectomy is the least radical surgical treatment method. This procedure is only indicated for patients with an early stage primary tumor that is located in the middle of the common hepatic duct, and which is not accompanied by invasion or metastasis.

(3) Prognosis of proximal cholangiocarcinoma

The resectability and curability of proximal cholangiocarcinomas has significantly improved with major hepatectomy. Launois et al[63] reviewed past literatures and found that there was a positive correlation between the resectability rate and the proportion of patients who received hepatectomy. This was further confirmed by Makuuchi et al[29] who showed that there was significant positive correlation between the major hepatectomy rate and curative resection rate. Early reports from the 1990's, when major hepatectomy that included caudate lobectomy was first introduced, have described 5-year survival rates of 25~35%, while reports after 2000 reported higher and improved survival rates of 35~40%.[29] Also, the initially high 10~20% postoperative hepatic dysfunction and mortality rates have been considered as one of the weaknesses of this procedure, but this rate has markedly decreased to approximately 5% after active employment of preoperative PTBD and PVE.[29]

2) Middle and distal bile duct cancer

The rate of lymph node metastasis in patients with middle and distal bile duct cancer is approximately 40%, and the resection rate is reported to be 40~90%. After radical resection, the 5-year survival rate is 20~30%, and known prognostic factors are histological tumor characteristics, lymph node metastasis status, and curability of surgery. Invasion characteristics of middle and distal cholangiocarcinoma, which are different from proximal tumors, are less frequent vertical invasion with submucosal spread and perineural invasion, and more frequent lymph node metastasis. Therefore, while it is crucial to attain negative resection margins in proximal tumors, extended lymph node dissection is of greater importance in middle and distal cholangiocarcinomas.

If preoperative studies demonstrate vascular invasion by the tumor, then successful radical resection is often difficult to achieve, but if the length of invaded portal vein is less than 2 cm, the combined resection with portal vein may be attempted. Also, while radical resection is considered to be contra-indicated in the presence of positive N2 level lymph nodes (hilar lymph nods, superior mesentericartery lymph nodes and celiac lymph nodes), Nagakawa et al[64] have shown a 14% 5-year survival rate after radical resection with extended lymph node dissection.

Pancreatoduodenectomy is commonly undertaken as standard radical surgery for middle and distal bile duct cancers. For middle bile duct cancer, it is occasionally difficult to achieve negative proximal resection margins with this procedure, and as it is anatomically proximate to the right hepatic artery and right portal vein, care should be taken as radical resection is sometimes difficult due to the presence of vascular invasion.

(1) Preoperative treatments

In the past, preoperative bile duct drainage for middle and distal bile duct cancer was conducted in order to reduce postoperative morbidities after pancreatoduodenectomy, but controversies existed as to whether drainage is necessary as reports showed significantly increased postoperative complications after bile duct drainage. In a study by Povoski et al[65] which analyzed 240 patients who underwent preoperative bile duct drainage and subsequent pancreatoduodenectomy, it was found that patients who received preoperative bile duct drainage were at significantly higher risk for postoperative intraabdominal infections such as abscess, and increased morbidities and mortalities, and suggesting therefore that preoperative bile duct drainage should be avoided if possible in patients with resectable peripancreatic cancers.

In another large study by Sohn et al[66] that reviewed 567 patients who received preoperative bile duct drainage and pancreatoduodenectomy, there was no significantly increased incidence of postoperative complications or mortality rates, but rather an increased number of patients who developed pancreatic fistula and wound infections. Therefore, as there is an increased risk for postoperative infection complications in patients who undergo preoperative bile duct drainage and pancreatoduodenectomy for middle and distal bile duct cancer, it is generally thought that such drainage should be avoided. In particular, endoscopic bile duct drainage may often lead to postoperative cholangitis, pancreatitis, bleeding and perforation, meaning that even more caution should be taken when considering this type of procedure. Preoperative bile duct drainage could be selectively performed prior to pancreatoduodenectomy in patients with severe cholangitis, severe pruritus due to jaundice, and in those patients for whom preoperative anticancer chemotherapy is planned.

(2) Surgical treatment of middle and distal cholangiocarcinoma

Because bile duct cancer is accompanied by early lymph node metastasis and longitudinal tumor invasion, radical bile duct resection without pancreato-duodenectomy is rarely performed in early stage patients without local invasion, but rather in most patients with middle and distal cholangiocarcinoma.

There are two differing standpoints regarding lymph node dissection during pancreatoduodenectomy: one is the classical dissection of lymph nodes surrounding the main tumor, and the other is extensive lymph node dissection. Yeo et al[67] of Johns Hopkins University studied 294 periampullary cancer patients who underwent pancreatoduodenectomy, and reported that there was no difference in long term survival between patients who received standard surgery with peripancreatic lymph node dissection and those who underwent extensive dissection with retroperitoneal lymph node dissection and distal gastrectomy. Also, according to the study, there was significantly increased incidence of complications such as temporal delays in emptying of the stomach and pancreatic fistula in the extensive lymph node dissection group (43% vs. 29%). However, in middle and distal cholangiocarcinoma patients, early metastasis to lymph nodes occurs, and up to 50% of patients are found to be with positive nodes at the time of surgery. If pancreatic invasion is present, the patterns of lymph node metastasis are the same as in pancreatic cancer. Therefore extensive lymph node dissection is performed, which includes lymph nodes in the hepatoduodenal ligament, lymph nodes around common hepatic artery, lymph nodes around superior mesenteric artery and paraaortic lymph nodes. Paraaortic lymph node metastasis is present in approximately half of the patients with pancreas invasion, and since the prognosis is poor for these patients, it is generally accepted that extended radical resection be avoided when intraoperative paraaortic lymph nodes are found to be positive for metastasis.

Until the 1970's, classical pancreatoduodenectomy had been the standard surgery for middle and distal cholangiocarcinomas. However, in order to reduce complications that arose after gastrectomy and also in an effort to improve the quality of life, Traverso et al (1978) proposed pylorus preserving pancreatoduodenectomy. Subsequent researchers observed that there was no significant difference in regards to complication rates and long term survival rates between the above two surgical methods.[68-70] Presently, pylorus preserving pancreatoduodenectomy is the standard surgery for the treatment of patients with middle and distal cholangiocarcinomas (Fig. 6). Classical pancreatoduodenectomy is currently limited to three categories of patients; those with suspected tumor invasion in the duodenal bulb, those with a history of peptic ulcers in the duodenum or distal stomach and those with middle cholangiocarcinomas with gross invasion in the surrounding tissues.

Reconstruction methods of the remnant stomach or duodenum, bile duct and pancreas after pancreatoduodenectomy are dependent on whether the resected pancreas is anastomosed to the jejunum or to the stomach, in what sequence the pancreas-bile duct-duodenum is going to be anastomosed, and by what method is the pancreas and intestine going to be joined together.

According to a study in 2001 by the Japanese Pancreatic Surgery Club (JPSC), out of a total of 3109 cases of pancreatoduodenectomy, there were 2483 (82.9%) patients who underwent pancreaticojejunostomy, and 511 (17.1%) who underwent pancreaticogastrostomy. One thousand five hundred and two of the pancreatico-jejunostomy patients and 106 of the pancreaticogastrostomy patients received mucosa-to-mucosa anastomosis, while the rest of them underwent anastomosis by the dunking method. In another similar review, Yeo et al[71] observed that out of a total of 650 cases of pancreatoduodenectomy, pancreaticojejunostomy was performed in 71%, and pancreaticogastrostomy in 29% of the cases.

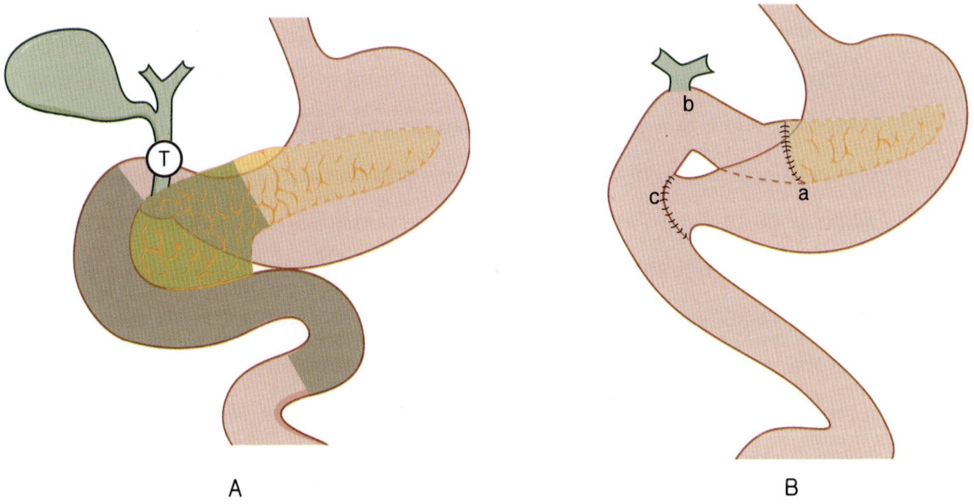

Fig. 6 Pylorus preserving pancreatoduodenectomy

A: Preoperative picture; B: postoperative picture after reconstruction. Green area, Tissues to be resected; T, tumor; a, pancreaticojejunostomy; b, hepaticojejunostomy; c. duodenojejunostomy.

Postoperative pancreatic fistula after pancreaticointestinal anastomosis is a significant cause of morbidity and mortality after pancreatoduodenectomy, and occurs in 5~15% of patients. While the majority of patients are successfully managed by conservative measures, severe complications such as sepsis and bleeding occur in 5% of patients. Risk factors for pancreatic fistula development are small calibered pancreatic duct (<4mm in diameter) and soft pancreas. Other authors have also reported the amount of intraoperative blood loss and duration of operation. Yeo et al[72] observed in a randomized prospective study of 145 pancreatoduodenectomy patients that there was no significant difference in pancreatic fistula rates between pancreaticojejunostomy and pancreaticogastrostomy patients.

The sequence of anastomosis of the pancreas, duodenum, and bile ducts after pylorus preserving pancreatoduodenectomy also varies, and most often the Traverso method is employed, in which the sequence of anastomosis is pancreas-bile duct-duodenum. This method may have a disadvantage in that since the duodenojejunostomy is accomplished last, there is a possibility of iatrogenic A-loop formation. A method introduced in 1960 by Imanaga, in which after end-to-end anastomosis of the remnant duodenum and jenunum, anastomosis is performed in pancreas-duodenum order, which does not result in A-loop formation, and is considered to be an extremely physiological reconstruction since ingested food is mixed with pancreas juice and bile at the proximal jejunum. In addition, postoperative endoscopic evaluation of the bile duct and pancreatic duct is facilitated. While there is concern of an increased risk for marginal ulcers and reflux cholangitis compared to the Traverso method, it was shown by Hishinuma et al that in a study of 55 patients who received reconstruction by the Imanaga method, that there was no observed increased incidence of marginal ulcers or reflux cholangitis compared to the Traverso method.

In summary, there are various methods of reconstruction after pancreato-duodenectomy. It is therefore difficult to determine which one is superior to the others. It is considered that careful patient selection and tailored surgery for each individual patient is an important aspect of this question.

3) Diffuse type of extrahepatic cholangiocarcinoma

In patients where there is longitudinal tumor spread from the hepatic duct to the intrapancreatic bile duct, or wherein massive lymph node metastasis presents not only around the bile duct but also involves the posterior aspect of the pancreatic head, the only option is to perform extended surgery such as hepatopancreatoduodenectomy (HPD) to achieve radical therapy. As the status of the lymph nodes is an important prognostic factor, radical resection may not be a definitive indication in the presence of multiple lymph node metastases. Hospital mortality rates have been reported to be a very high 35% by Nimura et al[73], while the 5 year survival rates after this radical resection were dismal (not exceeding 6%). The main reasons for mortality after HPD are postoperative liver failure and leakage of the pancreatojejunostomy site caused by bleeding from a major artery. To overcome these problems, Miyagawa et al[74] performed PTBD followed by PVE and staged reconstruction of the pancreaticojejunostomy in twelve consecutive cases of HPD, and showed that all patients recovered without any mortality cases. Considering the fact that diffuse advanced extrahepatic cholangiocarcinoma is accompanied by high mortality and low survival rates, caution should be exercised when selecting HPD as a treatment modality. The ideal indication for this procedure would be a grossly resectable Bismuth type 2 proximal cholangiocarcinoma with superficial spreading to the right and left hepatic duct and the intrapancreatic part of the common bile duct.

4) Extrahepatic cholangiocarcinoma with vascular invasion

There still exists a controversy as to whether major hepatectomy with combined vascular resection and reconstruction is suitable for radical resection for patients with extrahepatic cholangiocarcinoma that invades the portal vein or hepatic artery. In the past, vascular invasion of extrahepatic cholangiocarcinoma meant an unresectable tumor, but recent reports have shown favorable outcomes after major hepatectomy followed by portal vein resection and reconstruction. Neuhaus et al[75] reported a 5-year survival rate of 65% after curative resection of hilar cholangiocarcinoma patients with portal vein resection and reconstruction. However, their case series showed a postoperative mortality rate of 17%, which was in agreement with other previous rates of 10~20%. Recent reports have demonstrated marked improvement in survival for patients who underwent preoperative PVE before major hepatectomy with portal vein resection.[39,40,52]

There is as yet insufficient evidence that supports the clinical significance of major hepatectomy with hepatic artery reconstruction for cholangiocarcinoma patients. Since the cholangiocarcinoma that invades the hepatic artery is usually a locally far advanced tumor, combined resection of hepatic artery is less frequently performed compared to combined resection of portal vein. Even though some recent data have shown an acceptable postoperative mortality rate of 0~8% after major hepatectomy with reconstruction of the hepatic artery,[76,77] a lot more still largely holds that this procedure is more dangerous than major hepatectomy without reconstruction. Thus, major hepatectomy with reconstruction of hepatic artery should be advocated if the tumor can be resected without residual tumor at any surgical margin.[29]

3. Liver Transplantation for Cholangiocarcinoma

Cholangiocarcinoma patients who may be eligible for liver transplantation include those with intrahepatic cholangiocarcinomas and proximal extrahepatic cholangiocarcinoma, both of whom hepatectomy is essential in order to attain curative treatment for the cholangiocarcinoma.

Studies in the early 1990 had observed that the 5-year survival rates for liver transplantation patients with unresectable intrahepatic cholangiocarcinoma and unresectable proximal bile duct cancer were a very poor 0~23% and 0~17%, respectively.[78-82] Therefore, due to such hopeless outcomes of liver transplantation for unresectable cholangiocarcinomas, most institutions have excluded cholangiocarcinoma patients as candidates for transplantation.[83-86] As a result, only conservative treatments are available for patients with unresectable cholangiocarcinomas. Therefore, most patients experience early death due to cachexia and sepsis arising from cholangitis.

In a recent large scale study by a group from Spain, it was reported that in patients who received liver transplantation for unresectable cholangiocarcinomas without hematogenous spread, the 1, 3 and 5-year survival rates for proximal bile duct cancer and intrahepatic cholangiocarcinomas were 82%, 53%, 30%, and 77%, 65%, 42%, respectively. While these figures may have some oncological significance,[87-89] they are still a far cry from success rates for general liver transplantation. Since there is moreover a shortage of brain dead donors, liver transplantation for cholangiocarcinomas remains a subject of debate.

A German group, Neuhaus et al[90,91] showed a 5-year survival rate of 40% in unresectable cholangiocarcinoma patients who underwent a procedure combining liver transplantation and pancreatoduodenectomy, the so-called extended bile duct resection, while Gores et al[92] from the United States followed up primary sclerosing cholangitis patients, which is one of the risk factors for intrahepatic cholangiocarcinoma in Western countries, with Positron emission tomography (PET) and serum CA 19-9 (greater than 100 U/ml) to attempt early detection of intrahepatic cholangiocarcinoma. It was shown in the latter series that the two screening methods resulted in a sensitivity and specificity of 75% and 80% which were significantly higher than the early detection rate for endoscopic brush cytology. In addition, researchers from the Mayo Clinic administered preoperative chemoradiotherapy for 3 ~4 weeks in such early detected intrahepatic cholangiocarcinoma and proximal bile duct cancer. Two to 6 weeks later, all patients underwent an exploratory laparotomy to evaluate for disease spread outside the bile ducts and liver. Celiac and peripancreatic lymph nodes and nodes along the distal common bile duct and the hepatic artery were removed to confirm local extension. The liver hilum was not dissected, and the perihilar nodes were not removed. Patients were activated for the United Network for Organ Sharing (UNOS) waiting list at the time of the negative exploratory laparotomy. The final result was 38 liver transplantations, and the reported 1, 3 and 5-year survival rates were 92%, 82% and 82%, respectively. It was concluded that liver transplantation was not contraindicated absolutely for patients with unresectable intrahepatic cholangiocarcinoma and proximal bile duct cancer.[93-95] In summary, the conclusions stated by the above two studies from the German Neuhause group and the United States Mayo group need to be ascertained further by different institutions.

Jonas et al[96] commented that a 5-year survival rate of 40~60% after liver transplantation for unresectable proximal bile duct cancer and intrahepatic cholangiocarcinoma is a significant finding with respect to oncological aspect, but also opinionated that this procedure is still under debate due to the shortage of deceased donor organs. Living donor liver transplantation for unresectable cholangio-carcinomas, which has become widespread since 2000, has been proposed as a modality that may simultaneously reflect positive oncological viewpoints and that which may be able to solve the shortage problem of deceased donor organs.

In conclusion, as the majority of patients with intrahepatic cholangiocarcinoma or proximal bile duct cancer are not accompanied by liver cirrhosis, radical bile duct resection with major hepatectomy should be considered as the treatment of choice. This modality should also be a strongly advised even if the tumor directly invades the liver parenchyma or if there is partial invasion of the vessels or of the lymph nodes. In cases involving the presence of multiple hepatic metastases, direct invasion of surrounding organs, or hematogenous spread to other organs, conservative or symptomatic treatment should be advised. In selected patients with possible stage 1 or 2 cholangiocarcinoma, the location of the tumor may make it surgically unresectable while the presence of medical disease of the liver or bile duct may exclude major hepatectomy, or the major hepatectomy alone may not be able to adequately treat the cancer. It is thought that in such patients, deceased donor liver transplantation may afford comparable oncological outcomes with respect to conservative treatment results, but at present, the shortage of deceased donor organs has not fully supported liver transplantation as a treatment modality in patients with unresectable cholangiocarcinoma. Therefore, in order to improve survival rates, it is suggested that extended bile duct resection and living donor liver transplantation be advised for unresectable intrahepatic cholangiocarcinoma or proximal bile duct cancer after informing them of a presumed long term survival rate (20~40%) and obtaining consent as such, or, for cholangiocarcinoma with preoperative chemoradiotherapy after screening and early detection in specific patients with bile duct disease who are at risk of cholangiocarcinoma.

Reference

1. Lazaridis KN, Gores GJ. Cholangiocarcinoma. In: Boyer TD, Wright TL, Manns MP. Zakim and Boyer's Hepatology: Textbook of Liver Disease. 5th edi. Canada: Saunder Elsevier, 2006:1133-1146.
2. Khan SA, Davidson BR, Goldin R, et al. Guidelines for the diagnosis and management of cholangiocarcinoma. Gut 2002;51(suppl 6):1-9.
3. Lang H, Sotiropoulos GC, Fruhauf NR, et al. Extended hepatectomy for intrahepatic cholangiocellular carcinoma. Ann Surg 2005;241:134-143.
4. Jarnagin WR, Shoup M. Surgical management of cholangiocarcinoma. Semin Liver Dis 2004;24:189-199.
5. Robles R, Figueras J, Turrion VS, et al. Spanish experience in liver transplantation for hilar and peripheral cholangiocarcinoma. Ann Surg 2004;239:265-271.
6. Jonas S, Mittler J, Pascher A, et al. Extended indications in living-donor liver transplantation: bile duct cancer. Transpl 2005;80:S101-S104.
7. Nakeeb A, Pitt HA, Sohn TA, et al. Cholangiocarcinoma: a spectrum of intrahepatic , perihilar and distal tumors. Ann Surg 1996;224:463-473.
8. Patel T. Increasing incidence and mortality of primary intrahepatic Cholangiocarcinoma in the United States. Hepatology 2001;33:1353-1357.

9. Berdah SV, Delpero JR, Garcia S, et al. A western surgical experience of peripheral cholangiocarcinoma. Br J Surg 1996;83:1517-1521.

10. Chu KM, Lai EC, Al-Hadeedi S, et al. Intrahepatic cholangiocarcinoma. World J Surg 1997;21:301-305.

11. Weimann A, Varnholt H, Schlitt HJ, et al. Retrospective analysis of prognostic factors after liver resection and transplantation for cholangiocarcinoma. Br J Surg 2000;87:1182-1187.

12. Lee HS. Korean Sciety of Liver Surgeons. Surgical treatment of primary liver cancer in Korea. In: Korean Foundation for Cancer Research. The proceedings of 10th Seoul international cancer symposium. 1997: 11.

13. Lee KW. Treatment of intrahepatic cholangiocarcinoma. In: The Korean Society of Gastroenterology. Primary liver cancer. 1st edi. Seoul: Gunja, 2001:177-182.

14. Nakajima T, Kondo Y, Miyazaki M, Okui K. A histopathologic study of 102 cases of intrahepatic cholangiocarcinoma: histologic classification and modes of spreading. Hum Pathol 1988;19:1228-1234.

15. Yamamoto J, Kosuge T, Takayama T, et al. Surgical treatment of intrahepatic cholangiocarcinoma: four patients surviving more than five years. Surgery 1992;111: 617-622.

16. Ohashi K, Nakajima Y, Tsutsumi M, et al. Clinical characteristics and proliferating activity of intrahepatic cholangiocarcinoma. J Gastroenterol Hepatol 1994;9:442-446.

17. Yamanaka N, Okamoto E, Ando T, et al. Clinicopathologic spectrum of resected extraductal mass-forming intrahepatic cholangiocarcinoma. Cancer 1995;76:2449-2456.

18. Sasaki A, Aramaki M, Kawano K, et al. Intrahepatic peripheral cholangiocarcinoma: mode of spread and choice of surgical treatment. Br J Surg 1998;85:1206-1209.

19. The Liver Cancer Study Group of Japan. Primary liver cancer in Japan. Ann Surg 1990;211:277-287.

20. Terada T, Kida T, Nakanuma Y, Kurumaya H, Doishita K, Takayanagi N. Intrahepatic cholangiocarcinomas associated with nonbiliary cirrhosis. A clinicopathologic study. J Clin Gastroenterol 1994;18:335-342.

21. Yamamoto M, Takasaki K, Nakano M, Saito A. Minute nodular intrahepatic cholangiocarcinoma. Cancer 1998;82:2145-2149.

22. Madariaga JR, Iwatsuki S, Todo S, Lee RG, Irish W, Starzl TE. Liver resection for hilar and peripheral cholangiocarcinomas: A study of 62 cases. Ann Surg 1998;227:70-79.

23. Yamamoto M, Takasaki K, Yoshikawa T. Lymph node metastasis in intrahepatic cholangiocarcinoma. Jpn J Clin Oncol 1999;29:147-150.

24. Tsuji T, Hiraoka T, Kanemitsu K, Takaamori H, Tanabe D, Tashiro S. Lymphatic spreading pattern of intrahepatic cholangiocarcinoma. Surgery 2001;129:410-407.

25. Aishima S, Kuroda Y, Nishihara Y, et al. Proposal of progression model for intrahepatic cholangiocarcinoma: Clinicopathologic differences between hilar type and peripheral type. Am J Surg Pathol 2007;31:1059-1067.

26. Shimada K, Sano T, Sakamoto Y, Esaki M, Kosuge T, Ojima H. Clinical impact of the surgical margin status in hepatectomy for solitary mass-forming type intrahepatic cholangiocarcinoma without lymph node metastasis. J Surg Oncol 2007;96:160-165.

27. Gulluoglu MG, Ozden I, Poyanli A, Cevikbas U, Ariogul O. Intraductal growth-type mucin-producing peripheral cholangiocarcinoma associated with biliary papillomatosis. Ann Diagnostic Pathology 2007;11:34-38.

28. Suh KS, Roh HR, Koh YT, Lee KU, Park YH, Kim SW. Clinicopathological features of the intraductal growth type of peripheral cholangiocarcinoma. Hepatology 2000;31:12-17.

29. Seyama Y, Makuuchi M. Current surgical treatment for bile duct cancer. World J Gastroenterol 2007;13:1505-1515.

30. Bhuiya MR, Nimura Y, Kamiya J, et al. Clinicopathologic studies on perineural invasion of bile duct carcinoma. Ann Surg 1992;215:344-349.

31. Ogura Y, Takahashi K, Tabata M, Mizumoto R. Clinicopathological study on carcinoma of the extrahepatic bile duct with special focus on cancer invasion on the surgical margins. World J Surg 1994;18:778-784.

32. Sakamoto E, Nimura Y, Hayakawa N, et al. The pattern of infiltration at the proximal border of hilar bile duct carcinoma: a histologic analysis of 62 resected cases. Ann Surg 1998;227:405-411.

33. Ebata T, Wadanabe H, Ajioka Y, Oda K, Nimura Y. Pathological appraisal of lines of resection for bile duct carcinoma. Br J Surg 2002;89:1260-1267.

34. Kayahara M, Nagakawa T, Ohta T, Kitagawa H, Tajima H, Miwa K. Role of nodal involvement and the periductal soft-tissue margin in middle and distal bile duct cancer. Ann Surg 1999;229:76-83.

35. Kosuge T, Yamamoto J, Shimada K, Yamasaki S, Makuuchi M. Improved surgical results for hilar cholangiocarcinoma with procedures including major hepatic resection. Ann Surg 1999;230:663-671.

36. Nimura Y, Hayakawa N, Kamiya J, et al. Combined portal vein and liver resection for carcinoma of the biliary tract. Br J Surg 1991;78:727-731.

37. Ebata T, Nagino M, Kamiya J, Uesaka K, Nagasaka T, Nimura Y. Hepatectomy with portal vein resection for hilar cholangiocarcinoma: audit of 52 consecutive cases. Ann Surg 2003;238:720-727.

38. Chamberlain RS, Blumgart LH. Hilar cholangiocarcinoma: a review and commentary. Ann Surg Oncol 2000;7:55-66.

39. Kawasaki S, Imammura H, Kobayashi A, Noike T, Miwa S, Miyagawa S. Results of surgical resection for patients with hilar bile duct cancer: application of extended hemihepatectomy after biliary drainage and hemihepatic portal vein embolization. Ann Surg 2003;238:84-92.

40. Seyama Y, Kubota K, Sano K, et al. Long-term outcome of extended hemihepatectomy for hilar bile duct cancer with no mortality and high survival rate. Ann Surg 2003;238:73-83.

41. Hemming AW, Reed AI, Fujita S, Foley DP, Howard RJ. Surgical management of hilar cholangiocarcinoma. Ann Surg 2005;241:693-699.

42. Blamey SL, Fearon KC, Gilmour WH, Osborne DH, Carter DC. Prediction of risk in biliary surgery. Br J Surg 1983;70:535-538.

43. Gundry SR, Strodel WE, Knol JA, Eckhauser FE, Thompson NW. Efficacy of preoperative biliary tract decompression in patients with obstructive jaundice. Arch Surg 1984;119:703-708.

44. Pitt HA, Gomes AS, Lois JF, Mann LL, Deutch LS, Longmire WP Jr. Does preoperative percutaneous biliary drainage reduce operative risk or increase hospital cost? Ann Surg 1985;201:545-553.

45. Hochwald SN, Burke EC, Jarnagin WR, Fong Y, Blumgart LH. Association of biliary stenting with increased postoperative infectious complication in proximal cholangiocarcinoma. Arch Surg 1999;134:261-266.

46. Cherqui D, Benoist S, Malassagne B, Humeres R, Rodriguez V, Fagniez PL. Major liver resection for carcinoma in jaundiced patients without preoperative biliary drainage. Arch Surg 2000;135:302-308.

47. Mansfield SD, Barakat O, Charnley RM, et al. Management of hilar cholangiocarcinoma in the North of England: pathology, treatment, and outcome. World J Gastroenterol 2005;11:7625-7630.

48. Sakata J, Shirai Y, Wakai T, Nomura T, Sakata E, Hatakeyama K. Catheter tract implantation metastases associated with percutaneous biliary drainage for extrahepatic cholangiocarcinoma. World J Gastroenterol 2005;11:7024-7027.

49. Makuuchi M, Takayasu K, Takuma T, et al. Preoperative transcatheter embolization of the portal venous branch for patients receiving extended lobectomy due to the bile duct carcinoma. J Jpn surg Assoc 1984:45:1558-1564.

50. Makuuchi M, Thai BL, Takayasu K, et al. Preoperative portal embolization to increase safty of major hepatectomy for hilar bile duct carcinoma: a preliminary report. Surgery 1990;107:521-527.

51. Kubota K, Makuuchi M, Kusaka K, et al. Measurement of liver volume and hepatic functional reserve as a guide to decision-making in resectional surgery for hepatic tumor. Hepatology 1997;26:1176-1181.

52. Kondo S, Hirano S, Ambo Y, et al. Forty consecutive resections of hilar cholangiocarcinoma with no postoperative mortality and no positive duct margins: results of a prospective study. Ann Surg 2004;240:95-101.

53. Imamura H, Shimada R, Kubota M, et al. Preoperative portal vein embolization: an audit of 84 patients. Hepatology 1999;29:1099-1105.

54. Takayama T, Makuuchi M. Preoperative portal embolization: is it useful? J Hepatobiliary Pancreat Surg 2004;11:17-20.

55. Mizumoto R, Suzuki H, Surgical anatomy of the hepatic hilum with special reference to the caudate lobe. World J Surg 1988;12:2-10.
56. Nimura Y, Hayakawa N, Kamiya J, Kondo S, Shionoya S. Hepatic segmentation with caudate lobe resection bile duct carcinoma of the hepatic hilus. World J Surg 1990;14:535-543.
57. Ogura Y, Mizumoto R, Tabata M, Matsuda S, Kusuda T. Surgical treatment of carcinoma of the hepatic duct confluence: analysis of 55 resected carcinomas. World J Surg 1993;17:85-92.
58. Sugiura Y, Nakamura S, Lida S, et al. Extensive resection of the bile ducts combined with liver resection for cancer of the main hepatic duct junction: a cooperative study of the Keio Bile Duct Cancer Study Group. Surgery 1994;115:445-451.
59. Shimada K, Sano T, Sakamoto Y, Kosuke T. Safty and effectiveness of left hepatic trisegmentectomy for hilar cholangiocarcinoma. World J Surg 2005;29:723-727.
60. Nagino M, Kamiya J, Arai T, Nishio H, Ebata T, Nimura Y. "Anatomic" right hepatic trisectionectomy (extended right hepatectomy) with caudate lobectomy for hilar cholangiocarcinoma. Ann Surg 2006;243:28-32.
61. Miyazaki M, Ito H, Nakagawa K, et al. Segments I and IV resection as a new approach for hepatic hilar cholangiocarcinoma. Am J Surg 1998;175:229-231.
62. Nagino M, Nimura Y, Kamiya J, et al. Segmental liver resection for hilar cholangiocarcinoma. Hepatogastroenterology 1998;45:7-13.
63. Launois B, Terblanche J, Lakehal M, et al. Proximal bile duct cancer: high resectability rate and 5-year survival. Ann Surg 1999;230:266-275.
64. Nagakawa T, Kayahara M, Ikeda S et al. Biliary cancer treatment: results from the Biliary Tract Cancer Registry in Japan. J Hepatobiliary Pancreat Surg 2002;9:569-575.
65. Povoski SP, Karpeh MS, Conlon KC, Blumgart LH, Brennan MF. Association of preoperative biliary drainage with postoperative outcome following pancreatoduodenectomy. Ann Surg 1999;230:131-142.
66. Sohn TA, Yeo CJ, Cameron JL, Pitt HA, Lillemoe KD. Do biliary stents increase postpancreaticoduodenectomy complications? J Gastrointest Surg 2000;4:258-268.
67. Yeo CJ, Cameron JL, Sohn TA et al. Pancreaticoduodenectomy with or without extended retroperitoneal lymphadenectomy for periampullary adenocarcinoma: Comparison of morbidity and mortality and short-term outcome. Ann Surg 1999;299:613-624.
68. Seiler CA, Wagner M, Sadowski C, Kulli C, Buchler MW. Randomized prospective trial of pylorus-preserving vs. classic duodenopancreatectomy (Whipple procedure): initial clinical results. J Gastrointest Surg 2000;4:443-452.
69. Tran KT, Smeenk HG, Van Eijck CH, et al. Pylorus-preserving pancreaticoduodenectomy versus standard Whipple procedure: a prospective, randomized, multicenter analysis of 170 patients with pancreatic and periampullary tumors. Ann Surg 2004;240:738-745.

70. Yeo CJ, Cameron JL, Lillemoe KD, Sohn TA, et al. Pancreaticoduodenectomy with or without distal gastrectomy and extended retroperitoneal lymphadenectomy for periampullary adenocarcinoma, part 2: randomized controlled trial evaluating survival, morbidity, and mortality. Ann Surg 2002;236:355-366.

71. Yeo CJ, Cameron JL, Sohn TA et al. Six hundred fifty consecutive pancreaticoduodenectomies in the 1990s. Ann Surg 1997;226:248-260.

72. Yeo CJ, Cameron JL, Maher MM et al. A prospective randomized trial of pancreaticogastrostomy versus pancreaticojejunostomy after pancreaticoduodenectomy. Ann Surg 1995;222:588-592.

73. Nimura Y, Hayakawa N, Kamiya J, et al. Hepatopancreatduodenectomy for advanced carcinoma of the biliary tract. Hepatogastroenterology 1991;38:170-175.

74. Miyagawa S, Makkuuchi M, Kawasaki S, et al. Outcome of major hepatectomy with pancreatoduodenectomy for advanced biliary malignancies. World J Surg 1996;20:77-80.

75. Neuhaus P, Jonas S, Bechstein WO, et al. Extended resections hilar cholangiocarcinoma. Ann Surg 1999;230:808-818.

76. Yamanaka N, Yasui C, Yamanaka J, et al. Left hemihepatectomy with microsurgical reconstruction of the right-sided hepatic vasculature. A strategy for preserving hepatic function in patients with proximal bile duct cancer. . Langenbecks Arch Surg 2001;386:364-368.

77. Sakamoto Y, Sano T, Shimada K, et al. Clinical significance of reconstruction of the right hepatic artery for biliary malignancy. Langenbecks Arch Surg 2006;391:203-208.

78. Pichlmayr R, Weimann A, Klempnauer J, et al. Surgical treatment in proximal bile duct cancer. A single center experience. Ann Surg 1996;224:628-638.

79. Iwatsuki S, Todo S, Mash JW, et al. Treatment of hilar cholangiocarcinoma (Klatskin tumors) with hepatic resection or transplantation. J Am Coll Surg 1998;187:358-364.

80. Chung SW, Greig PD, Cattral MS, et al. Evaluation of liver transplantation for high-risk indications. Br J Surg 1997;84:189-195.

81. Jonas S, Mittler J, Pascher A, et al. Extended indications in living-donor liver transplantation: bile duct cancer. Transpl 2005;80:S101-S104.

82. Neuhaus P, Jonas S, Bechstein WO, et al. Extended resections for hilar cholangiocarcinoma. Ann Surg 1999;230:808-819.

83. Strong RW. Transplantation for liver and biliary cancer. Semin Surg Oncol 2000;19:189-199.

84. Goldstein RM, Stone M, Tillery GW, et al. Is liver transplantation indicated for cholangiocarcinoma? Am J Surg 1993;166:768-772.

85. Busuttil RW, Farmer DG. The surgical treatment of primary hepatobiliary malignancy. Liver Transpl Surg 1996;2(5 suppl 1):114-130.

86. Pichlmayr R, Weimann A, Oldhafer KJ, et al. Role of liver transplantation in the treatment of unresectable liver cancer. World J Surg 1995;19:807-813.

87. Neuhaus P, Jonas S. Surgery for hilar cholangiocarcinoma-German experience. J Hepatobiliary pancreat Surg 2000;7:142-147.

88. Gores GJ. Early detection and treatment of cholangiocarcinoma. Liver Transpl 2000;6:S30-S34.

89. Rea DJ, Heimbach JK, Rosen CB et al. Liver transplantation with neoadjuvant chemoradiation is more effective than resection for hilar cholangiocarcinoma. Ann Surg 2005;242:451-461.

90. De Vreede I, Steers JL, Burch PA, et al. Prolonged disease-free survival after orthotopic liver transplantation plus adjuvant chemoirradiation for cholangiocarcinoma. Liver transpl 2000;6:309-316.

91. Jarnagin WR, Shoup M. Surgical management of cholangiocarcinoma. Semin Liver Dis 2004;24189-199.

92. Nimura Y, Hayakawa N, Kamiya J, Kondo S, Shionoya S. Hepatectomy with caudate lobe resection for bile duct carcinoma of the hepatic hilus. World J Surg 1990;14:535-543.

93. Anderson CD, Pinson CW, Berlin J, Chari RS. Diagnosis and treatment of cholangiocarcinoma. Oncologist 2004;24:189-99.

94. Nakeeb A, Tran KQ, Black MJ, et al. Improved survival in resected biliary malignancies. Surgery 2002;132:555-563.

95. Lillemore KD, Cameron JL. Surgery for hilar cholangiocarcinoma: the Johns Hopkins approach. J Hepatobiliary Pancreat Surg 2000;7:115-121.

96. Heimbach JK, Haddock MG, Alberts SR, et al. Transplantation for hilar cholangiocarcinoma. Liver Transpl 2004;10:S65-S68.

X·II
Chemotherapy

Cholangiocarcinoma refers to malignant tumors arising from epithelial cells lining the biliary tract. Cholangiocarcinoma is one of the most lethal cancers defying long-term control of disease. Like most other malignant tumors, a complete surgical resection with negative margins on histology is the only way to expect cure of this tumor. Unfortunately less than 30% of patients with cholangiocarcinoma are candidates for curative resection.[1] Besides, the high recurrence rate after curative surgery is another factor leading to dismal outcome of this disease.[2]

As a result, most patients with cholangiocarcinoma are potential candidates for systemic chemotherapy. The role of systemic chemotherapy in the palliation of cholangiocarcinoma is not defined yet. Likewise, there is no convincing evidence that postoperative adjuvant chemotherapy has survival advantage. Despite the poor response rate of cholangiocarcinoma to chemotherapy, systemic chemotherapy remains as the only viable anticancer treatment option in large proportion of the patients during the course of the disease.

1. Systemic Chemotherapy

Patients having locally advanced or metastatic disease are candidates for palliative systemic chemotherapy. So far, no single agent or combination regimen has achieved significant survival advantage. During the period of 70s through 90s, 5-fluorouracil and mitomycin have been the main chemotherapeutic agents for cholangiocarcinoma. Though earlier studies reported encouraging response rate of 47% with single agent MMC chemotherapy in biliary cancer, later studies could not reproduce comparable outcomes.[3] In an EORTC trial of MMC for advanced biliary tract cancers, the objective response rate was only 10% in 30 patients.[4]

Subsequent phase I or II studies were carried out using 5-fluorouracil alone or in combination with other agents in a small number of patients. One of the largest studies was carried out by Eastern Cooperative Oncology Group (ECOG) and reported 10% of partial response rate and 6.3 months of median survival by 5-fluorouracil alone in 30 patients with advanced gallbladder or bile duct cancer.[5] A series of following studies with either 5-fluorouracil alone or combination chemotherapy reported similar outcomes (Table 1).[6-14]

In a clinical trial using 5-fluorouracil and leucovorin, tumor response rate was 32%.[8] Another trial of combination chemotherapy using 5-fluorouracil, leucovorin, and cisplatin reported tumor response rate of 34%.[13] These result suggest that addition of leucovorin to 5-fluorouracil modestly increase tumor response rate. Median survival, however, was not prolonged by addition of leucovorin.

A series of subsequent clinical trials of 5-fluorouracil combined with streptozotocin, methyllomustine, m-amsacrine, doxorubine, or mitomycin C did not show any survival advantages compared to 5-fluorouracil alone. Tumor response rate by 5-fluorouracil plus cisplatin was 24%.[10] In a clinical trial, 5-fluorouracil, cisplatin, and epirubicin combination chemotherapy produced 40% of tumor response rate and 11 months of median survival rate.[8] Subsequent trials with same regimen, however, did not reveal consistent outcomes.[12] In a trial of combination chemotherapy with interferon-a plus 5-fluorouracil, an overall tumor response rate of 34% was achieved with a median survival of 12 months.[7] Addition of cisplatin or doxorubicin to this regimen increased toxicity without improvement of response rate.[15]

Most of the clinical trials of chemotherapy for biliary tract cancers were carried out in the form of phase I or II single-armed regimen in a small number of patients. Thus any single trial was not large enough to draw meaningful conclusion. This limitation attributes to the relative rarity of biliary tract cancer. Moreover, majority of the patients with biliary tract cancers are not suitable for systemic chemotherapy due

Table 1. Chemotherpay for patients with biliary tract cancer.

Regimen	N	Response Rate (%)	Median survival (months)	References
5FU	30	10	6.3	Falkson et al[5]
5FU/streptomycin	26	8	3	Falkson et al.[5]
5FU/methyl-CCNU	31	10	8	Falkson et al.[5]
5FU	18	0	NR	Takada et al.[6]
5-FU/mitomycin C/doxorubicin	18	0	NR	Takada et al.[6]
5-FU/leucovorin/hydroxyurea	30	30	8	Gebbia et al.[7]
5FU/leucovorin	28	32	6	Choi et al.[8]
5FU/cisplatin	25	24	10	Ducreux et al.[10]
5FU/epirubicin/cisplatin	20	40	11	Ellis et al.[11]
Gemcitabine	19	16	6.5	Raderer et al.[14]
Gemcitabine	32	22	11.5	Penz et al.[24]
Gemcitabine	39	36	6.5	Arroyo et al.[28]
Gemcitabine	13	8	16.0	Mezger et al.[31]
Gemcitabine/5FU	22	36	11	Gebbia et al.[30]
Gemcitabine/cisplatin	11	50	11.3	Carraro et al.[33]
Gemcitabine/cisplatin	40	27.5	9	Thongparsert et al.[35]
Gemcitabine/oxaliplatin	33	36	15.4	Andre et al.[36]
Gemcitabine/docetaxel	43	9	11	Kuhn et al.[38]
Gemcitabine/irinotecan	14	14	NR	Bhargava et al.[39]
Gemcitabine/capecitabine	17	33	NR	Knox et al.[37]

to their medical condition such as obstructive jaundice, cholangitis, and deranged liver function. In those patients with biliary obstruction and cholangitis, adequate palliative biliary drainage holds the first priority.

Anyway, most of the drugs of 70s to early 90s appear to be not effective for biliary tract cancers. In a review of 65 trials of systemic chemotherapy for biliary tract cancers carried out before 2000, none of the trials achieved significant survival benefit.[16]

Newer agents developed in late 90s and early 2000s include oral 5-fluorouracil such as capecitabine and S-1, taxane, CPT11, gemcitabine, and targeted agents such as erlotinib and bevacizumab. Uracil-tegafur, capecitabine, and S-1 belong to oral 5-

fluorouracil prodrugs and have been evaluated in advanced biliary tract cancers. Uracil-tegafur, when administrated with leucovorin, achieved 14% of tumor response rate with median survival of 5 months in 14 patients.17 Capecitabine possesses relative tumor selectivity, producing 125 times higher concentration in tumor cells than normal cells. In 18 patients with cholangiocarcinoma, capecitabine stabilized tumor in 28% with a partial response rate of 6% and a median survival of 8.1 months.[18] When combined with cisplatin, capecitabine produced an overall response rate of 21.4% and a median survival of 9.1 months.[19] S1 also has been tried in 19 patients and achieved a response rate of 21.1% and a median survival of 8.3 months.[20]

Taxanes such as paclitaxel and docetaxel seem to have minimal activity against biliary tract cancer.[21,22] Likewise, irinotecan, a topoisomerase inhibitor exerted minimal activity with a response rate of 8% in 36 patients with biliary tract cancer.[23]

The most promising anticancer drug for cholangiocarcinoma is gemcitabine which has showed obvious response in patients with pancreatic cancer. In a series of single agent chemotherapy with gemcitabine in patients with biliary tract cancer, overall response rate has been reported to be around 30% (8-60%) with a median survival of 10 months.[24-30] Clinical trials of gemcitabine-base combination chemotherapy also revealed variable results with overall response rates in the range of 27.5~50% and median survival rates in the range of 5~11.3 months.[31-36] Compared to gemcibine alone, gemcitabine-based combination chemotherapy achieved slightly better or similar response. Cisplatin was one of the most commonly combined drugs with gemcitabine and produced overall response rates of 27.5~50% and median survivals of 5~11.3 months.[33-35] When capecitabine was combined with capecitabine, it was well-tolerated in patients with deranged liver function and showed 30% of overall response rate.[37] Oxaliplatin, when combine with gemcitabine, also achieved similar response rate of 35.5%.[36] Irinotecan and docetaxel which were not very effective in biliary tract cancer produced negligible additive effect by combination with gemcitabine.[38,39] Though currently there are no published data regarding targeted agents such as erlotinib, an EGFR antagonist or bevacizumab, a VEGF blocker in biliary tract cancers, clinical trials using those targeted agents are under consideration.

Considering that blood vessels feeding biliary tree branch from hepatic artery, intraarterial chemotherapy through hepatic artery has theoretical advantage over conventional intravenous administration because this route can avoid first pass metabolism by the liver. In a clinical trial, intraarterial chemotherapy achieved more than 50% of response rate.[40] However, the enrolled patients were too small to generalize the outcome.

Currently, there is no standard chemotherapeutic regimen for metastatic biliary tract cancer. Though gemcitabine has been known to be the most active agent, there is no confirmative evidence that systemic chemotherapy using gemcitabine chemotherapy provides better survival compared to best supportive care. Newer anticancer agents are under development and some of them are awaiting evaluation. Incessant efforts should be exerted to find effective newer agents or combinations by carrying out clinical trials, and patients should be encouraged to enroll in treatment protocols.

2. Postoperative Adjuvant Therapy

Available data are still lacking to determine the role of adjuvant chemotherapy alone in patients with biliary tract cancers. Likewise systemic chemotherapy for advanced biliary tract cancers, most studies of adjuvant setting are small, retrospective, and single-centered. In a recent trial relative large number of 139 patients were randomly assigned as surgery alone and surgery plus adjuvant chemotherapy using 5-fluorouracil and mitomycin.[41] There was no difference in the rate of lymph node involvement. According to the results, there was no difference in survival rate, survival time, and recurrence rate between surgery alone and adjuvant group.

Adjuvant radiotherapy is a viable adjuvant therapy for patients who underwent surgical resection of bile duct cancer. This is based on the finding that most cases of recurrence after curative surgery occur at locoregional area. Adjuvant radiotherapy might kill the residual tumors at surgical bed. In fact adjuvant radiotherapy seems to improve survival by preventing locoregional recurrence. In a clinical trial, intraoperative or postoperative radiation therapy significantly improved 5-year survival rate, median survival, and recurrence rate in patients with Klatskin tumor.[42]

Though the survival advantage of adjuvant radiation was obvious when resection margin harbors microscopic residual tumor cells, it was not evident in patients in whom radical resection was carried out.

The role of adjuvant radiotherapy is not definite for gallbladder cancer. In a clinical trial of Mayo clinic, postoperative external beam irradiation in 21 patients with gallbladder cancer improved survival in radical resection group.[43] In Duke's trial, however, there was no difference in survival between radical group and residual tumor group.[44] These inconsistent data probably result from the small size of enrolled patients, thus large prospective study is needed to define the role of radiotherapy in gallbladder cancer.

Most often radiotherapy was combined with chemotherapy to enhance the effect of irradiation. 5-fluorouracil, the most common drug combined with radiotherapy, has been known as radiosensitizer. In a series of clinical trials, postoperative adjuvant combination chemoradiotherapy revealed survival benefit, especially when resection margin was positive for microscopic residual tumor cells.[45-48] In a trial, 5-fluorouracil-based adjuvant chemoradiotherapy was carried out for 84 patients with resected extrahepatic bile duct cancer. When enrolled patients were categorized into radical resection, microscopic residual tumor, and gross remnant tumor, 5 year survival rates were 36%, 35%, and 0% respectively.[48] Likewise adjuvant radiotherapy, benefit of chemoradiation is not obvious in patients who underwent radical surgery. However, there are still lacking prospective randomized trial of chemoradiation. In a retrospective comparative study, there was no survival benefit by chemoradiation compared to radiation alone.[49]

3. Preoperative Adjuvant Therapy

Neoadjuvant therapy indicated for locally advanced biliary tract cancer in which curative resection is not amenable due to involvement of vessels or ducts beyond the scope of surgical resection. This is based on the results of prior clinical trials in pancreas or colon cancer in which downstaging by chemoradiation or radiation therapy leads to curative surgery.[50,51] Neoadjuvant therapy has several theoretical advantages. First, eradication of tumor cells at tumor periphery will decrease spreading of tumor during surgical manipulation or contact, second, detection of metastatic foci during therapy can prevent unnecessary surgery, third tumor cell at preoperative state are more vulnerable to chemoradiation than postoperative state due to sufficient oxygen supply.[52] Improvement of patient's general condition is utmost important because combination of chemotherapy and radiotherapy would increase treatment-related toxicity. Palliative biliary drainage along with nutritional support should be preceded before initiation of chemoradiotherapy.

In a trial, neoadjuvant chemoradiation induced complete remission in 3 of 9 patients with extrahpatic bile duct cancer.[53] In another clinical trial, 39 patients with gallbladder cancer were randomly assigned as surgery alone or neoadjuvant chemoradiation followed by surgery.[54] Among the 20 patients of 5-fluorouracil-based chemoradiation group, radical resection was performed in 14 patients resulting in 5 long-term survival patients. However, there was no statistical difference of survival rate between two groups. A recent trial reported favorable response rate of 24% by gemcitabine-based chemoradiation in 42 patients with bile duct, gallbladder, or pancreas cancer.[55] In spite of promising result of neoadjuvant therapy there are no large, randomized studies. Neoadjuvant chemoradiation is currently practiced in a few specialized centers to selected patients.

Conclusion

Advanced biliary tract cancer is still an embarrassing disease showing poor response to conventional chemotherapy. Though gemcitabine is known to be the most single active anticancer drug, standard chemotherapeutic regimen has not been determined yet. Moreover there is no convincing evidence that chemotherapy improves survival. In adjuvant setting, active chemoradiotherapy seems to achieve survival benefit especially for patient with margin-positive surgery.

Incessant efforts should be exerted to find optimal regimen and to develop newer agents effective for biliary tract cancer. Together, those new regimens or drugs should be validated by large randomized clinical trials.

Reference

1. Khan SA, Davidson BR, Goldin R, et al. Guidelines for the diagnosis and treatment of cholangiocarcinoma: Consensus document. Gut 2002;51 (suppl VI):1-9.
2. Mittal B, Deutsch M, Iwatsuki S. Primary cancer of extrahepatic biliary passages. Int J Radiat Oncol Biol Phys 1985;11:849-854.
3. Crooke ST, Bradner WT. Mitomycin C: a review. Cancer Treat Rev 1976; 3:121-139.
4. Taal BG, Audisio RA, Bleiberg H, et al. Phase II trial of mitomycin C (MMC) in advanced gall-bladder and biliary tree carcinoma. An EORTC gastrointestinal tract cancer cooperative group. Ann Oncol 1991;4: 607-612.
5. Falkson G, Maclntyre JM, Moertel CG. Eastern Cooperative Oncology Group experience with chemotherapy for inoperable gallbladder and bile duct cancer. Cancer 1984;54: 965-969.
6. Takada T, Kato H, Matsushiro T. Comparison of 5-fluorouracil, doxorubicin and mitomycin C with 5-fluorouracil alone in the treatment of pancreatic-biliary carcinomas. Oncology 1994;51:396-400.
7. Gebbia V, Majello E, Testa A, et al. Treatment of advanced adenocarcinomas of the exocrine pancreas and the gall bladder with 5-fluorouracil, high dose levofolinic acid and oral hydroxyurea on a weekly schedule. Results of a multicenter study of the Southern Italy Oncology Group (G.O.I.M.). Cancer 1996;78:1300-1307.
8. Choi CW, Choi IK, Seo JH, et al. Effects of 5-fluorouracil and leucovorin in the treatment of pancreatic-biliary tract adenocarcinomas. Am J Clin Oncol 2000;23:425-428.
9. Patt YZ, Jones DV Jr, Hoque A, et al. Phase II trial of intravenous fluorouracil and subcutaeous interferon alfa-2b for biliary tract cancer. J Clin Oncol 1996;14:2311-2315.
10. Ducreux M, Rougier P, Fandi A, et al. Effective treatment of advanced biliary tract canrcinoma using 5-fluorouracil continuous infusion with cisplatin. Ann Oncol 1998;9: 653-656.
11. Ellis PA, Norman A, Hill A, et al. Epirubicin, cisplatin and infusional 5-fluorouracil (5-FU) (ECF) in hepatobiliary tumours. Eur J Cancer 1995;31A:1594-1598.
12. Lee MA, Woo IS, Kang JH, et al. Epirubicin, cisplatin and protracted infusion of 5-FU (ECF) in advanced intrahepatic cholangiocarcinoma. Cancer Res Clin Oncol 2004;130: 346-350.
13. Taieb J, Mitry E, Boigo V, et al. Optimization of 5-fluorouracil (5-FU)/cisplatin combination chemotherapy with a new schedule of leucovorin, 5-FU and cisplatin (LV5FU2-P regimen) in patients with biliary tract carcinoma. Ann Oncol 2002;13:1192-1196.
14. Raderer M, Hejna MH, Valencak JB, et al. Two consecutive phase II studies of 5-fluorouracil/leucovorin/mitomycin C and of gemcitabine in patients with advanced biliary cancer. Oncology 1999;56:177-180.

15. Patt YZ, Hassan MM, Lozano RD, et al. Phase II trial of cisplatin, interferon alpha-2b, doxorubicin, and 5-fluorouracil for biliary tract cancer. Clin Cancer Res 2001;7:3375-3380.

16. Hejna M, Pruckmayer M, Raderer M. The role of chemotherapy and radiation in the management of biliary cancer: A review of the literature. Eur J Cancer 1998;34:977-986.

17. Chen JS, Yang TS, Lin YC, Jan YY. A Phase II trial of tegafur?uracil plus leucovorin (LV) in the treatment of advanced biliary tract carcinomas. Jpn J Clin Oncol 2003;33:353-356.

18. Patt YZ, Hassan MM, Aguayo A, et al. Oral capecitabine for the treatment of hepatocellular carcinoma, cholangiocarcinoma, and gallbladder carcinoma. Cancer 2004;101:578-586

19. Kim TW, Chang HM, Kang HJ, et al. Phase II study of capecitabine plus cisplatin as first-line chemotherapy in advanced biliary cancer. Ann Oncol 2003;14:1115-1120.

20. Ueno H, Okusaka T, Ikeda M, et al. Phase II study of S-1 in patients with advanced biliary tract cancer. Br J Cancer 2004;91:1769-1774.

21. Jones DV, Lozano R, Hoque A, et al. Phase II study of paclitaxel therapy for unresectable biliary tree carcinomas. J Clin Oncol 1996;14:2306-2310.

22. Pazdur R, Royce ME, Rodrigues GI, et al. Phase II trial of docetaxel for cholangiocarcinoma. Am J Clin Oncol 1999;22:78-81.

23. Fishkin PA, Alberts SR, Burgart LJ, et al. CPT-11 for bile duct and gall bladder carcinoma. A Phase II North Central Cancer Treatment Group Study. Int J Gastrointest Cancer 2002;32:110-114.

24. Penz M, Kornek GV, Raderer M, et al. Phase II trial of two-weekly gemcitabine in patients with advanced biliary tract cancer. Ann Oncol 2001;12:183-186.

25. von Delius S, Lershc C, Schulte-Frohlinde E, Mayr M, Schmid RM, Eckel F. Phase II trial of weekly 24-hour infusion of gemcitabine in patients with advanced gallbladder and biliary tract carcinoma. BMC Cancer 2005;12:61

26. Kubicka S, Rudolf KL, Tietze MK, et al. Phase II study of systemic gemcitabine chemotherapy for advanced unresectable hepatobiliary carcinomas. Hepatogastroenterology 2001;48:783-789.

27. Valencak J, Kornek GV, Raderer M, et al. Gemcitabine for the treatment of advanced biliary tract carcinomas: Evaluation of two different dose regimens. Onkologie 1999;22:498-501.

28. Arroyo G, Gallardo J, Rubio B. Gemcitabine (GEM) in advanced biliary tract cancer (ABTC). Experience from Chile and Argentina in phase II trials. Proc Am Soc Clin Oncol 2001;20:157a (Abstr 626).

29. Park JS, Oh SY, Kim SH, et al. Single-agent gemcitabine in the treatment of advanced biliary tract cancers: a phase II study. Jpn J Clin Oncol 2005;35:68-73.

30. Gebbia V, Giuliani F, Maiello E, et al. Treatment of inoperable and/or metastatic biliary tree carcinomas with single agent gemcitabine or in combination with levofolinic acid and

infusional fluorouracil: results of a multicenter phase II study. J Clin Oncol 2001;19: 4089-4091.

31. Mezger J, Sauerbruch T, Ko Y, et al. A phase II trial of gemcitabine in gallbladder and biliary tract carcinomas. Oncologie 1998;21:232-234.
32. Alberts SR, Al-Khatib H, Mahoney MR, et al. Gemcitabine, 5-flurouracil, and leucovorin in advanced biliary tract and gallbladder carcinoma: a North Cancer Treatment Group phase II trial. Cancer 2005;103:111-118.
33. Carraro S, Servienti PJ, Bruno MF. Gemcitabine and cisplatin in locally advanced or metastatic gallbladder and bile duct adenocarcinomas. Proc Am Soc Clin Oncol 2001;20:146B (Abstr 2333).
34. Doval DC, Sekhon JS, Gupta SK, et al. A phase II study of gemcitabine and cisplatin in chemotherapy-naïve, unresectable gallbladder cancer. Br J Cancer 2004;90:1516-1520.
35. Thongparsert S, Napapan S, Charoentum C, Moonprakan S. Phase II study of gemcitabine and cisplatin as first line chemotherapy in inoperable biliary tract carcinoma. Ann Oncol 2005;16:279-281.
36. Andre T, Tournigand C, Rosmorduc O, et al. Gemcitabine combined with oxaliplatin (GEMOX) in advanced biliary tract adenocarcinoma: a GERCOR study. Ann Oncol 2004;15:1339-1343.
37. Knox J, Hedley D, Oza A, et al. Combining gemcitabine and capecitabine in patients with advanced biliary cancer: A phase II trial. J Clin Oncol 2005;23:2332-2338
38. Kuhn R, Hribaschek A, Eichelmann K, et al. Outpatient therapy with gemcitabine and docetaxel for gallbladder, biliary, and cholangiocarcinomas. Invest New Drugs 2002;20:351-356.
39. Bhargava P, Jani CR, Savarese DM, et al. Gemcitabine and irinotecan in locally advanced or metastatic biliary cancer: preliminary report. Oncology (Huntingt) 2003;17 (9 suppl 8):23-26.
40. Cantore M, Rabbi C, Guadagni S, Zamagni D, Aitini E. Intra-arterial hepatic chemotherapy combined with continuous infusion of 5-fluorouracil in patients with metastatic cholangiocarcinoma. Ann Oncol 2002;12:1687-1688.
41. Takada T, Amano H, Yasuda H, et al. Is postoperative adjuvant chemotherapy useful for gallbladder carcinoma? A phase III multicenter prospective randomized controlled trial in patients with resected pancreaticobiliary carcinoma. Cancer 2002;95:1685-1695.
42. Gonzalez D, Gerard MA, Maners AE. Results of radiation therapy in carcinoma of the proximal bile duct. Semin Liver Dis 1990;10:131-141.
43. Kresl JJ, Schild SE, Henning GT, et al. Adjuvant external beam radiation therapy with concurrent chemotherapy in the management of gallbladder carcinoma. Int J Radiat Oncol Biol Phys 2002;52:167-175.

44. Czito BG, Hurwitz HI, Clough RW, et al. Adjuvant external beam radiation therapy with concurrent chemotherapy after resection of primary gallbladder carcinoma: A 23 year experience. Int J Radiat Oncol Biol phys 2005;62:1030-1034.

45. Robertson JM, Lawrence TS, Andrews JC, et al. Long-term results of hepatic artery fluorodeoxyuridine and conformal radiation therapy for primary hepatobiliary cancers. Int J Radiat Oncol Biol Phys 1997;37:325-330.

46. Whittington R, Neuberg D, Tester WJ, et al. Protracted intravenous fluorouracil infusion with radiation therapy in the management of localized pancreaticobiliary carcinoma: a phase I Eastern Cooperative Oncology Group Trial. J Clin Oncol 1995;13:227-232.

47. Serafini FM, Sachs D, Bloomston M et al. Location, not staging, of cholangiocarcinoma determines the role for adjuvant chemoradiation therapy. Am Surg 2001;67:839-843;discussion 843-844.

48. Kim S, Kim SW, Bang YJ, et al. Role of postoperative radiotherapy in the management of extrahepatic bile duct cancer. Int J Radiat Oncol Biol Phys 2002;54:414-419.

49. Figueras J, Llado L, Valls C, et al. Changing strategies in diagnosis and management of hilar cholangiocarcinoma. Liver Transpl 2000;6:786-794.

50. Pilpich MV, Millar HH. Preoperative irradiation in carcinoma of the pancreas. Cancer 1980;46:1945-1949.

51. Gerard A, Buyse M, Nordlinger B, et al. Preoperative radiotherapy as adjuvant treatment in rectal cancer: Final results of a randomized study of the European organization for research and treatment of cancer (EORTC). Ann Surg 1988;208:606-614.

52. De Aretxabala X, Roa I, Berrios M, et al. Chemoradiotherapy in gallbladder cancer. J Surg Oncol 2006;93:699-704.

53. McMasters KM, Tuttle TM, Leach SD, et al. Neoadjuvant chemoradiation for extrahepatic cholangiocarcinoma. Am J Surg 1997;174:605-609.

54. de Aretxabala X, Roa I, Burgos L, et al. Pre operative chemoradiation in gallbladder cancer. Am Surg 1999;65:241-246.

55. Lin L, Picus J, Drebin JA, et al. A phase II study of alternating cycles of split course radiation therapy and gemcitabine chemotherapy for inoperable pancreatic or biliary tract carcinoma. Am J Clin Oncol 2005;28:234-241.

X·III
Radiotherapy for Cholangiocarcinoma

Introduction

Cholangiocarcinoma, the primary cancer arising from the epithelial cells of the bile ducts, is a rare malignant tumor with an estimated incidence of 0.01~0.8%. Histologically, well-differentiated adenocarcinoma is most common in cholangiocarcinoma. Traditionally, cholangiocarcinoma tumors were classified simply as intrahepatic, perihilar, or distal based on their location within the biliary tree. Approximately 60~70% of cholangiocarcinomas occur at the hepatic duct bifurcation (Klatskin tumors), 20~30% occur in the distal common bile duct, and 5~10% are peripheral, arising within the liver.[1,2]

Cholangiocarcinomas frequently spread by direct extension through the bile duct and the abundant submucosal lymphatic network. These tumors also commonly invade the surrounding structures including the perineural, periductal spaces, and portal tracts.[3] Lymph node metastasis of cholangiocarcinoma depends on the location of the primary tumor and occurs in half of the patients. Intrahepatic and perihilar cholangiocarcinomas spread mainly to the nodes in the hepatoduodenal ligament, and the pancreaticoduodenal nodes are more often involved in the distal bile duct tumor.[4-6]

Cholangiocarcinomas are highly fatal because of late clinical presentation with local invasion and proximity to vital structures. Most patients with biliary cancers present with unresectable or metastatic disease, and the overall 5-year survival rate is less than 10%. Cancer cachexia, liver failure, and recurrent sepsis, secondary to biliary obstruction, can contribute to high mortality.[7,8]

A complete surgical resection with histologically negative resection margins remains the only potentially curative treatment modality for patients with cholangiocarcinoma. Unfortunately, only 10% to 35% of patients are potential candidates for surgical resection at presentation.[9] Some investigators have reported that more aggressive surgical approaches can improve the survival rate for patients with resectable cholangiocarcinoma.[10,11] However, there have been minimal improvements in the long-term survival rate over the past decade. Survival rates are still disappointing after curative resection; 5-year survival rates after resection range from 10% to 40%, depending on the site of the primary tumor.[12-16]

With surgical resection, the proximal and distal margins are often narrow or microscopically positive because of luminal extension to both the right and left hepatic ducts. Also, the radial margins are similar because of the early radial extension of the disease to critical structures, such as the portal vein and the hepatic arteries.[11, 15,17-19] Even in patients undergoing complete gross resection, there is approximately 50% local recurrence, which usually causes biliary obstruction, sepsis, and/or liver failure.[9-11,14,20,21] Due to this pattern of recurrence after surgery, radiotherapy has been proposed as a local treatment modality with or without chemotherapy. In order to improve local and regional disease control as well as the survival rate, radiotherapy has been attempted with a variety of procedures such as brachytherapy or intraoperative radiotherapy. Unfortunately, there have not been any randomized trials studying the role of radiotherapy in cholangiocarcinoma because of the low incidence of disease. Although the benefits of radiotherapy are still controversial, retrospective data suggest improved survival rates in the postoperative setting.[19,22-25] For patients with unresectable cholangiocarcinoma, the purpose of treatment is to palliate symptoms such as obstructive jaundice, biliary tract infection, pain, and ascites. Survival rates are very poor, ranging from 2 to 3 months in patients receiving medical management alone and 6 to 12 months for those undergoing palliative treatment such as bypass surgery, stent insertion, or radiotherapy with or without chemotherapy.[26-31]

1. Intrahepatic Cholangiocarcinoma

Intrahepatic cholangiocarcinoma (or peripheral cholangiocarcinoma) accounts for 5% to 10% of all biliary tract cancers and is the second most common following hepatocellular carcinoma, constituting 10% to 20% of primary liver cancer.[32] Intrahepatic cholangiocarcinoma appears within the second bifurcation of the intrahepatic bile duct. The resectability in all patients is only 30% to 50% because of the presentation of advanced clinical features.[33,34] After resection, the 5-year survival rate is still low, ranging from 8% to 47%. A negative surgical resection margin is the most important indicator for patient survival. Bilobar distribution, lymph node involvement, vascular invasion, and distant metastases were found to be poor prognostic factors.[27,35,36] The patterns of failure after the resection of intrahepatic cholangiocarcinoma are primarily in the liver (56%), regional lymph node (20%) and peritoneal seeding (24%).[37] Treatment options are determined by the local extent of the cancer and vascular invasion, as well as underlying liver function. Surgical resection is the only curative treatment modality in selected patients without the portal structure or main hepatic artery involvement of disease. There are no convincing data that adjuvant chemotherapy or radiation therapy is capable of increasing survival rates and reducing tumor recurrence. Most reports of adjuvant therapy for intrahepatic cholangiocarcinoma have been small retrospective studies. The role of postoperative adjuvant radiotherapy with or without chemotherapy in the management of intrahepatic cholangiocarcinoma is controversial.[38,39] Until now, in patients with residual tumors after surgical resection, radiotherapy with or without chemotherapy is one of the additional modalities suggested in the NCCN guidelines. In patients with unresectable disease, radiation therapy, or the combination of radiotherapy and chemotherapy, remains the only treatment option, even though survival is uniformly unsuccessful with a patient survival of only 3~6 months. Palliative radiotherapy contributes only to biliary decompression.

2. Hilar Cholangiocarcinoma

Hilar (or perihilar) cholangiocarcinoma is the most common biliary tract cancer and accounts for 65% to 70% of biliary tract tumors.[2] Perihilar tumors, also known as Klatskin tumors, involve the bifurcation of the hepatic duct.1 Bismuth and colleagues classified these tumors into four categories according to the tumor extension into the intrahepatic bile ducts. Bismuth type I tumors involve only the proximal common hepatic duct below the confluence of the left and right hepatic ducts. Type II tumors involve the confluence but do not extend into the right or left segmental hepatic ducts. Type IIIa and IIIb tumors involve the confluence and also extend into the segmental right and the left hepatic ducts, respectively. Type IV tumors are multicentric or involve the confluence and both the right and left hepatic ducts.[40] Regional lymph node metastases commonly appear in up to 35% of cases.[4]

3. Resectable Hilar Cholangiocarcinoma

Surgical resection is feasible in approximately 25% to 79% of patients.[41] The main prognostic factors are histological margin status and lymph node involvement. The 5-year survival rates are greater in patients with a negative margin (19~47%) than in those with a positive margin 0~12%.[3,36,42-44] The 3-year survival rate was 55% for patients without node involvement, 32% for patients with regional node metastasis, and 12% for patients with paraaortic node metastasis.[4] After complete surgical resection, the most common treatment failure is local recurrence, which is related to a patient's mortality.[45] Many authors have advocated postoperative radiotherapy alone or in combination with chemotherapy as a strategy for local control and prolonged survival. Although this approach offers a theoretical rationale, there are no prospective, randomized trials in the available literature on adjuvant radiotherapy following resection of cholangiocarcinoma. Single-institution studies have attempted to clarify the role of adjuvant external beam radiotherapy in resected patients. However, the benefit of postoperative radiotherapy is not conclusive because the available literature is limited to retrospective studies.[46]

Several studies have demonstrated a survival benefit for postoperative adjuvant radiotherapy of hilar cholangiocarcinomas (Table 1). The European Organization for the Research and Treatment of Cancer (EORTC) reported a survival improvement with postoperative radiotherapy (external beam radiotherapy with or without intraluminal brachytherapy) following surgical resection. There was improvement in the median survival length and in 1- and 3-year survival rates (19.0 versus 8.25 months; 85% versus 36%; 31% versus 10%, respectively; P=0.0005).[22] Japanese investigators reported similar results in patients with histological margin-positive resections for locally advanced Klatskin tumors. The patients who were treated with postoperative radiotherapy (intraoperative radiotherapy and/or external beam radiotherapy) had significantly longer median survival lengths and higher 5-year survival rates than patients who underwent resection alone (32 months versus 10 months; 33.9% versus 13.5%, respectively; P=0.01). Also, this study reported a higher locoregional control rate in the adjuvant radiotherapy group (79.2%) than in the resection-alone group (31.2%).[19] In one of the recent retrospective series from the Netherlands, 91 patients with resectable hilar cholangiocarcinoma were treated with postoperative radiotherapy using external beam radiotherapy with or without brachytherapy. The median survival was superior in the adjuvant radiation group

Table 1. Results of postoperative radiotherapy

Author	Treatment	N	R0 (%)	Median survival (months)	P
Gonzalez et al.[22]	RES alone	17	-	8.25	<0.01
	RES+EBRT±BT	38	-	19	
Todoroki et al.[19]	RES alone	21	1 (4)	10	0.01
	RES+IORT and/or EBRT	42	1 (2)	32	
Gerhards et al.[47]	RES alone	20	2 (10)	8	<0.01
	RES+EBRT±BT	71	11 (15)	24	
Pitt et al.[38]	RES alone	17	-	20	NS
	RES+EBRT	14	-	20	
Sagawa et al.[48]	RES alone	30	13 (43)	20	NS
	RES+EBRT±BT	39	21 (53)	23	

Abbreviations: R0=no residual tumor after surgery, RES=resection, EBRT=external beam radiotherapy, BT=brachytherapy, IORT=intraoperative radiotherapy compared to the resection alone group (24 vs. 8 months, respectively, p<0.01).[47] In contrast, a retrospective analysis from Johns Hopkins suggests that postoperative adjuvant radiation therapy does not improve survival. They reported a similar median survival of 20 months. However, the radiotherapy group was more likely to have vascular invasion and the number of patients in the study was too small.[38] No firm conclusions can be drawn from these data in terms of the role of postoperative radiotherapy. Sagawa et al. also reported a negative outcome for postoperative radiotherapy in patients who underwent resection, demonstrating a survival of 23 months compared to 20 months, respectively.[48] Given the potential radiosensitization effect of 5-fluorouracil, the combination of adjunctive radiation and chemotherapy should theoretically be more effective than either method alone. However, the true effect of adjuvant chemoradiotherapy following surgical resection remains as unclear as that of radiation alone. Currently, according to the NCCN guidelines, chemoradiotherapy is recommended in the patients with residual disease after surgical resection or lymph node metastasis.

4. Unresectable Hilar Cholangiocarcinoma

Around 80% of the patients with hilar cholangiocarcinoma are candidates for palliative management. Of these patients, those with locally advanced unresectable cholangiocarcinoma may be candidates for palliative radiotherapy. In this setting, the first aim of management is quality of life and the relief of symptoms, and the second aim is to prolong survival. Endoscopic biliary drainage is the preferred modality and provides long-term relief from pruritis, cholangitis, pain, and jaundice. Percutaneous biliary drainage provides comparable results when endoscopic drainage is not available. Surgical cholangiojejunostomy provides biliary drainage also but is limited in its effects on morbidity and mortality. Radiotherapy has been used following biliary stent insertion for better durable palliation in terms of longer mean survival, fewer stent occlusions, and a superior quality of life.[49,50] The prognosis of advanced unresectable disease is dismal. The median survival is 9~12 months in patients who are treated with external beam radiation therapy with doses of 45~50 Gy alone, with the addition of an intraluminal brachytherapy boost or in combination with chemotherapy. External beam radiotherapy is the most commonly used type of radiotherapy. However, delivery dose is limited because of surrounding radiosensitive organs such as the liver, kidneys, and small intestine. In addition, the usual cause of death after radiotherapy for locally advanced cholangiocarcinoma is associated with local persistence of disease. Thus, radiation dose intensification using brachytherapy, intraoperative radiotherapy, and radiosensitization by chemotherapy have been applied (Table 2).

Several small retrospective studies have reported the survival benefit of radiotherapy for patients with unresectable cholangiocarcinoma compared to that for patients receiving no treatment or stenting alone. Grove et al. reported a significantly increased median survival in patients who received radiotherapy after biliary duct dilatation versus those who underwent surgical decompression alone (12.2 vs. 2.2 months, respectively; P=0.05).[29] Tollenaar et al. reported a similar increase in median survival length with the use of external beam radiotherapy after surgical decompression, compared with the survival after surgical decompression alone (16 versus 3 months, respectively, p<0.001).[31] Millela et al. reported a survival advantage

Table 2. Results of external beam radiotherapy with intraluminal brachytherapy or intraoperative radiotherapy in locally advanced cholangiocarcinoma

Author	Treatment	N	Median survival (months)	P
Grove et al.[29]	Stent alone	9	2.2	0.05
	Stent+EBRT	19	12.2	
Tollenaar et al.[31]	RES	39	3	<0.001
	RES+EBRT	16	16	
Milella et al.[30]	EBRT	10	11.5	-
	EBRT+BT	12	14	-
	No EBRT	89	3.6	
Alden et al.[26]	No EBRT	24	5.5	0.01
	EBRT±BT±5-FU	24	12	
Shin et al.[59]	EBRT	17	5	0.06
	EBRT+BT	14	9	
Monson et al.[56]	IORT+EBRT	13	16.5	

Abbreviations are the same as in Table 1, FU=fluorouracil

in patients with unresectable disease who underwent palliative radiotherapy. The median survival was greater in the radiotherapy groups than in the percutaneous biliary drainage alone group. The investigators also reported an improved quality of life in patients who underwent radiotherapy.[30]

In intraluminal brachytherapy, radioactive sources inside percutaneous transhepatic catheters within the lumen of the duct are placed in proximity to the tumor for delivery of a high dose to the tumor. In contrast, normal tissues receive lower doses of radiation because the delivered dose is confined to an area near the source. For intraoperative radiotherapy, surrounding normal tissues can be moved physically and shielded directly from the radiation field. These modalities can deliver a boost dose of 10~25 Gy to external beam radiotherapy. Although there have not been any randomized trials to compare external beam radiotherapy alone with brachytherapy or intraoperative radiotherapy plus external beam radiotherapy, some studies have suggested enhanced survival as well as durable palliation for patients undergoing a combination treatment. A 2-year survival of 10~20% and median survival length of 12 to 14 months has been reported in several studies with this combination.[26,27,30,49,51-58] The previously mentioned study by Millela reported a slightly higher median survival rate in patients treated with brachytherapy (14 versus 11.5 months).[30] Shin et al. reported a prolongation of the median time to tumor recurrence in the brachytherapy with the external radiotherapy group compared to that in the no brachytherapy group (9 months vs. 5 months, respectively; p=0.06). The overall 2-year survival rate was also better in the patient group receiving brachytherapy (21% vs. 0%; p=0.015).[59] However, the main limitation of this combination is a high incidence of complications such as duodenal stenosis, intestinal bleeding, portal vein obstruction, cholangitis, and ascites. The high radiation doses could be dangerous or could even be detrimental to the prognosis.[60] These toxicities may be avoidable with currently available three-dimensional brachytherapy planning techniques. Monson et al. reported improved survival data in 14 patients who were treated with a combination of intraoperative radiotherapy and external beam radiotherapy. For these patients, the median survival length was 18.5 months and the 1- and 5-year survival rates were 69% and 7%, respectively.[56]

The combination of radiotherapy and chemotherapy is theoretically the most attractive modality for relieving pain and biliary obstruction, and to achieve long-term survival for the management of unresectable cholangiocarcinoma. The most active agents include 5-fluorouracil, gemcitabine, docetaxel and oxaliplatin.[61] In a neoadjuvant setting, McMasters and colleagues reported promising results from nine patients who underwent preoperative chemoradiotherapy before curative resection. Three patients experienced a complete pathologic response, and the rate of margin-free resection was 100% in all nine patients.[25] Foo et al. suggested the importance of a simultaneous administration of 5-fluorouracil with external beam radiotherapy. Superior 5-year survival rate was reported in the combination treatment of 5-fluorouracil, external beam radiotherapy and brachytherapy compared with that without 5-fluorouracil (22% vs. 8%, respectively).[53] Brunner et al. compared stenting and chemoradiation. The median survival time for patients with CRT was 22.7 months, and the median survival time for stenting alone was 9.3 months. ($p = 0.058$).[62] In a recent study, Deodato et al. reported encouraging results. In 21 patients who received 5-fluorouracil and external beam radiation therapy with or without intraluminal brachytherapy, the median duration of local control, disease-free survival and overall survival were 44.5 months, 16.3 months, and 23.0 months, respectively, and the 5-year survival was 18.0%.[63] With advances in radiotherapy techniques, precise radiotherapy can deliver a high dose to the tumor, thereby saving the normal tissue. In addition, new molecular target agents will improve survival. The combination treatment consisting of high precision radiotherapy and a molecular target agent will provide a new paradigm for cholangiocarcinoma treatment.

5. Distal Bile Duct Cholangiocarcinoma

Primary distal bile duct adenocarcinoma represents approximately 20~30% of all cholangiocarcinomas and is usually treated with pancreaticoduodenectomy (Whipple procedure). The goal of treatment is to achieve a margin-negative resection. Patients with distal duct carcinoma have a relatively higher chance of curative resection (up to 56%) compared to patients with proximal duct carcinoma.[14] The prognosis for patients with distal duct carcinoma is also better than that for patients with proximal duct carcinoma.[64] A multiple-case series demonstrated 20~54% 5-year survival rates in selected patients who underwent curative resections.[14,65,66] The role of postoperative radiotherapy is also unclear. Alden et al. reported that postoperative radiotherapy did not improve survival in patients with distal duct carcinoma after complete resection.[67] In a recent study, however, Hughes et al. found that adjuvant chemoradiation seems to improve local control and overall survival. Thirty-four patients with distal common bile duct cholangiocarcinoma were treated with pancreaticoduodenectomy followed by adjuvant radiation therapy with concurrent and maintenance 5-fluorouracil-based chemotherapy. In these patients, the median survival was 37 months, with a 5-year survival rate of 35%. When compared to historical controls treated with pancreaticoduodenectomy only from the same institution, patients receiving adjuvant therapy showed a significantly longer survival (37vs.22 months, $P<0.05$).[68,69] These data support the use of adjuvant chemoradiation following pancreaticoduodenectomy for the treatment of distal cholangiocarcinoma.

6. Radiotherapy

If the radiation dose-limiting organ near the tumor can be avoided, a high dose of radiotherapy can be delivered to the tumor, exposing the surrounding normal organ to an acceptable level of exposure. With the improvement of radiation-treatment planning using imaging techniques, tumor volume and nearby normal organs can be precisely rendered on the CT slice for the delivery of sophisticated high-dose external beam radiotherapy without an increase complication risk. In patients who undergo surgical resection, surgical clip placement at the time of surgery is useful in delineating the postoperative target volume. In unresectable cholangiocarcinoma, the extent of the tumor within the bile duct can be delineated on the planning CT scan based on a dynamic CT scan, percutaneous cholangiography, MRCP and/or PET scan. In general, gross tumor volume and potential lymphatic drainage areas are the objectives of radiation treatment. The optimal radiation dose and schedule for adjuvant and definitive treatment of cholangiocarcinoma is unknown. However, in practice, the target volume is treated by 45 to 50 Gy in 1.8- to 2-Gy fractions given 5

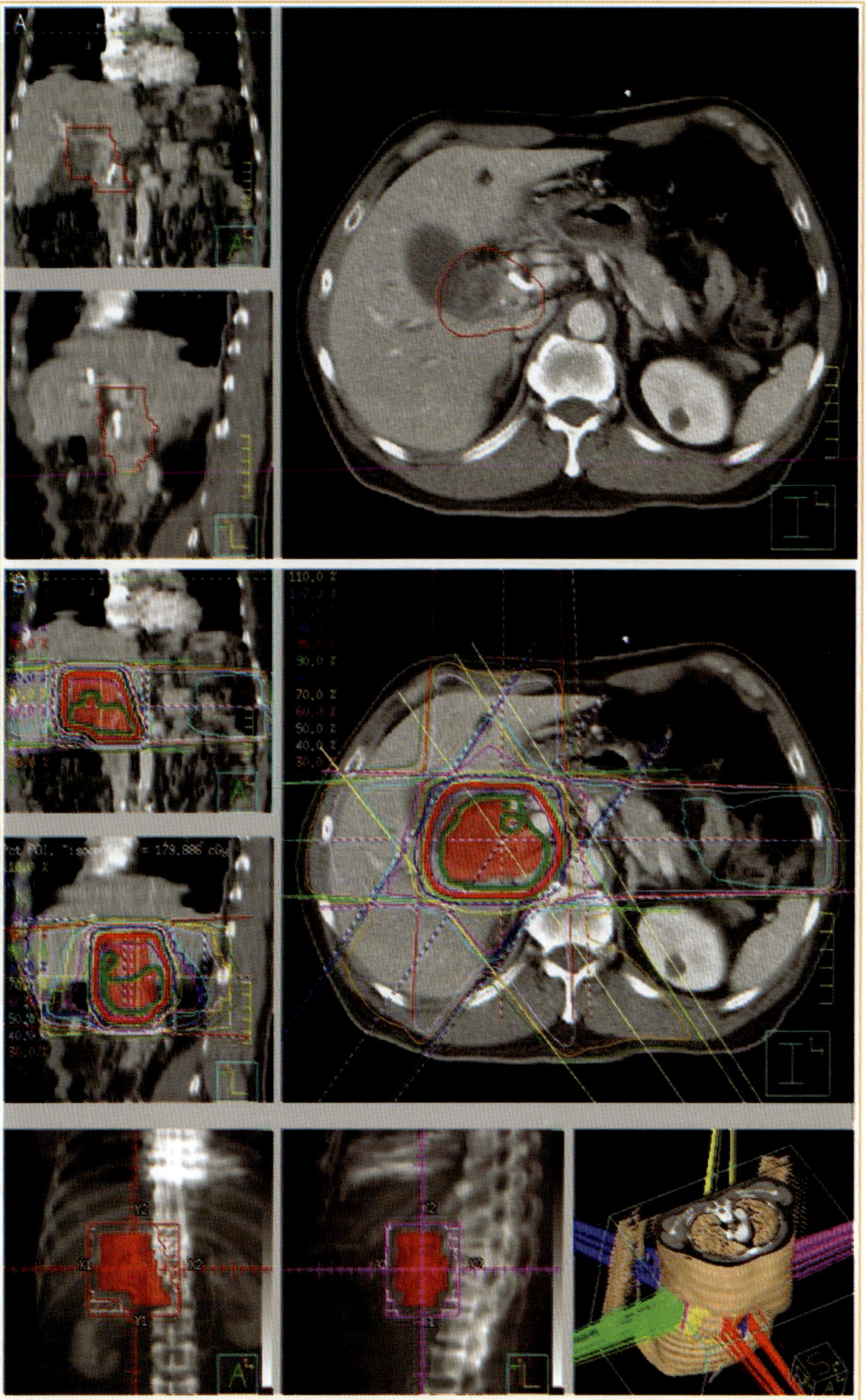

Fig. 1 Radiation treatment planning using computed tomography

A: The target volume was delineated on every CT slice as well as on the surrounding normal organ including liver, stomach, duodenum, kidneys, colon, and spinal cord. B: Beam arrangement and dose distribution were evaluated by a radiation oncologist.

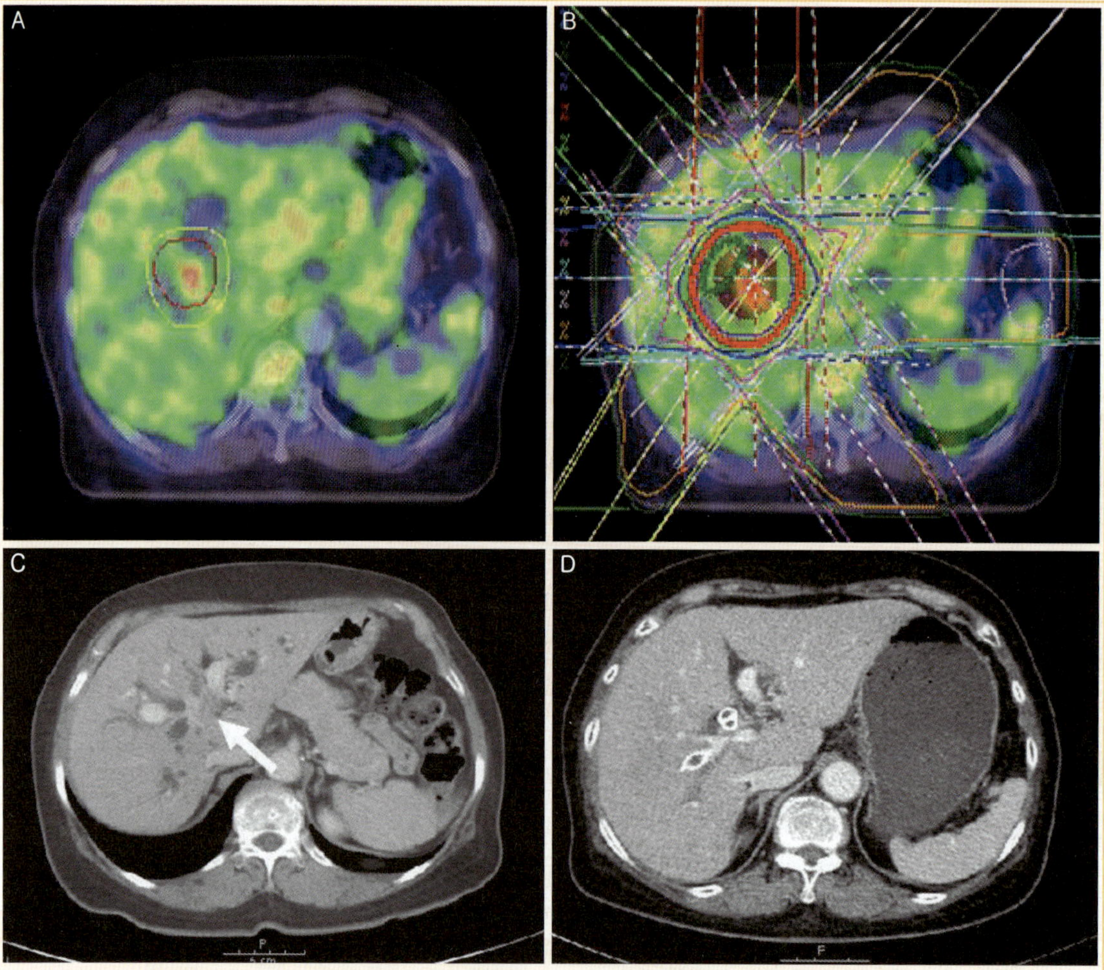

Fig. 2 A 72-year-old female with hilar cholangiocarcinoma was treated with concurrent chemoradiotherapy (50.4Gy in 28 fractions with 5 fluorouracil and gemcitabine, monthly). 3D conformal radiotherapy was performed

A: Target volume was delineated with PET image fusion. B: Beam arrangement was determined based on the dose distribution to the tumor and normal tissues. C: A hilar mass was observed at diagnosis (white arrow). D: All hilar lesions nearly disappeared on a CT scan performed 1 month after concurrent chemoradiotherapy. At the beginning of treatment, CA 19-9 was found to be elevated (> 20,000 U/ml). After 1 month, CA 19-9 reduction (89 U/ml) was observed.

days a week (Fig. 1, 2). With the recent improvements in precision with radiotherapy techniques, 4-dimensional planning, 3D brachytherapy planning, intensity modulated radiotherapy and respiratory-gated therapy have the theoretical potential to escalate the radiation dose and improve therapeutic efficacy.

Summary

Although the data on the use of radiotherapy for treating cholangiocarcinoma is not sufficient and there have not been any controlled randomized trials, it seems that local failure is the main recurrence pattern after curative resection, and some studies have reported an improvement in the survival of patients receiving postoperative radiotherapy. In various reports, for patients with unresectable cholangiocarcinoma, radiotherapy offers palliation of symptomatic disease and results in improved survival. Until now, radiotherapy results with or without chemotherapy have been disappointing. Recent advances in radiotherapy technique, however, allow for the precise delivery of a high dose of radiation with acceptable morbidity. Three-dimensional conformal therapy, four-dimensional planning, 3D brachytherapy planning, intensity-modulated radiotherapy, and respiratory gated therapy have the theoretical potential to improve therapeutic outcomes. With novel molecular target agents, a combinatorial therapy seems promising and warrants further investigation.

Reference

1. Klatskin G. Adenocarcinoma of the hepatic duct at its bifurcation within the porta hepatis. An unusual tumor with distinctive clinical and pathological features. Am J Med 1965;38:241-256.
2. Nakeeb A, Pitt HA, Sohn TA, Coleman J, Abrams RA, Piantadosi S, et al. Cholangiocarcinoma. A spectrum of intrahepatic, perihilar, and distal tumors. Ann Surg 1996;224:463-465.
3. Klempnauer J, Ridder GJ, von Wasielewski R, Werner M, Weimann A, Pichlmayr R. Resectional surgery of hilar cholangiocarcinoma: A multivariate analysis of prognostic factors. J Clin Oncol 1997;15:947-954.
4. Kitagawa Y, Nagino M, Kamiya J, Uesaka K, Sano T, Yamamoto H, et al. Lymph node metastasis from hilar cholangiocarcinoma: Audit of 110 patients who underwent regional and paraaortic node dissection. Ann Surg 2001;233:385-392.
5. Tsuji T, Hiraoka T, Kanemitsu K, Takamori H, Tanabe D, Tashiro S. Lymphatic spreading pattern of intrahepatic cholangiocarcinoma. Surgery 2001;129:401-407.

6. Yoshida T, Aramaki M, Bandoh T, Kawano K, Sasaki A, Matsumoto T, et al. Para-aortic lymph node metastasis in carcinoma of the distal bile duct. Hepatogastroenterology 1998;45:2388-2391.

7. Rea DJ, Munoz-Juarez M, Farnell MB, Donohue JH, Que FG, Crownhart B, et al. Major hepatic resection for hilar cholangiocarcinoma: Analysis of 46 patients. Arch Surg 2004;139:514-523.

8. Shaib Y, El-Serag HB. The epidemiology of cholangiocarcinoma. Semin Liver Dis 2004;24:115-125.

9. Kopelson G, Harisiadis L, Tretter P, Chang CH. The role of radiation therapy in cancer of the extra-hepatic biliary system: An analysis of thirteen patients and a review of the literature of the effectiveness of surgery, chemotherapy and radiotherapy. Int J Radiat Oncol Biol Phys 1977;2:883-894.

10. Iwasaki Y, Todoroki T, Fukao K, Ohara K, Okamura T, Nishimura A. The role of intraoperative radiation therapy in the treatment of bile duct cancer. World J Surg 1988;12:91-98.

11. Miyazaki M, Ito H, Nakagawa K, Ambiru S, Shimizu H, Shimizu Y, et al. Aggressive surgical approaches to hilar cholangiocarcinoma: Hepatic or local resection? Surgery 1998;123:131-136.

12. Klempnauer J, Ridder GJ, Werner M, Weimann A, Pichlmayr R. What constitutes long-term survival after surgery for hilar cholangiocarcinoma? Cancer 1997;79:26-34.

13. Kusano T, Tamai O, Miyazato H, Isa T, Shiraishi M, Muto Y, et al. Surgical treatment for proximal bile duct carcinoma. Int Surg 1998;83:119-123.

14. Nagorney DM, Donohue JH, Farnell MB, Schleck CD, Ilstrup DM. Outcomes after curative resections of cholangiocarcinoma. Arch Surg 1993;128:871-879.

15. Nimura Y, Kamiya J, Nagino M, Kanai M, Uesaka K, Kondo S, et al. Aggressive surgical treatment of hilar cholangiocarcinoma. J Hepatobiliary Pancreat Surg 1998;5:52-61.

16. Todoroki T, Kawamoto T, Koike N, Takahashi H, Yoshida S, Kashiwagi H, et al. Radical resection of hilar bile duct carcinoma and predictors of survival. Br J Surg 2000;87:306-313.

17. Ahrendt SA, Cameron JL, Pitt HA. Current management of patients with perihilar cholangiocarcinoma. Adv Surg 1996;30:427-452.

18. Ogura Y, Kawarada Y. Surgical strategies for carcinoma of the hepatic duct confluence. Br J Surg 1998;85:20-24.

19. Todoroki T, Ohara K, Kawamoto T, Koike N, Yoshida S, Kashiwagi H, et al. Benefits of adjuvant radiotherapy after radical resection of locally advanced main hepatic duct carcinoma. Int J Radiat Oncol Biol Phys 2000;46:581-587.

20. Kopelson G, Galdabini J, Warshaw AL, Gunderson LL. Patterns of failure after curative surgery for extra-hepatic biliary tract carcinoma: Implications for adjuvant therapy. Int J Radiat Oncol Biol Phys 1981;7:413-417.

21. Willett CG, Warshaw AL, Convery K, Compton CC. Patterns of failure after pancreaticoduodenectomy for ampullary carcinoma. Surg Gynecol Obstet 1993;176:33-38.

22. Gonzalez Gonzalez D, Gerard JP, Maners AW, De la Lande-Guyaux B, Van Dijk-Milatz A, Meerwaldt JH, et al. Results of radiation therapy in carcinoma of the proximal bile duct (klatskin tumor). Semin Liver Dis 1990;10:131-141.

23. Kresl JJ, Schild SE, Henning GT, Gunderson LL, Donohue J, Pitot H, et al. Adjuvant external beam radiation therapy with concurrent chemotherapy in the management of gallbladder carcinoma. Int J Radiat Oncol Biol Phys 2002;52:167-175.

24. Mahe M, Romestaing P, Talon B, Ardiet JM, Salerno N, Sentenac I, et al. Radiation therapy in extrahepatic bile duct carcinoma. Radiother Oncol 1991;21:121-127.

25. McMasters KM, Tuttle TM, Leach SD, Rich T, Cleary KR, Evans DB, et al. Neoadjuvant chemoradiation for extrahepatic cholangiocarcinoma. Am J Surg 1997;174:605-609..

26. Alden ME, Mohiuddin M. The impact of radiation dose in combined external beam and intraluminal ir-192 brachytherapy for bile duct cancer. Int J Radiat Oncol Biol Phys 1994;28:945-951.

27. Cameron JL, Pitt HA, Zinner MJ, Kaufman SL, Coleman J. Management of proximal cholangiocarcinomas by surgical resection and radiotherapy. Am J Surg 1990;159:91-98.

28. Garner PD, Hall LD, Johnstone PA. Palliation of unresectable hilar cholangiocarcinoma. J Surg Oncol 2000;75:95-97.

29. Grove MK, Hermann RE, Vogt DP, Broughan TA. Role of radiation after operative palliation in cancer of the proximal bile ducts. Am J Surg 1991;161:454-458.

30. Milella M, Salvetti M, Cerrotta A, Cozzi G, Uslenghi E, Tavola A, et al. Interventional radiology and radiotherapy for inoperable cholangiocarcinoma of the extrahepatic bile ducts. Tumori 1998;84:467-471.

31. Tollenaar RA, van de Velde CJ, Taat CW, Gonzalez Gonzalez D, Leer JW, Hermans J. External radiotherapy and extrahepatic bile duct cancer. Eur J Surg 1991;157:587-589.

32. Altaee MY, Johnson PJ, Farrant JM, Williams R. Etiologic and clinical characteristics of peripheral and hilar cholangiocarcinoma. Cancer 1991;68:2051-2055.

33. Chen MF, Jan YY, Jeng LB, Hwang TL, Wang CS, Chen SC, et al. Intrahepatic cholangiocarcinoma in taiwan. J Hepatobiliary Pancreat Surg 1999;6:136-141.

34. Chu KM, Fan ST. Intrahepatic cholangiocarcinoma in hong kong. J Hepatobiliary Pancreat Surg 1999;6:149-153.

35. Jarnagin WR, Shoup M. Surgical management of cholangiocarcinoma. Semin Liver Dis 2004;24:189-199.

36. Su CH, Tsay SH, Wu CC, Shyr YM, King KL, Lee CH, et al. Factors influencing postoperative morbidity, mortality, and survival after resection for hilar cholangiocarcinoma. Ann Surg 1996;223:384-394.

37. Yamamoto M, Takasaki K, Otsubo T, Katsuragawa H, Katagiri S. Recurrence after surgical resection of intrahepatic cholangiocarcinoma. J Hepatobiliary Pancreat Surg 2001;8: 154-157.

38. Pitt HA, Nakeeb A, Abrams RA, Coleman J, Piantadosi S, Yeo CJ, et al. Perihilar cholangiocarcinoma. Postoperative radiotherapy does not improve survival. Ann Surg 1995;221:788-797.

39. Yeo CJ, Pitt HA, Cameron JL. Cholangiocarcinoma. Surg Clin North Am 1990;70: 1429-1447.

40. Bismuth H, Nakache R, Diamond T. Management strategies in resection for hilar cholangiocarcinoma. Ann Surg 1992;215:31-38.

41. Tsao JI, Nimura Y, Kamiya J, Hayakawa N, Kondo S, Nagino M, et al. Management of hilar cholangiocarcinoma: Comparison of an american and a japanese experience. Ann Surg 2000;232:166-174.

42. Jarnagin WR, Fong Y, DeMatteo RP, Gonen M, Burke EC, Bodniewicz BJ, et al. Staging, resectability, and outcome in 225 patients with hilar cholangiocarcinoma. Ann Surg 2001;234:507-517.

43. Lillemoe KD, Cameron JL. Surgery for hilar cholangiocarcinoma: The johns hopkins approach. J Hepatobiliary Pancreat Surg 2000;7:115-121.

44. Nakeeb A, Tran KQ, Black MJ, Erickson BA, Ritch PS, Quebbeman EJ, et al. Improved survival in resected biliary malignancies. Surgery 2002;132:555-563.

45. Jarnagin WR, Ruo L, Little SA, Klimstra D, D'Angelica M, DeMatteo RP, et al. Patterns of initial disease recurrence after resection of gallbladder carcinoma and hilar cholangiocarcinoma: Implications for adjuvant therapeutic strategies. Cancer 2003;98:1689-1700.

46. Czito BG, Anscher MS, Willett CG. Radiation therapy in the treatment of cholangiocarcinoma. Oncology (Williston Park) 2006;20:873-888.

47. Gerhards MF, van Gulik TM, Gonzalez Gonzalez D, Rauws EA, Gouma DJ. Results of postoperative radiotherapy for resectable hilar cholangiocarcinoma. World J Surg 2003;27:173-179.

48. Sagawa N, Kondo S, Morikawa T, Okushiba S, Katoh H. Effectiveness of radiation therapy after surgery for hilar cholangiocarcinoma. Surg Today 2005;35:548-552.

49. Ishii H, Furuse J, Nagase M, Kawashima M, Ikeda H, Yoshino M. Relief of jaundice by external beam radiotherapy and intraluminal brachytherapy in patients with extrahepatic cholangiocarcinoma: Results without stenting. Hepatogastroenterology 2004;51:954-957.

50. Shinchi H, Takao S, Nishida H, Aikou T. Length and quality of survival following external beam radiotherapy combined with expandable metallic stent for unresectable hilar cholangiocarcinoma. J Surg Oncol 2000;75:89-94.

51. Buskirk SJ, Gunderson LL, Schild SE, Bender CE, Williams HJ, Jr., McIlrath DC, et al. Analysis of failure after curative irradiation of extrahepatic bile duct carcinoma. Ann Surg 1992;215:125-131.

52. Busse PM, Stone MD, Sheldon TA, Chaffey JT, Cady B, McDermott WV, et al. Intraoperative radiation therapy for biliary tract carcinoma: Results of a 5-year experience. Surgery 1989;105:724-733.

53. Foo ML, Gunderson LL, Bender CE, Buskirk SJ. External radiation therapy and transcatheter iridium in the treatment of extrahepatic bile duct carcinoma. Int J Radiat Oncol Biol Phys 1997;39:929-935.

54. Kamada T, Saitou H, Takamura A, Nojima T, Okushiba SI. The role of radiotherapy in the management of extrahepatic bile duct cancer: An analysis of 145 consecutive patients treated with intraluminal and/or external beam radiotherapy. Int J Radiat Oncol Biol Phys 1996;34:767-774.

55. Kuvshinoff BW, Armstrong JG, Fong Y, Schupak K, Getradjman G, Heffernan N, et al. Palliation of irresectable hilar cholangiocarcinoma with biliary drainage and radiotherapy. Br J Surg 1995;82:1522-1525.

56. Monson JR, Donohue JH, Gunderson LL, Nagorney DM, Bender CE, Wieand HS. Intraoperative radiotherapy for unresectable cholangiocarcinoma—the Mayo Clinic experience. Surg Oncol 1992;1:283-290.

57. Morganti AG, Trodella L, Valentini V, Montemaggi P, Costamagna G, Smaniotto D, et al. Combined modality treatment in unresectable extrahepatic biliary carcinoma. Int J Radiat Oncol Biol Phys 2000;46:913-919.

58. Vallis KA, Benjamin IS, Munro AJ, Adam A, Foster CS, Williamson RC et al. External beam and intraluminal radiotherapy for locally advanced bile duct cancer: Role and tolerability. Radiother Oncol 1996;41:61-66.

59. Shin HS, Seong J, Kim WC, Lee HS, Moon SR, Lee IJ, et al. Combination of external beam irradiation and high-dose-rate intraluminal brachytherapy for inoperable carcinoma of the extrahepatic bile ducts. Int J Radiat Oncol Biol Phys 2003;57:105-112.

60. Gonzalez Gonzalez D, Gouma DJ, Rauws EA, van Gulik TM, Bosma A, Koedooder C. Role of radiotherapy, in particular intraluminal brachytherapy, in the treatment of proximal bile duct carcinoma. Ann Oncol 1999;10 Suppl 4:215-220.

61. Verderame F, Russo A, Di Leo R, Badalamenti G, Santangelo D, Cicero G, et al. Gemcitabine and oxaliplatin combination chemotherapy in advanced biliary tract cancers. Ann Oncol 2006;17 Suppl 7:vii 68-72.

62. Brunner TB, Schwab D, Meyer T, Sauer R. Chemoradiation may prolong survival of patients with non-bulky unresectable extrahepatic biliary carcinoma. A retrospective analysis. Strahlenther Onkol 2004;180:751-757.

63. Deodato F, Clemente G, Mattiucci GC, Macchia G, Costamagna G, Giuliante F, et al. Chemoradiation and brachytherapy in biliary tract carcinoma: Long-term results. Int J Radiat Oncol Biol Phys 2006;64:483-488.

64. Bortolasi L, Burgart LJ, Tsiotos GG, Luque-De Leon E, Sarr MG. Adenocarcinoma of the distal bile duct. A clinicopathologic outcome analysis after curative resection. Digestive Surgery 2000;17:36-41.

65. Fong Y, Blumgart LH, Lin E, Fortner JG, Brennan MF. Outcome of treatment for distal bile duct cancer. Br J Surg 1996;83:1712-1715.

66. Wade TP, Prasad CN, Virgo KS, Johnson FE. Experience with distal bile duct cancers in U.S. Veterans affairs hospitals: 1987-1991. J Surg Oncol 1997;64:242-245.

67. Alden ME, Waterman FM, Topham AK, Barbot DJ, Shapiro MJ, Mohiuddin M. Cholangiocarcinoma: Clinical significance of tumor location along the extrahepatic bile duct. Radiology 1995;197:511-516.

68. Hughes MA, Frassica DA, Yeo CJ, Riall TS, Lillemoe KD, Cameron JL, et al. Adjuvant concurrent chemoradiation for adenocarcinoma of the distal common bile duct. Int J Radiat Oncol Biol Phys 2007;68:178-182.

69. Yeo CJ, Sohn TA, Cameron JL, Hruban RH, Lillemoe KD, Pitt HA. Periampullary adenocarcinoma: Analysis of 5-year survivors. Ann Surg 1998;227:821-831.

X·IV
Photodynamic Therapy for Cholangiocarcinoma

Introduction and Rational of Local Tumor Ablation in Cholangiocarcinoma

Cholangiocarcinomas are characterized by a usually slow growth rate and a low propensity for metastasis. Because of late symptoms and their close proximity to important vascular structures in the hilum of the liver and their tendency to grow into perineural tissue, however, these tumors are only seldom curative resectable at time of diagnosis.[1,2] About 80% of hilar CCs exhibit predominantly a longitudinal growth pattern along the biliary tree, most as highly desmoplastic tumors with infiltration of adjacent nerve plexus and lymphatics.[3,4] Most hilar CCs are locally confined, and 10 to 20% show distant metastases (liver, peritoneum) at the time of diagnosis.[4] Nevertheless, 70 to 80% of hilar CCs are nonresectable because of infiltration of the second-order bile duct branches or encasement of the vascular supply in both lobes.[3,5] The prognosis is poor. Even with an aggressive surgical approach only 33% to 50% are resectable[5,6], and in only 28% are negative histologic margins obtained.[5] There seems to be a significant survival advantage for patients with negative margins. The median survival time in a recent study by Burke et al[5] was 40 months overall in all resected patients, 22 months in those with positive margins, and greater than 60 months in those with negative margins.

In nonresectable cholangiocarcinoma usually the only therapeutic strategy is to improve cholestasis by endoscopic or percutaneous drainage or biliary bypass.

Although these procedures do not influence tumor growth and it is not clear if they increase survival, they significantly improve emotional functions and ameliorate symptoms like fatigue, diarrhea, anorexia, pruritus, jaundice, and sleep pattern.[7] They do carry some risk, however, of procedure-related morbidity and mortality. Early morbidity and 30-day mortality are significantly higher with surgical procedures, whereas long-term complications occur more frequently with endoscopic therapy.[8] Because long-term complications are of minor importance by reported poor median survival time of 147 and 182 days, respectively, the interventional techniques should be preferred.

In the majority of patients with tumor stenoses in the distal and middle part of the bile duct cholestasis can be relieved quickly. Palliative intervention is limited in proximal bile duct cancers. Independent of the type of stricture, technically successful endoprosthesis placement is possible in 84% to 96% of these patients.[9,10] A successful drainage (bilirubin decrease>30% to 50%) is only achieved, however, in 69% to 91% of Bismuth type I and II stenosis and 15% to 73% in Bismuth type III and IV tumors. This is reflected in the survival time of these patients: 149 to 160 days for Bismuth type I, 84 to 131 days for Bismuth type II, and 62 to 70 days for Bismuth type III strictures.[9,11]

Although metal stent insertion improves occlusion rates and reduces the number of therapeutic interventions, median survival time is not ameliorated.[12] Attempts to affect tumor growth are made with radiotherapy or chemotherapy. Until now, however, no randomized prospective studies concerning the effect of these already long-used additional therapies are yet available. The only retrospective comparative study of palliative radiation therapy showed no significantly improved median survival time (300 versus 210 days) between endoscopic biliary stenting alone or additional external-beam radiotherapy and internal ^{192}Ir brachytherapy.[13] A survival advantage in the radiotherapy group was observed in the first 9 months. The median hospital stay was 50 days with radiotherapy versus only 7 days with endoprosthesis alone.

A treatment modality for local ablation of the primary tumor could improve the outcome of curative as well as palliative therapies. Palliative brachytherapy with only 192-iridium (dose of 35 Gy in 1-cm distance) did not prolong median survival time (4.3 to 5 months)[14], but, when combined with external beam radiotherapy (30 Gy), resulted in median survival times of 10 to 10.5 months.[13] Another modality for local tumor ablation of CC is PDT.

1. Photodynamic Therapy (PDT)

PDT is a new, promising topical therapy with the aim to destroy tumor tissue selectively. After administration of a photosensitizer, illumination with light at an appropriate wavelength is performed. This leads to a photochemical reaction, particularly of type II with generation of cytotoxic singlet oxygen or other oxygen-derived free radicals.[15,16] These toxic products interact with a number of cellular components like microsomes, mitochondria, nucleus, cell membranes, and so forth. The initial trigger is not yet known.[17,18] The selective sensitivity of the tumor microvasculature to PDT seems to play an additional important role.[19]

1) Photosensitizing agents

There are a variety of candidate photosensitizing agents for use in PDT, based upon modifications of porphyrin, chlorine, and chlorophyll (Table 1). Their macro-molecular nature contributes to preferential localization within and delayed clearance from neoplastic tissues.

Phorphyrin-based photosensitizers, such as hematoporphyrin derivatives and its partly purified commercial preparation, porfimer sodium (Photofrin®), have been the most commonly used sensitizers. Photofrin accumulates in CC cells with a tumor to normal tissue fluorescence ratio of 2:1 after 24 and 48 h administration.[20] Photofrin preferentially accumulates in CC cells, reaching peak values during the first 2 days. Porfimer sodium (Photofrin, Axcan Scandipharm Inc, Birmingham, Ala), is a mixture of oligomers of up to 8 porphyrin units and is photoactivated by light at both 630 nm and 515 nm wavelengths. It is a freeze-dried brownish powder, requiring reconstitution in 5% dextrose or 0.9% NaCl before use. After reconstitution, porfimer sodium should be protected from bright light and administered immediately. Dosing is usually 2 mg/kg given via slow intravenous (IV) infusion over 3 to 5 minutes. After

Table 1. Photosensitizers in Photodynamic Therapy

Photosensitizer	?Nm (peak)	Typical absorption coefficient*	Skin Phototoxicity	Comments
Porfimer sodium (Photofrin)	630	10000	4~6 weeks	Good tissue penetration, but prolonged skin photosensitivity
5-aminolevulinic acid (5-ALA)	632	<5000	1~2 days	Specific mucosal photosensitization, very limited penetration (2 mm) when used orally
Meta-tetrahydroxyphenylchlorin (mTHPC)	652	10000	1~2 weeks	Biological effect similar to PDT with porfimer sodium, smaller required light dose
Lutetium texaphyrin	732	42000	<3 days	Very good tissue penetration, rapid uptake and clearance, narrow treatment window 4~6 h after injection
Benzoporphyrin derivative	690	35000		Transient skin phototoxicity, approved for macular degeneration treatment
Zinc II Phthalocyanine	675~700	100000	1~2 days	Excellent tissue penetration and light absorption
Aluminum sulfonated Phthalocyanine	675	100000	1~2 days	Hydrophobic formulation with excellent tumor selectivity and cytotoxicity
Tin etiopurpurin (SnET2)	660	28000		Transient skin phototoxicity, deeper penetration than HpD

*Absortion of light cm^{-1} mol^{-1} L^{-1}

administration it is cleared from most tissues over 40 to 72 hours but retained for longer intervals in tumors, skin, and the reticuloendothelial system. Hence, light application is usually scheduled at 40 to 50 hours after administration. Porfimer sodium is contraindicated in patients taking other potential photosensitizing agents, including fluoroquinolones, griseofulvin, some hypoglycemic agents, phenothiazines, sulfonamides, sulfonylurea, tetracyclines, and thiazides. There is no published experience with overdosage of porphyrin sodium, and the effect of overdosage on duration or intensity of photosensitivity is not known. Porphyrin sodium is not dialyzable. Laser light applications should be withheld in the event of overdosage.

2) Light sources

Several commercial laser light sources can deliver appropriate wavelength light for application in the gastrointestinal tract. The diode laser system (Ceralas PDT 633; CeramOptec, Bonn, Germany), a 630 nm red light laser system, is the available light source in our center. It delivers up to 2000 mW of energy at the tip of the delivery fiber.

3) Light delivery devices

One challenge in the endoscopic application of PDT is the delivery and even distribution of adequate doses of light to the tissue being treated. For hollow cylindrical organs, such as the bile duct, light must be diffused evenly and circumferentially in a perpendicular orientation to the long axis of the fiber guide.

4) Treatment regimens

Total light dose of 160 to 180 J/cm are used for cholangiocarcinoma. To avoid generating a direct thermal effect of light on the tissue, a power density of 400 mW/cm is usually not exceeded. The relationship between total light dose in J/cm, power output from the diffusing fiber in watts, diffuser length in cm, and treatment time can be expressed as follows:

Light dose (J/cm)
= [power output from diffuser (W) x treatment time (s)] /diffuser length (cm)

2. PDT of Cholangiocarcinoma

Wong et al[21] showed a reduction of up to 60% of tumor volume after PDT with hematoporphyrin and with chlorine in nude mice inoculated with a human cholangiocarcinoma cell line. In vivo the first hint for its beneficial treatment came from a single case report of McCaughan et al.[22]

A translucent ERC cannular (triple lumen for guidewire, diffuser and contrast injection) is inserted into the tumor stenosis through which a 400-μm thin quartz fiber with a cylindrical light diffuser and radiopaque markers at the tip (Optiguide DCYL

200 series, QLT Phototherapeutics Inc., Vancouver, British Columbia) is placed under fluoroscopic guidance across the tumor stenosis. An alternative technique uses preloaded catheter.[23] After positioning a 0.035-inch guidewire proximal to the biliary stricture, the preloaded catheter is advanced over the guidewire using the monorail technique and positioned into the stricture. The guidewire is then withdrawn, and the diffuser tip with its radiopaque markers is positioned across the stricture. However, the peroral transpapillary transpapillary approach of PDT has some limitations with regard to appropriate application and patient follow-up. Although flexible tip diffusing fibers are usually employed, they may be rendered ineffective as a result of partial or complete fracture of the laser diffuser tip caused by bending during cannulation via the peroral route. In comparison, percutaneous cholangioscopy-guided PDT can provide an effective, homogeneous irradiation of the targeted lesion with the possibility of direct visual control. It is easily performed and can be monitored repeatedly without periodic peroral endoscopy, similarly to the merits of brief application and less pain associated with the routine exchange of stents in PTBD treatment.[24] PDT site is usually obstruction temporarily due to swelling and coagulation necrotic change within 1 week after PDT, therefore, insertion of exchangeable plastic endoprostheses or external drainage tube.

3. Results of Palliative PDT for Cholangiocarcinoma

In a pilot study,[25] Ortner et al performed PDT in patients with nonresectable cholangiocarcarcinoma Bismuth type III and IV who failed endoprostheses placement and had the poorest prognosis. Two days after intravenous application of a hematoporphyrin derivative Photofrin II, intraluminal photoactivation was performed cholangioscopically. Red light at 630 nm was emitted by an argon-dye laser and laser fibers of 400 μm core diameter with flexible cylindrical diffuser tips of 2.5 and 4 length were used. With output of 800 mW the light flux was 310 and 190 mW/cm^2, and by changing irradiation time the resulting dose was 180 J/cm^2. Bilirubin serum levels declined from 318±72 to 103±35 μmol/L (p=0.0039) with no significant increase during the 2 monthly follow-ups. Quality of life indices improved dramatically

(Karnofsky index 32.3%±8.13% to 68.9%±6.1%, p=0.0078; World Health Organization index 3.2±0.36 to 1.7±0.4, p=0.016; performance rating scale 13.6±1.6 to 5±0.93, p=0.0078) and remained stable during follow-up. Thirty-day mortality was 0%, 1-year survival was 77.7%, and median survival time was 439 days. In recently the prospective, open-label, randomized, multicenter study with a group sequential design compared PDT in addition to stenting (group A) with stenting alone (group B) in patients with nonresectable cholangiocarcinoma was reported.[26] PDT resulted in prolongation of survival (group A: n=20, median 493 days; group B: n=19, median 98 days; P<0.0001). It also improved biliary drainage and quality of life. Authors concluded that PDT, given in addition to best supportive care, improves survival in patients with NCC. The study was terminated prematurely because PDT proved to be so superior to simple stenting treatment that further randomization was deemed unethical. Similar results were obtained by our study.[27] Twenty patients who were treated with endoscopic biliary drainage alone (Group A) and 27 patients treated with PDT under percutaneous cholangioscopy and additional percutaneous biliary drainage (Group B) were analyzed retrospectively. The mean bilirubin level declined effectively

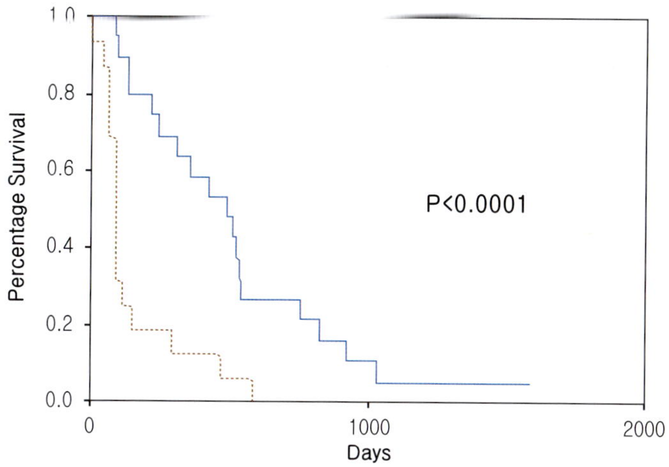

Fig. 1 Kaplan-Meier Survival Curve (ITT)

Kaplan-Meier survival curve of randomized patients treated with PDT plus stenting (group A, n = 20) and of patients with stenting alone (group B, n=19). Survival was longer in group A compared with group B (P=0.0001).

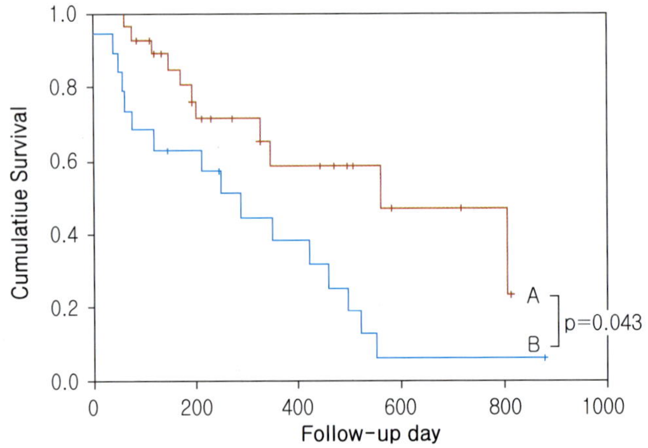

Fig. 2 Cumulative survival curve of patients with stenting alone (group A) and of patients treated PDT plus external biliary drainage (group B)

Kaplan-Meier estimate of survival function showed that median survival was 288.0±71.15 days in group A, 558.0±178.79 days in group B. Survival with PDT plus biliary drainage was superior than that in patients with endoscopic biliary drainage alone (p=0.0143). *Cheon YK, et al. Korean J Gastroentrol, 2004.*

in both group after treatment. One-year survival was 28% in group A, 52% in group B ($p<0.05$). Median survival time was 288 days in group A, 558 days in group B ($p=0.0143$, fig. 2).

4. Follow-up and Evaluation of PDT Efficacy

Evaluation of the therapeutic effects of PDT for patients with BDC presents a number of challenges. Ortner et al.[25] evaluated the therapeutic effect of PDT in cases of advanced BDC by comparing the tumor length before and after PDT using the 'mother baby' cholangioscopic technique; however, it has been argued that their assessment was insufficiently objective. Although the authors[26] reported reduced serum bilirubin levels after PDT, plastic biliary endoprostheses were inserted in all patients following the PDT procedure, making it difficult to assess the direct effect of PDT in reducing serum bilirubin. However, the PDT group might have mainly benefited from the number of ERCP sessions. For this reason, we do not consider the serum bilirubin level to be an objective parameter for assessing response to PDT. Ductal cholangiocarcinomas characteristically spread along or within the intrahepatic bile ducts, making it difficult to define the response to PDT based on changes in the tumor mass by CT. Similarly, it may be difficult to obtain objective results when the evaluation of the response to PDT is based solely on the extent of reopening of an occluded segment of bile duct, as has been done in some studies.[28] Previously, we assessed the thickness of the tumor mass before and after PDT treatment, measuring the thickest part of the tumor before the treatment and every month thereafter.[24] The mean thickness of the bile duct masses, as measured by IDUS, decreased from 8.7±3.7 mm before PDT to 7.1±2.0 mm at 1 month (P=0.176), to 7.1±2.4 mm (P=0.157) at 2 months, and declined significantly to 5.8±2.0 mm (P=0.046) 3 months after PDT.

In murine cancer models, some investigators have found that serum IL-6 levels correlate with tumor burden,[29,30] though this remains to be demonstrated clinically. Goydos et al.[30] reported that serum IL-6 levels were correlated with the tumor burden as measured by CT in patients with cholangiocarcinoma; 2 wk after tumor resection in 3 of 15 patients, IL-6 levels had dropped to undetectable levels in two patients and by almost tenfold in the third. I prospectively measured serum IL-6 levels in patients with BDC (N=26: 14 patients treated with PDT, 12 with biliary drainage alone), hepatocelluar carcinoma (HCC, N=26), and healthy adults (N=23). Serum IL-6 levels

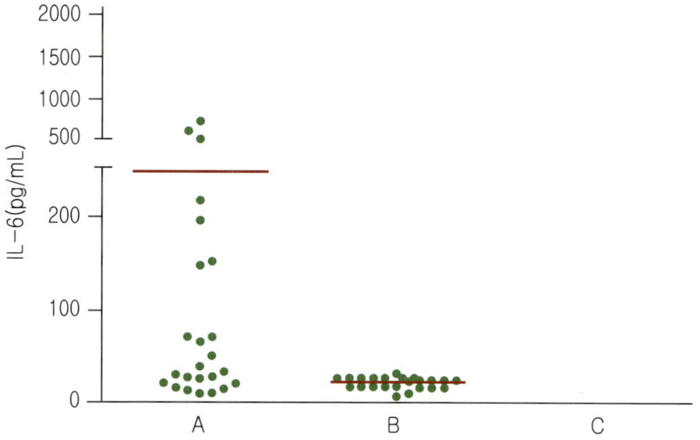

Fig. 3 Distribution of serum IL-6 levels in patients with bile duct cancer, hepatocellular carcinoma, and normal adults
Group A, bile duct cancer; group B, hepatocellular carcinoma; group C, healthy adults.

Table 2. Accuracy of the Tested Tumor Markers for the Diagnosis of Bile Duct Cancer

	Sensitivity	Specificity	Accuracy	PPV	NPV
IL-6>25.8 pg/mL	73%	92%	84%	83%	87%
CA 19-9>100 U/mL	52%	100%	85%	100%	80%

PPV=positive predictive value; NPV=negative predictive value

were measured by an enzyme-linked immunosorbent assay. Patients with clinical conditions known to increase IL-6 levels were excluded.[31] IL-6 was detected in all patients with BDC and HCC, and in 6 of 23 healthy adults. Median and mean levels of IL-6 were higher in patients with BDC than in both other groups ($P<0.001$, Fig. 3). Using a 25.8 pg/mL cutoff, IL-6 provided a diagnostic sensitivity of 73% and a specificity of 92%; positive and negative predictive values were 83% and 87%, respectively (Table 2). Serum levels of IL-6 were correlated with tumor burden in BDC patients. One month after treatment of BDC with PDT, the mean IL-6 level decreased significantly from 282.1±121.8 to 38.2±9.9 pg/mL ($P=0.008$, Fig. 4).

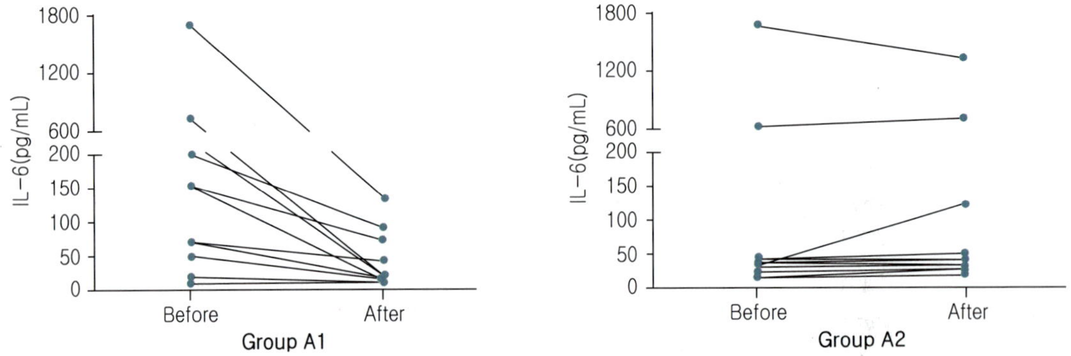

Fig. 4 Seruminterleukin-6 (IL-6) levels before and one month after photodynamic therapy (PDT) or stenting
(A) Group A1: patients treated with PDT; (B) Group A2: patients treated with endoscopic biliary drainage alone.

5. Sunlight Avoidance

The step-by-step instructions for how to "bleach out" the porfimer accumulated in the skin must be strictly followed. Following Berr's experience[32] on the 4th day after administration of porfimer patients start to expose some areas of skin (e.g., face, hands, and calves) completely for 10 minutes to mild evening sunlight before sunset. If tolerated without frank erythema, they can re-expose the same areas to sunlight for 10 minutes starting an hour earlier on the next day, check the effect, and continue on for the next days until they tolerate bright sunlight at noon. If unexposed to sunlight the skin's photosensitivity will persist for 5 or more months.

Conclusion

PDT seems to be a promising therapeutic approach for nonresectable cholangiocarcacinoma. It combines the aim to treat cholestasis and to reduce tumor growth. It is now necessary to strengthen these data in an extended randomized multicenter study. If the results are confirmed one could think of trying new photosensitizers with greater penetration depth and shorter photosensitivity, or using better drug targeting or combination therapies to induce more tumor necrosis. PDT

Table 3. Results of Photodynamic Therapy for nonresectable cholangiocarcinoma in Cancer Palliation

Author	n	Drug Dose (mg/kg)	Time interval (h)	Light Dose (J/cm^2)	Objective tumor response (%)	Follow-up (months)	Major complications
Ortner (25)	39	Photofrin (2)	48	180 j/cm^2	Median survival	41	2 cholangitis
Cheon (27)	47	Photofrin (2)	48	180~240 j/cm	Median survival prolongation	18	none
Shim CS (24)	24	Photofrin (2)	48	180~240 j/cm	Median survival prolongation	18	none

has a role to treat unresectable cholangiocarcacinoma as follows; (1) nonresectable hilar CC with unrelieved cholestasis; (2) inoperable co-morbid patient with respectable hilar CC; (3) Borderline respectable of hilar CC (neoadjuvant PDT for purging of intrahepatic ducts from tumor cells beyond the tumor margins); and (4) prolonging the patency of metal stent.

Reference

1. Kremer B, Henne-Bruns D, Vogel I, Grimm H, Soehendra N. Impact of staging on treatment of biliary carcinoma. Endoscopy 1993;25:92-99.
2. Klempnauer J, Ridder GJ, Werner M, et al. What constitutes long term survival after surgery for hilar cholangiocarcinoma? Cancer 1997;79:26-34.
3. de Groen PC, Gores GJ, LaRusso NF, et al. Biliary tract cancers, N Engl J Med 1999;341:1368-1378.
4. Hensen DE, Albores-Saavedra J, Corle D. Carcinoma of the extrahepatic bile ducts. Histologic types, stage of disease, grade and survival rates. Cancer 1992;70:1498-1501.
5. Burke EC, Jarmagin WR, Hochwald SN, et al. Hilar cholnagiocarcinoma: patterns of spread, the importance of hepatic resection for curative operation, and presurgical clinical staging system. Ann Surg 1998; 228:385-394.
6. Bhuiya MR, Nimura Y, Kamiya J, et al. Clinicopathologic factors influencing survival of patients with bile duct carcinoma: multivariate statistical analysis. World J Surg 1993;17:653-657.
7. Luman W, Cull A, Palmer KR. Quality of life in patients stented for malignant biliary obstructions. 1997;9:481-484.
8. Smith AC, Dowsett JF, Russell RC, et al. Randomized trial of endoscopic stenting versus surgical bypass in malignant low bile duct obstruction. Lancet. 1994;344:1655-1660.
9. Polydorou A, Cainms SR, Dowsett J, et al. Palliation of proximal malignant biliary obstruction by endoscopic endoprosthesis insertion. Gut 1991;32:685-689.
10. Ducreux M, Liguory CL, Lefebvre F, et al. Management of malignant hilar biliary obstruction by endoscopy. Results and prognostic factors. Dig Dis Sci 1992;37:778-783.
11. Chang WH, Kortan P, Haber GB. Outcome in patients with bifurcation tumors who undergo unilateral vs. bilateral hepatic duct drainage. Gastrointest Endosc 1998;47: 354-362.
12. Davids PH, Groen AK, Rauws EA, et al. Randomized trial of self-expanding metal stents versus polyethylene stents for distal malignant biliary obstruction. Lancet 1992;340: 1488-92.

13. Bowling TE, Galbraith SM, Hatfield AR, et al. A retrospective comparison of endoscopic stenting alone with stenting and radiotherapy in non-resectable cholangiocarcinoma. Gut 1996;39:852-855.
14. Molt P, Hopfan S, Watson R, et al. Intraluminal radiation therapy in the management of malignant biliary obstruction. Cancer 1986;57:536-544.
15. Weishaupt KR, Gomer CJ, Doughterty TJ. Identification of singlet oxygen as the cytotoxic agent in photoinactivation of a murine tumor. Cancer Res 1976;36:2326-2329.
16. Foote CS. Definition of type I and type II photosensitized oxidation. Photochem Photobiol. 1991;54:659.
17. Salet C, Moreno G. Photosensitization of mitochondria: Molecular and celluar aspects. J Photochem Photobiol B 1990;5:133-150.
18. Okunaka T, Eckhauser ML, Kato H. Correlation between photodynamic efficacy of different porphyrins and membrane portioning behavior. Lasers Surg Med 1992;12:98-103.
19. Henderson BW, Donovan JM. Release of prostaglandin E2 from cells by photodynamic treatment in vitro. Cancer Res 1989;49:6896-900.
20. Pahernik SA, Dellian M, Berr F, et al. Distribution and pharmacokinetics of Photofrin in human bile duct cancer. J Photochem Photobiol B 1998;47:58-62.
21. Wong M, Wang KK, Alexander Gl, et al. Cholorin E6 and hematophorphyrin derivative (HPD) on photodynamic therapy of a human cholangiocarcinoma model [abstract]. Gastroenterology 1996;110:595.
22. McCaughan JS, Mertens BF, Cho C, Barabash RD, Payton HW. Photodynamic therapy to treat tumors of the extrahepatic biliary ducts. A case report. Arch Surg 1991;126:111-113.
23. Rumalla A, Baron T, Wang K, et al. Endoscopic application of photodynamic therapy for cholangiocarcinoma. Gastrointest Endosc 2001;53:500-504.
24. Shim CS, Cheon YK, Cha SW, et al. Prospective study of the effectiveness of percutaneous transhepatic photodynamic therapy for advanced bile duct cancer and the role of intraductal ultrasonography in response assessment. Endoscopy 2005;37:425-33.
25. Ortner MA, Liebetruth J, Schreiber ST, et al. Photodynamic therapy of nonresectable cholangiocarcinoma. Gastroenterology 1998;114:536-42.
26. Ortner ME, Caca K, Berr F, et al. Successful photodynamic therapy for nonresectable cholangiocarcinoma: A randomized prospective study. Gastroenterology 2003;125:1355-63.
27. Cheon YK, Cho YD, Baek SH JH, et al. Comparison of survival of advanced hilar cholangiocarcinoma after biliary drainage alone versus photodynamic therapy with external drainage. Korean J Gastroenterol. 2004;44:280-7.
28. Berr F, Wiedmann M, Tannapfel A, et al. Photodynamic therapy for advanced bile duct cancer: Evidence for improved palliation and extended survival. Hepatology 2000;31:291-8.
29. Utsumi K, Takai Y, Tada T, et al. Enhanced production of IL-6 in tumor-bearing mice and determination of cells responsible for its augmented production. J Immunol 1990;145: 397-403.

30. Goydos JS, Brumfield AM, Frezza E, et al. Marked elevation of serum interleukin-6 in patients with cholangiocarcinoma: Validation of utility as a clinical marker. Ann Surg 1998; 227:398-404.

31. Cheon YK, Cho YD, Moon JH, et al. Diagnostic utility of interleukin-6 (IL-6) for primary bile duct cancer and changes in serum IL-6 levels following photodynamic therapy. Am J Gastroenterol. 2007;102:2164-70.

32. Berr F. Photodynamic therapy for cholangiocarcinoma. Semin Liver Dis 2004;24:177-187.

X·V
Endoscopic and Radiologic Palliation

Cholangiocarcinoma is divided into the extrahepatic and intrahepatic types, based on its anatomic location in the biliary tract and the extrahepatic type is divided as hilar (Klatskin) and distal tumors according to the anatomic location. Hilar tumors are further described according to the Bismuth classification based on the degree of the proximal tumor extension within the intrahepatic biliary tract.[1] Intrahepatic tumors can be found with a large peripheral mass, a cystic lesion or an intraductal tumor with segmental bile duct dilatation. They do not usually cause extensive bile duct dilatation, so jaundice, as a primary symptom, is rare. Extrahepatic tumors account for two-thirds of all the cholangiocarcinoma and usually present with obstructive jaundice due to obstruction at the hilum or common bile duct level.

The best available potentially curative therapy for cholangiocarcinoma is complete surgical resection.[2,3] Unfortunately, a majority of these patients with advanced cases are not good candidates for such curative therapy. Therefore, these patients may benefit from palliative therapy. Median survival for unresectable cholangiocarcinomas is lower without biliary drainage than with,[4-6] and bacterial cholangitis or liver failure often contributes to death. The aims of palliation in these patients are to relieve the obstructive cholestasis and its associated morbidities like pruritus, cholangitis and pain, to avoid liver failure due to progressive biliary obstruction, and to improve quality of life through minimal invasive therapy, cost-effectiveness, low procedure-related complications, and fewer hospital stays.[7] Palliation of obstructive cholestasis can be achieved successfully through two major non-surgical routes; One is a percutaneous route via percutaneous transhepatic cholangiography (PTC) and the other is an endoscopic route via endoscopic retrograde cholangio-pancreatography (ERCP).

Depending on the level of biliary stricture of the cholangiocarcinomas being distal or hilar lesions, the strategy of palliative treatment differs.

Palliation for Distal Extrahepatic Cholangiocarcinoma

The majority of distal extrahepatic cholangiocarcinomas are inoperable, and therefore restoring biliary flow with relief of jaundice and pruritus is the primary aim in the palliation of obstructive cholestasis due to distal lesions. Biliary drainage via the endoscopic route in these patients offers the advantages of physiologic bile drainage without externally exposed drainage tubes and has been proved to be more non-invasive and comfortable for the patients than that via the percutaneous route, mostly due to reduced frequency of bile leak, infection and hemorrhage following puncture of the liver.[8,9] So ERCP is used as the primary procedure for palliative endoscopic stenting of malignant distal bile duct obstruction.

1. Endoscopic Palliation with Biliary Stents

Endoscopic biliary drainage with biliary stent placement has now become the main and least invasive palliative modality for achieving adequate symptom relief and perhaps may provide a survival benefit in patients with obstructive cholestasis due to distal extrahepatic cholangiocarcinoma.[10] Endoscopic route via ERCP in these patients has several advantages over percutaneous route via PTC. The duodenum and the papilla can be directly inspected to check for tumor infiltration under endoscopic view of ERCP, cytological or biopsy samples can be easily obtained via endoscopic channel and subsequent placement of a biliary stent can be performed to relieve the obstructive cholestasis. So most stents in these patients are inserted endoscopically.

The two main types of commercially available biliary stents are the plastic stents and the self-expandable metal stents (SEMSs). Biliary stents are inserted successfully in approximately 90~95% of patients with distal extrahepatic cholangiocarcinoma and the procedure is more often successful in patients with distal rather than hilar lesions.[10]

When contemplating endoscopic palliation of obstructive jaundice, important variables that need to be considered include location and extent of the biliary obstruction, potential need for repeated interventions, plastic versus metal stents, and the life expectancy of the patient.[11]

1) Technique of endoscopic stenting

After cannulating the bile duct and injecting contrast medium under ERCP, careful consideration of biliary imaging allows detailed planning and successful execution of the palliative procedure. If endoscopic palliation of obstructive jaundice is contemplated, a decision should be made regarding the size and type of biliary stent. Whatever stent is to be used, a standard 0.035-inch guidewire through the catheter is inserted across the stricture to be stented into the bile duct and its tip passed into an intrahepatic duct. Although biliary sphincterotomy is usually required for access, it is not obligatory for placement of smaller diameter plastic stents and uncovered SEMSs in transpapillary positions. Relief of jaundice due to distal cholangiocarcinoma requires introduction of large 10-12 Fr plastic stents or SEMSs inserted with a duodenoscope with a 3.8 mm or 4.2 mm working channel. While plastic stents are inserted using a three layer coaxial system, consisting of guide-wire, inner guiding catheter and pusher tube/stent (Fig. 1), SEMSs are placed over the standard guidewire. The stents must be positioned and released accurately through the tumor under fluoroscopic and endoscopic guidance. The distal part of the metal stent should protrude about 1 cm into

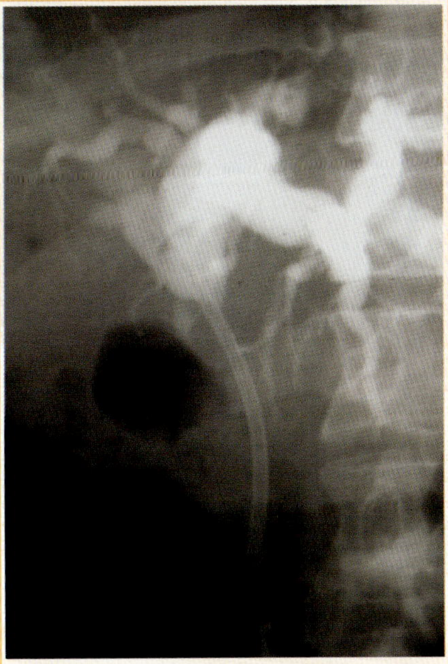

Fig. 1
Endoscopic placement of a 10-Fr plastic stent in a patient with malignant distal bile duct obstruction due to cholangiocarcinoma.

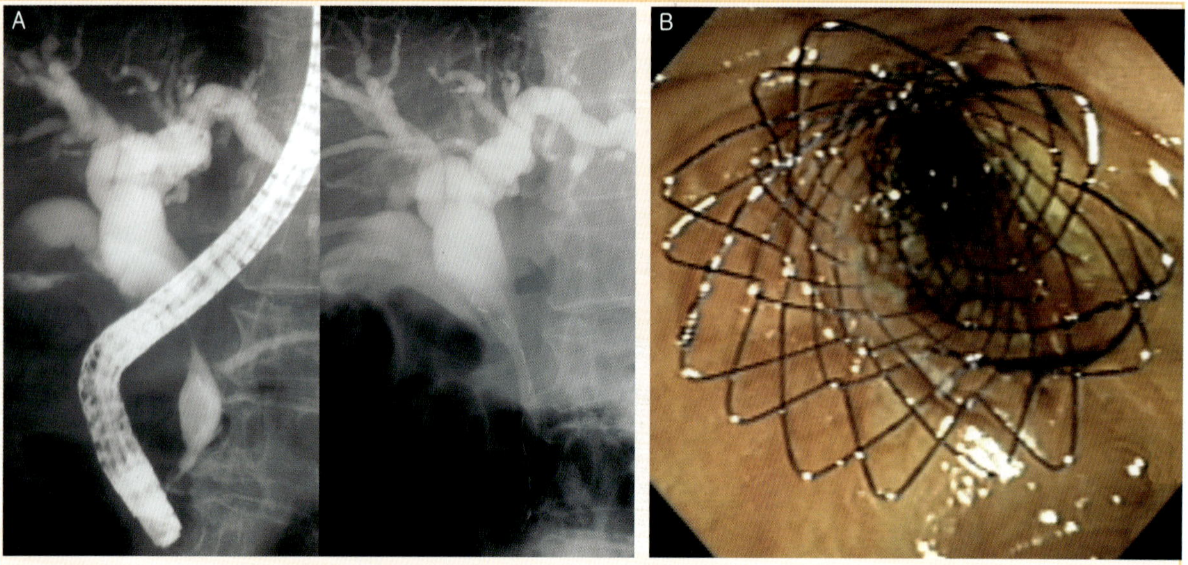

Fig. 2

Endoscopic placement of a 30-Fr uncovered metal stent in a patient with malignant distal bile duct obstruction due to cholangiocarcinoma.

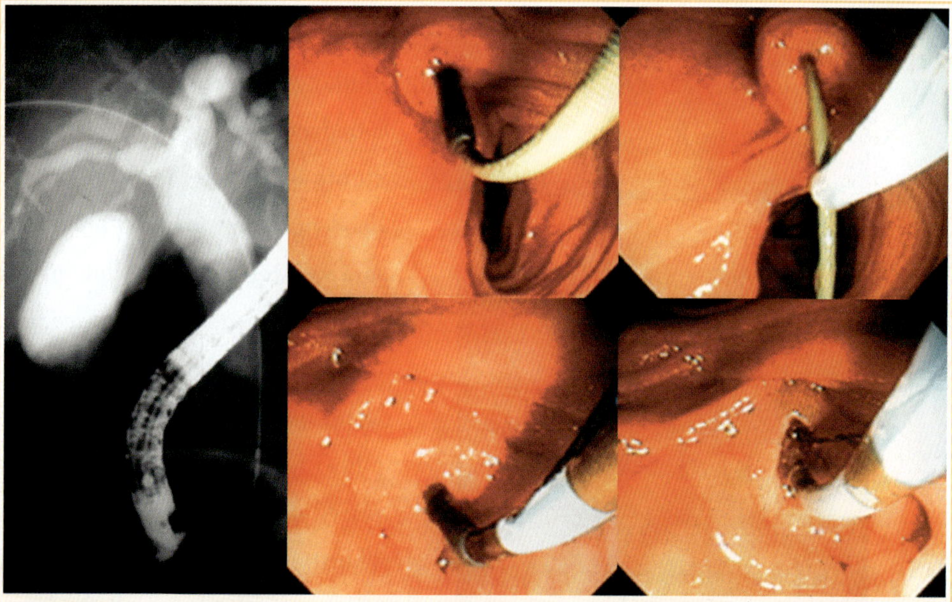

Fig. 3

Percutaneous endoscopic biliary stenting in a patient with malignant distal bile duct obstruction. It was performed in combination with the percutaneous-endoscopic methods for conversion of percutaneous biliary drainage into endoscopic biliary drainage. A long guidewire, which was inserted through the PTBD tube, was trapped by a basket in the duodenum and pulled out through the working channel of the duodenoscope, thereafter endoscopic stenting was undertaken in an ordinary method after endoscopic sphicterotomy.

the duodenum to allow easy endoscopic access, in case it is needed for the restoration of patency of occluded stents (Fig. 2).[9] If endoscopic stenting fails despite best efforts, percutaneous endoscopic biliary stenting (PEBS) is then performed as a combined percutaneous-endoscopic method for conversion of percutaneous biliary drainage into endoscopic biliary drainage (Fig. 3).

2) Plastic versus metal stents

Both plastic stents and SEMSs can be used for the palliation of distal cholangiocarcinoma. Plastic stents are relatively less expensive compared to SEMSs, and can be removed and replaced easily if they become occluded. However, the diameter of plastic stents is limited up to 12 Fr by the working channel size of the duodenoscope. Plastic stents have limited stent patency because they have a relatively narrow lumen and easily become occluded with biliary sludge and/or bacterial biofilm comprising of protein, bilirubin, bacteria and amorphous debris.[12] Stent occlusion usually leads to recurrent biliary obstruction with attendant jaundice and/or ascending cholangitis. Plastic stents of 10-11.5 Fr have patency rates of approximately 3 months but smaller diameter stents have significantly lower patency rates and should not be routinely placed for palliative drainage.[13] Two strategies have been employed related to plastic stent occlusion, including expectant management in episodes of stent occlusion and prophylactic scheduled exchange at 3-month intervals in order to prevent the risk of subsequent cholangitis. Prophyactic plastic stent changes improve symptom free survival compared to stent change at signs of stent occlusion. However, with prophylactic plastic stent changes, patients who live more than 6 months are least likely to be affected by the cost expenses and patient compliance for repeated stent changes is needed.[14] So plastic stents should be placed in patients who are likely to live less than 6 months.[15,16]

SEMSs were developed to overcome limitation of the diameter of plastic stents as they deliver a larger diameter stent up to 30 Fr or 10 mm, when deployed, using a relatively smaller delivery system of 7-8 Fr, facilitating easier passage across the biliary strictures. This larger diameter facilitates biliary flow and improves patency rates.[17] The comparison studies between plastic and SEMSs at ERCP conclude that the patency rates of SEMSs are superior to those of plastic stents for distal biliary obstruction, 10-12 months versus 3-4 months.[14,16-18] Because unresectable malignant biliary obstruction is typically associated with a survival of less than one year, SEMSs are intended to yield palliation of obstructive symptoms throughout the remaining lifespan of the patients.[17,19,20] Although SEMSs are more expensive and there is no significant difference in survival between plastic and SEMSs, They are chosen over plastic stents and are more cost-effective in patients who are likely to have a survival of more than 6 months.[21] This is due to superior stent patency, decreased need for repeated ERCP to manage recurrent jaundice, shorter hospital stays, reduced duration of antibiotic treatment, and fewer complications.[14,21] SEMSs may still eventually become occluded with tumor ingrowth, tumor overgrowth, epithelial hyperplasia or biliary sludge. Another major limiting factor of SEMSs is that they cannot be removed any other way than by operation. So tissue confirmation of cancer should always be obtained before placement of the SEMSs.[22]

3) Covered versus uncovered metal stents

Uncovered stents are made from stainless steel, cobalt based alloy, or a nickel-titanium (nitinol) alloy and are designed with a wire mesh. Covered stents were developed to overcome tumor ingrowth through the wire mesh and have non-porous covering membranes, such as polyurethane, silicone, or polytetrafluoroethylene (ePTFE) (Fig. 4). Although they prevent tumor ingrowth, overgrowth still remains a problem. The long-term durability of the covering membrane is sometimes problematic, because the covering membranes can be damaged during deployment or degradation due to reflux of the duodenal and gastric juices.[23] So tumor ingrowth in covered stents have the possibility of occurring through the tear of the covered membranes. Other potential problems of the covered stents include encrustation of bile, stent migration, or occlusion of the cystic duct, pancreatic duct, or lateral branches of the bile ducts. There was no significant difference in the incidence of cholecystitis between covered and uncovered metal stents.[24-26] Acute pancreatitis was revealed in 5.6 % to 6.1 % of patients after covered stent placement.[24,27-29] Each bare meshed end of covered stents with 5 mm in length allows embedding into the tissue to

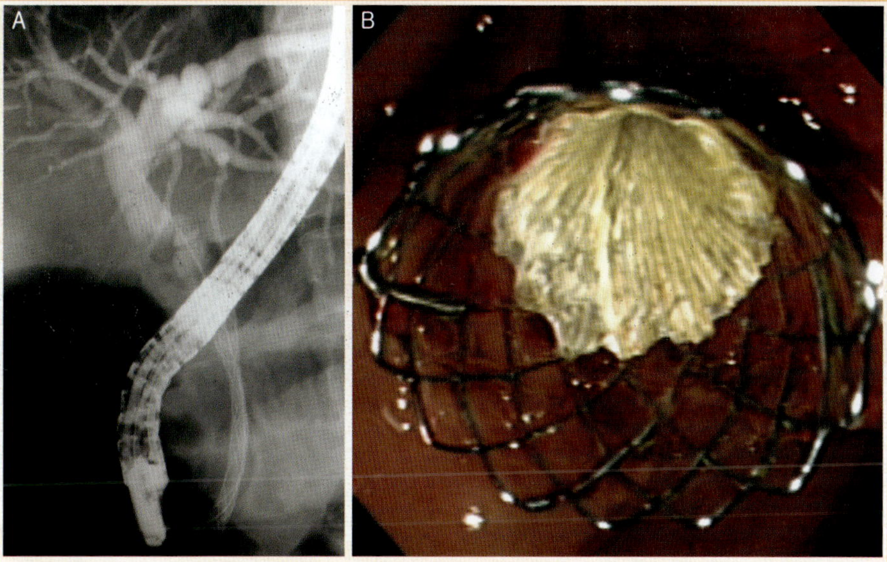

Fig. 4

Endoscopic placement of a 30-Fr covered metal stent with bare meshed ends in a patient with malignant distal bile duct obstruction due to cholangiocarcinoma.

reduce the risk of migration. They were originally introduced in an attempt to improve patency rates as compared with uncovered stents. However, the comparison studies between covered and uncovered Wallstents in unresectable distal malignant biliary obstruction failed to show a difference in stent patencies or complication rates,[24,30] except one study of covered versus uncovered diamond stents. Further well-designed large-scaled randomized prospective studies are needed to identify the benefits and indications for covered stents.

2. Percutaneous Palliation

When endoscopic biliary drainage fails or is unable to be performed, percutaneous transhepatic biliary drainage (PTBD) with or without percutaneous stenting may be a better off choice as an alternative palliation of the distal cholangiocarcinoma (Fig. 5). Failure of endoscopic drainage may be due to anatomical alterations, a periampullary diverticulum, duodenal obstruction by adjacent tumor, failure of deep cannulation into

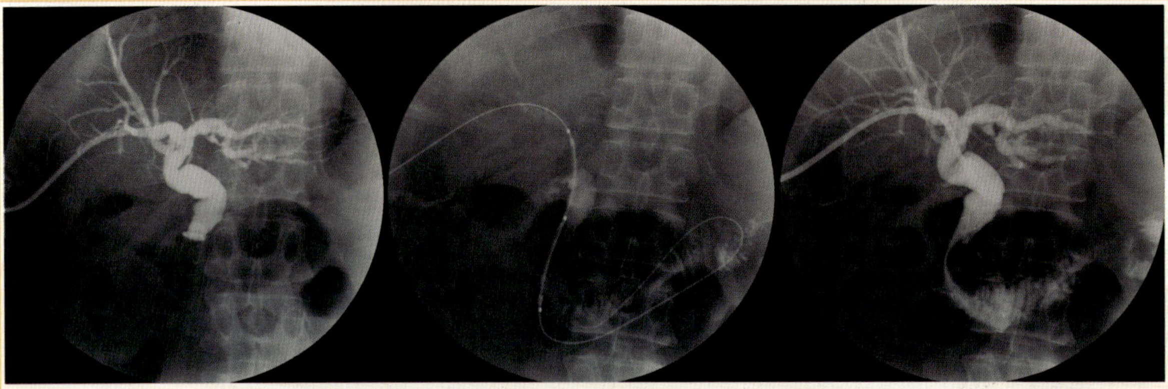

Fig. 5

Percutaneous biliary metal stenting in a patient with malignant distal bile duct obstruction. A metal stent assembly was inserted via the left side PTBD tract over a guidewire, which had been placed into the duodenum through the stenosis of the distal common bile duct, and then the metal stent was successfully deployed in a good position.

the common bile duct, or inability to advance the guidewire or insert a biliary stent through the biliary stricture.[31] PTBD procedures done under fluoroscopic and ultrasonographic guidance can reduce these complication rates, compared to those performed under only fluoroscopic guidance. In general, a bleeding tendency with a platelet count below 50,000/cm^3 and prothrombin time longer than 15 secs is considered an absolute contraindication of PTBD. Percutaneous drainage is not recommended for patients with advanced metastatic liver tumors, massive ascites or hepatic failure with a life expectancy of only days or weeks.[32] A major disadvantage of PTBD is due to the presence of a percutaneous tube, which could be uncomfortable for the patients and cause tube related-complications, such as hemorrhage, infection, bile leakage, pleural complications, and catheter blockage and migration. So external biliary drainage using the PTBD procedure is halted and internal drainage is percutaneously undertaken after removal of the percutaneous tube. SEMSs are generally preferable to plastic stents for internal drainage via percutaneous route and can be placed as a one-stage procedure in patients with unresectable distal cholangiocarcinoma. In one published prospective randomized trial comparing percuteneous and endoscopic stenting for palliation of inoperable malignant biliary obstructions, it was concluded that percutaneous placement of SEMSs was an alternative palliation to endoscopic placement of plastic stents.[33] Many non-comparative studies assessing the outcomes between percutaneous and endoscopic palliation for treatment of distal bile duct obstruction, stated that there were no significant differences in technical success, complication and mortality rates.[34-36] In patients in whom SEMSs protruding into the duodenum have become occluded, patency can usually be restored by endoscopic insertion of a plastic stent or SEMSs.

Palliation for Hilar Cholangiocarcinoma

Palliative treatment in patients with hilar cholangiocarcinoma clearly has an important role, because 80% of these are unresectable and a risk of recurrence is high even in those undergoing resection.[37,38] It represents a significantly greater challenge both technically and in decision making than that in patients with distal cholangiocarcinoma, because it is often difficult, needs a high degree of expertise, and carries a considerably high morbidity and mortality rate.[39] More than 90% of unresectable hilar cholangiocarcinomas have obstructive cholestasis and therefore restoration of bile flow is one of the main objectives of palliative treatment.[40] A median survival of 6-9 months for an unresectable hilar tumor implies that durable palliation should be one of the major objectives of treatment planning.[40] An ideal palliative procedure should be simple and effective in relieving obstructive cholestasis, have low procedure-related morbidity and mortality, and offer durable palliation.[22] In general, when appropriate expertise is available, ERCP is prefered to PTC for palliation of malignant hilar obstruction, because it allows definitive internal drainage in one procedure. However, the palliative management of hilar tumors is strongly dependent on individual expertise. Combined percutaneous and endoscopic procedures or percutaneous drainage alone are used in hilar tumors either after the failure of the endoscopic procedure or for further non-surgical intervention where obstructive cholestasis fails to be resolved after the endoscopic procedure.

1. Endoscopic Palliation with Biliary Stents

Endoscopic palliation has been considered as the treatment of choice if the hilar tumor is unresectable on preoperative evaluation. Endoscopic biliary drainage can be achieved with either plastic or metal stents, but patency rates of biliary stents are generally lower for hilar cholangiocarcinomas, compared with distal cholangiocarinomas.[41] The two questions which remain debatable are whether to use one or multiple stents, or plastic or metal stents for endoscopic palliation.

1) Technique

Important technical considerations during biliary stent insertion in hilar obstruction, include that initially it is imperative not to inadvertently inject contrast above the level of the hilar stricture into unintended multiple hepatic segments. A guidewire should be selectively inserted through the stricture into the bile duct of the desired hepatic segment, at which stage the contrast should be injected via a catheter which is passed deep over the guidewire into the targeted bile duct to get a selected unilateral cholangiogram. Finally a biliary stent is inserted over the guidewire. Dilatation may be helpful for hilar strictures particularly when bilateral stenting is being attempted. The left hepatic segments should be drained preferentially if a single stent is to be placed. This is due to the longer length of the left main heaptic duct before branching, which leads to larger volumes of the liver being able to be drained, resulting in a more effective drainage than the right. Since the right system is more variable with earlier branching and multiple segment obstructions are more common, a right sided stent is more likely to drain only a limited portion.

Bilateral stenting is technically challenging. The first stent is endoscopically placed in either the left or right hepatic duct whichever is more difficult to access first. The left stent is usually placed first as it is more difficult to access compared to the right stent. There are two techniques for endoscopic placement of bilateral metal stents; one is the 'side-by-side' (SBS) stenting technique and the other is the 'through-the-mesh' (TTM) stenting technique. The SBS technique is an endoscopic procedure for bilateral plastic or metal stenting with sequential delivery of two or more parallel plastic stents

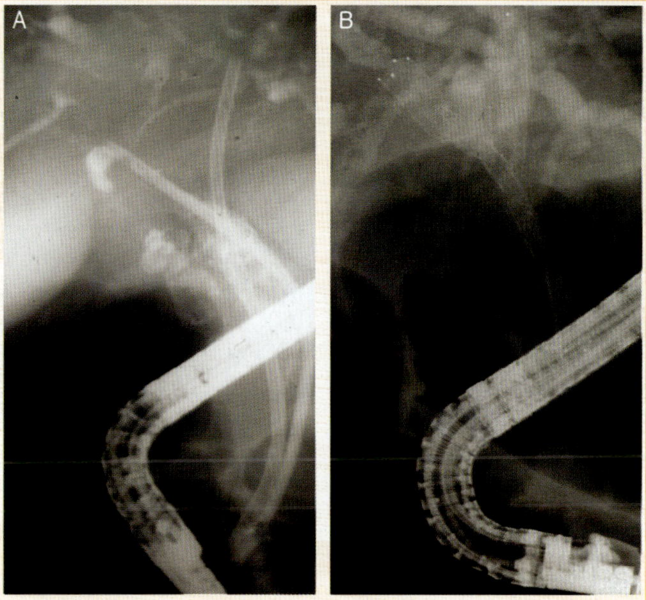

Fig. 6

Endoscopic placement of bilateral stenting using the 'side-by-side' stenting technique in patients with unresectable Bismuth type II malignant hilar obstruction. a. endoscopic biliateral plastic stenting, b. endoscopic biliateral metal stenting.

or SEMSs, to drain both intrahepatic bile ducts after multiple guidewire placements (Fig. 6). It can be extremely difficult or impossible despite best efforts in patients with unresectable hilar tumors. Once a metal stent is deployed endoscopically within the biliary tree, passage of a second metal stent alongside the initial stent is not technically easy because the first stent expands to completely occupy the bile duct lumen. So this technique usually demands prior dilatation. Advantage of the SBS technique is to allow access to both stents for endoscopic reintervention and easier recanalization in cases of subsequent stent occlusion.[9] However, it may be difficult when the stents do not traverse the papilla.

On the other hand, the TTM technique is alternative endoscopic procedure that allows bilateral metal stenting to be placed in a Y-configuration, in which a second stent traverses through the open-mesh wall of the initial stent to enter the opposite hepatic lobe. During this procedure, attempts to pass a second metal stent through the mesh of the indwelling initial conventional metal stent can be technically problematic, due to the tightly woven structure of the stent wire mesh. Even if a taper-tipped

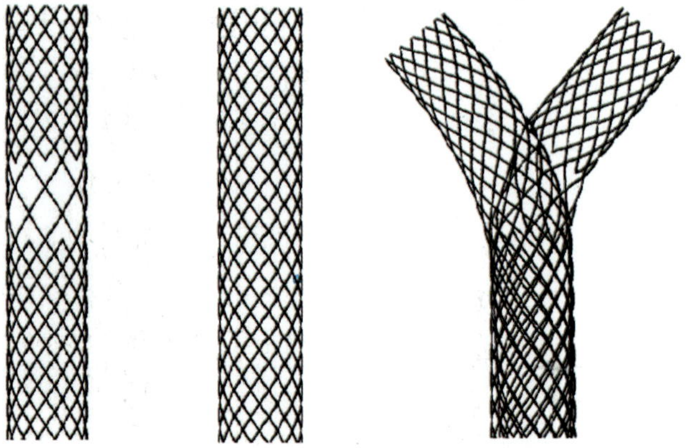

Fig. 7

Schema of 'Through-the-mesh' technique for endoscopic bilateral metal stenting using a biliary Y-stent with a wider-mesh portion in the center (left). The joining of the Y-stent and conventional metal stent (middle) through the wider-mesh portion of the Y-stent produces a Y-shaped arrangement (right).

catheter, hydrostatic balloon, or a 7 Fr Soehedra stent extractor is used to widen the smaller-mesh wall of the initial stent, it still proves difficult to permit passage of the second stent during an ERCP.[42]

For overcoming such technical difficulty in the TTM technique using conventional metal stents, several kinds of newly designed SEMSs have been recently introduced to facilitate passage of the second metal stent during bilateral stenting. One of them is a Y-stent (Y type biliary Niti-S stent, Taewoong Inc., Seoul, Korea) with a wider-mesh portion in the center and smaller-mesh portions on both ends. The joining of the Y-stent and conventional metal stent through the wider-mesh portion of the Y-stent produces a Y-shaped arrangement (Fig. 7). Y-stent being the first stent, is endoscopically placed through the hilar stricture into the intrahepatic bile duct, and then the second being a conventional biliary metal stent is advanced over the guidewire from the inside of the Y-stent through the central wider-mesh portion into the contralateral intrahepatic duct, and released to form a Y-shape. The large opening in the wider-mesh wall of the first Y-stent permits easy passage of the delivery catheter for the second stent and its wide expansion (Fig. 8). More than two metal stents, including multiple Y-stents, can be inserted in sequence using the TTM technique in order to drain multiple hepatic segments (Fig. 9). The two main drawbacks of this Y-

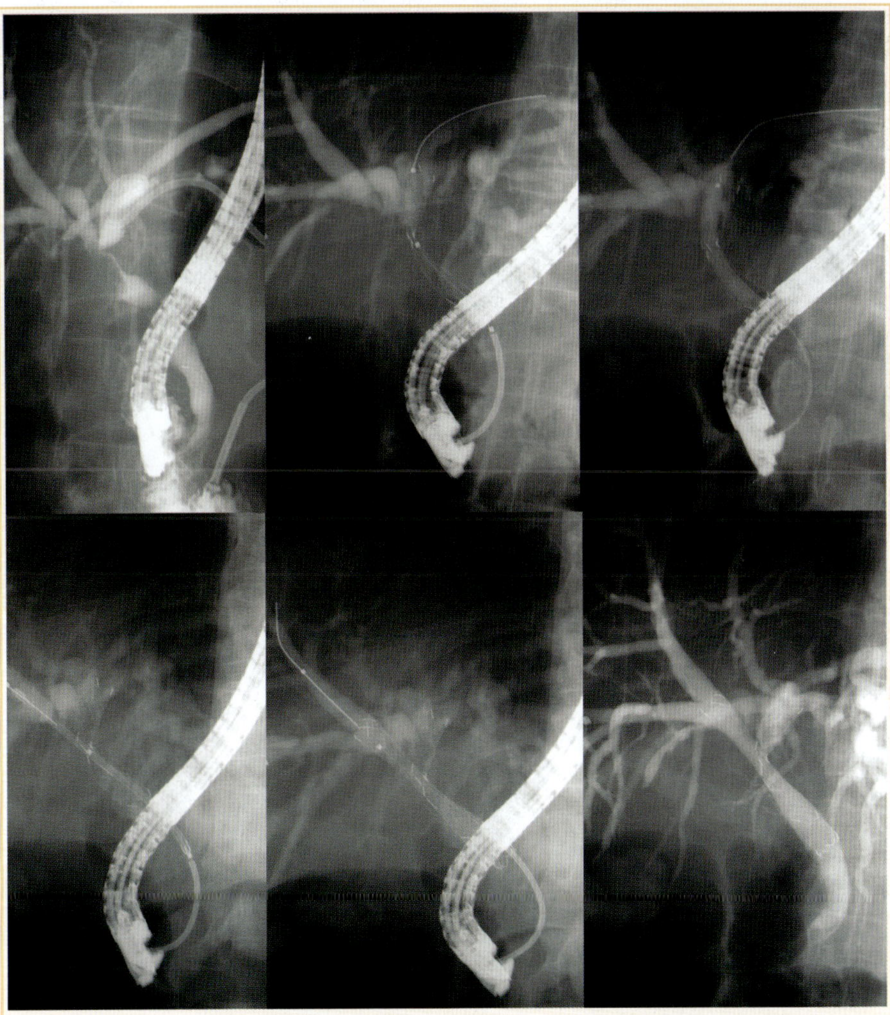

Fig. 8 Endoscopic placement of bilateral metal stenting using a biliary Y-stent in patients with unresectable Bismuth type II malignant hilar obstruction

The first stent, being a Y-stent, was endoscopically placed in the left hepatic duct which is usually more difficult to access first, and balloon dilatation was done to widen the opening of its central portion, thereafter a second stent, being a conventional biliary stent, was inserted through the open-mesh wall of the first stent to gain access to the opposite hepatic lobe, resulting in a Y-configuration.

stent are firstly, that later endoscopic access to both stents is often impossible after stent occlusion. Secondly, the wider-mesh structure in the center causes an increasing tendency of tumor ingrowth and poor stent expansion due to the weak radical force.

Other types of metal stents (M-Hilar stent and K-Hilar stent, Standard Sci-Tech Inc., Seoul, Korea) for bilateral stenting have just been developed to overcome the

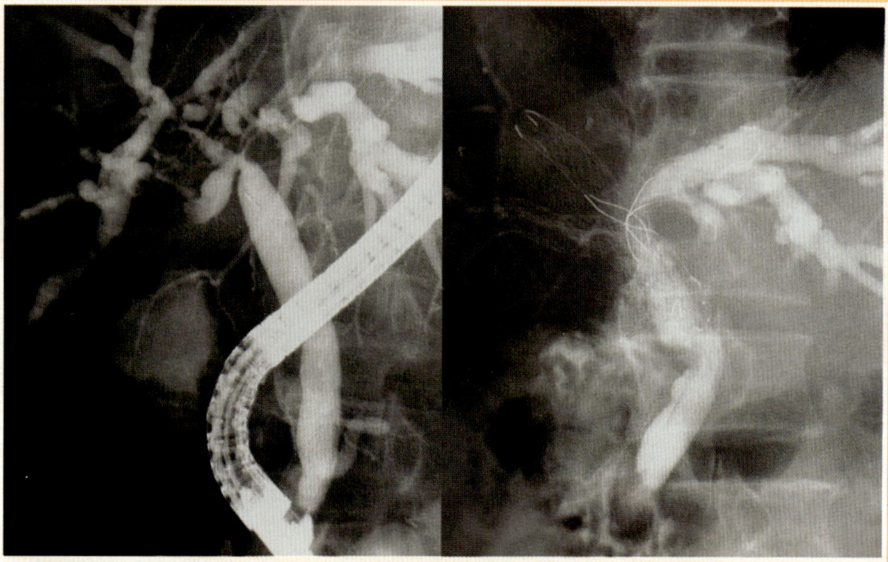

Fig. 9

Endoscopic placement of three metal stents using the 'through-the-mesh' stenting technique in a patient with Bismuth type IV malignant hilar obstruction. Two Y-stents in the left hepatic duct and right anterior intrahepatic bile duct, repsectively, and one Zilver stent in the right posterior intrahepatic bile duct were successfully inserted in sequence.

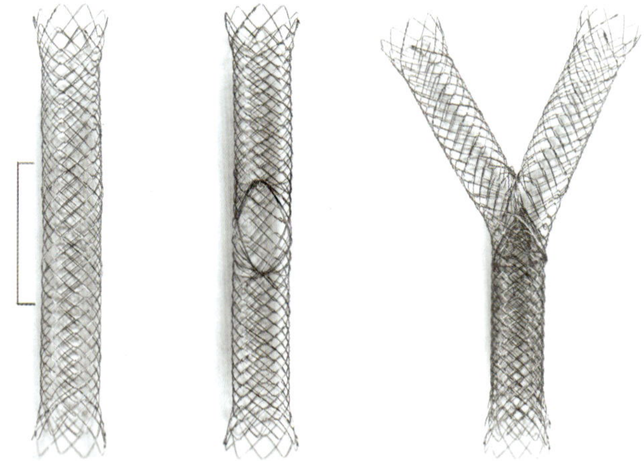

Fig. 10 Schema of 'Through-the-mesh' technique for endoscopic bilateral metal stenting using a biliary M-hilar (left) and K-hilar stent (middle)

The joining of both stents through the central-mesh portion of the M-hilar stent produces a Y-shaped arrangement (right). The M-hilar stent has been designed with a differently woven structure in the center (left, noted portion), which permits easy passage of the delivery catheter of the second stent, even though it has no wider-mesh portion. The K-hilar stent is another special stent with a large hole in the center of the stent. When this particular stent is used as the second stent during bilateral stenting, lumens of both stents are absolutely patent without blockage of the wire mesh.

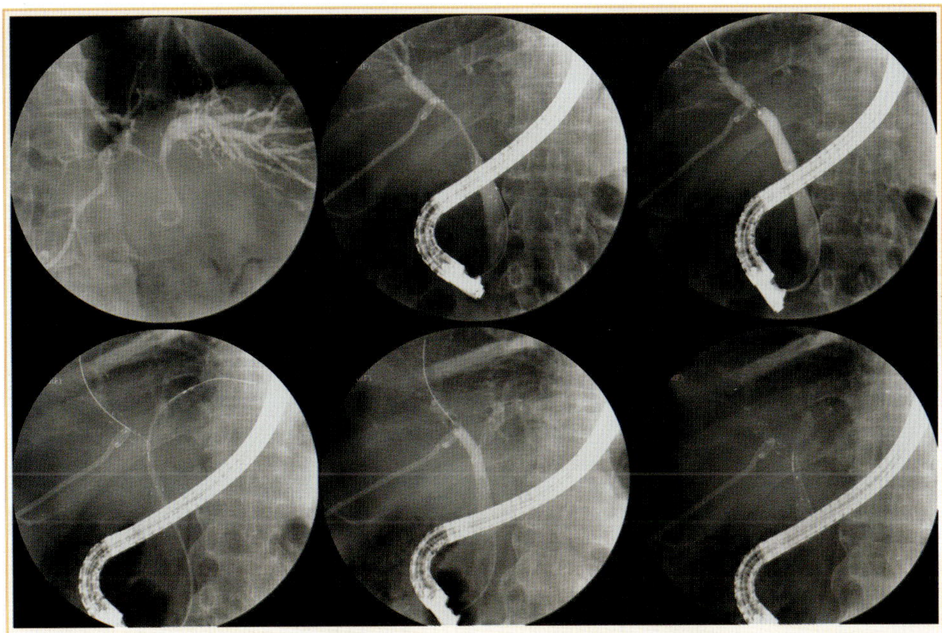

Fig. 11 Endoscopic placement of bilateral metal stenting using both biliary Bona-M and Bona-K stents in a patient with unresectable Bismuth type IIIa malignant hilar obstruction.

The first stent, being the Bona-M stent, was endoscopically placed in the right intrahepatic bile duct, and balloon dilatation was done to widen its lumen, thereafter a second stent, being the Bona-K stent, was inserted through the differently woven structure in the center of the first stent to gain access to the opposite hepatic lobe, resulting in a Y-configuration.

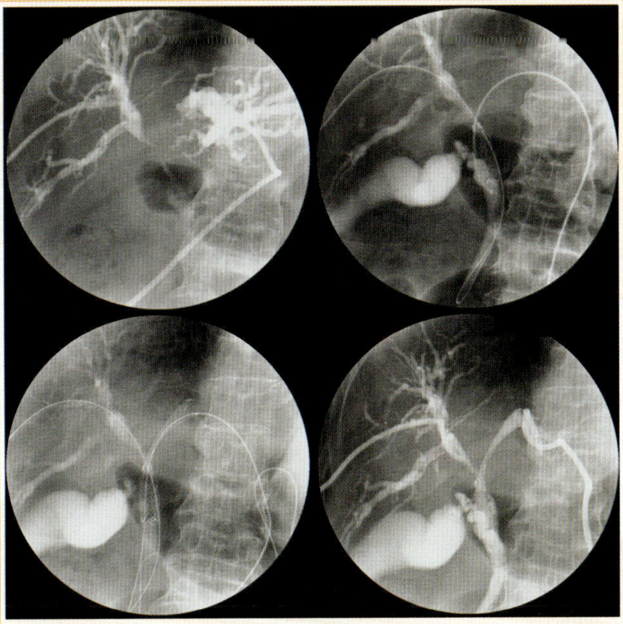

Fig. 12 Percutaneous placement of bilateral stenting using the 'side-by-side' stenting technique in patients with Bismuth type II malignant hilar obstruction

drawbacks of the Y-stent as described above. The M-Hilar stent has been designed with a differently woven structure in the center, which permits easy passage of the delivery catheter of the second stent, even though it has no wider-mesh portion. The K-Hilar stent is another special stent with a large hole in the center of the stent (Fig. 10). When this particular stent is used as the second stent during bilateral stenting, lumens of both stents are absolutely patent without blockage of the wire mesh (Fig. 11). So endoscopic re-intervention with plastic stents, is easily performed using these new Y-stents.

2) Unilateral versus bilateral biliary stents

Single stents are adequate for Bismuth type I hilar cholangiocarcinomas, which have strictures of the main bile duct below the confluence. However, there is significant controversy as to whether single or multiple stents should be inserted for Bismuth type II, III and IV hilar cholangiocarcinomas. The decision of whether to place single or multiple bilary stents depends on the location and extent of the stricture in the biliary tract as well as the degree of biliary contamination.[7] It is well known that only 25% of the liver volume needs to be drained for adequate palliation of obstructive cholestasis with improvement in biochemical parameters.[35,43] Therefore, a single bilary stent into one functional liver lobe for unilateral drainage should provide adequate palliation in a major portion of patients with hilar cholangiocarcinoma, and many studies have reported good results using a single stent in about 80% of patients with Bismuth type II and III hilar cholangiocarcinomas.[44,45] No difference in efficacy has been shown between single stent placement in the left or the right hepatic lobe.[46]

Sometimes, however, bilateral biliary stents may be needed for palliative drainage of both hepatic lobes when both sides are contaminated, when a non-dominant or atrophic lobe is inadvertently stented without efficacy, or if bilateral brachytherapy is scheduled.[47] Especially the vigorous opacification of multiple bile ducts of both hepatic lobes, to obtain detailed cholangiograms with contrast during ERCP, increases the necessity for biliateral stent insertion in hilar tumors, because cholangitis mainly arises from contaminated and undrained bile ducts. The necessity for the drainage of both systems during ERCP is really more to prevent postprocedure cholangitis than to have effective palliation. If both lobes are imaged with contrast during ERCP, bilateral stent insertion reduces the potential sequelae of cholangitis in undrained bile ducts. However, even in the most experienced hands, endoscopic placement of bilateral stents may be difficult or impossible, and failure of bilateral stenting after extensive contaminated contrast filling of multiple bile ducts may frequently lead to subsequent cholangitis. If contrast does not contaminate both sides or is sufficiently drained from unilateral bile duct after imaging both sides, then unilateral stenting should be enough and is substantially easier to perform endoscopic reintervention.

Several studies have attempted to address whether unilateral or bilateral drainage is preferred for palliation of obstructive jaundice in patients with hilar tumors.[6,45,48,49] Early studies have shown high rates of cholangitis following ERCP in large parts attributed to the contamination of the undrained segments which was caused by contrast injection without any planned limitations.[6,48] These studies showed that bilateral stent insertion was associated with an increased survival rate and reduced the risk of cholangitis, compared to unilateral drainage for Bismuth type II and III hilar lesions.[48] The highest survival rate was noted in patients with hilar tumors who had bilateral drainage, while the lowest survival rate in those who showed cholangiographic opacification of both lobes but only able to have unilateral drainage.[6] These results are believed to have been caused by inadvertent contrast injections into the undrained bile ducts and quite clearly show that failure to drain an opacified lobe leads to a significantly negative outcome, thus bilateral drainage being mandatory if both hepatic lobes are opacified. However, an unsuccessful attempt at bilateral drainage can lead to increased incidence of cholangitis and lower survival rates.[44,50] So ERCP in hilar tumors should only be undertaken in highly regarded institutions with high success rates for drainage of hilar obstruction.

Selectively targeted and planned endoscopic drainage guided by MRCP or CT imaging has recently been introduced to reduce inadvertent contrast injections into atrophied and/or unintended multiple hepatic segments, and thus resulting in a lower incidence of postprocedure cholangitis.[12,15,45,49,50] MRCP is widely known as a reliable and noninvasive diagnostic tool and shows equivalent imaging to that of ERCP in demonstrating the detailed anatomy of the biliary tree. Several advantages that MRCP has over ERCP include noninvasive diagnostic tool, no use of contrast medium and the delineation of missing ducts which are not visible in the endoscopic cholangiogram due to complete obstruction of the bile ducts. Cholangiograms obtained from MRCP provide a road map for the biliary endoscopist to define the biliary anatomy prior to ERCP, and results in them being able to choose the optimal hepatic lobe and bile ducts for effective drainage.[12,45,49,50] Nowadays MRCP has led to the unnecessary need for a diagnostic ERCP and is rapidly replacing its role for the delineation of the biliary tree, therefore ERCP is becoming an unnecessary procedure for such diagnostic purposes in hilar tumors. ERCP for hilar obstruction can be undertaken mainly for the therapeutic purpose of endoscopic intervention such as stenting into the targeted bile duct with the help of MRCP. Several studies have evaluated the role of MRCP-guided selective unilateral biliary stent placement for endoscopic palliation of hilar tumors, and showed that the use of MRCP to plan endoscopic stent placement, reduced the need to inject contrast into multiple segments during ERCP, and thus diminished the risk of postprocedure cholangitis.[15,49-51]

3) Plastic versus metal biliary stents

A plastic stent has been commonly used to achieve biliary drainage in patients with a malignant hilar stricture. However, the use of plastic stents for hilar tumor palliation revealed poor results in some series.[47,52] Plastic stents in the hilar stricture have limited stent patency due to their narrow lumen and a higher chance of stent clogging due to the longer length of the stent used. Stent occlusion frequently results in cholangitis with cholangitis rates as high as 20~40% reported for unilateral or biliateral plastic stents due to bacterial contamination of undrained bile ducts.[47,52] Other disadvantages of plastic stents include that it is technically difficult to place more than one 10 Fr stent at the initial setting and plastic stents in hilum are prone to distal migration.[7]

SEMSs are increasingly favored, although individually more expensive. A larger diameter of SEMSs may potentially result in improved stent patency as compared with that of plastic stents, thus needing fewer repeated procedures.[16,51,53] In addition, there are some theoretical advantages to the use of metal stents in hilar tumors, including the open-mesh design, which allows drainage of secondary branches through the side of the stent and is less likely to result in an obstructive segmental cholangitis.[54] When single lobe drainage is planned, insertion of an uncovered metal stent is preferred to prolong patency, and to avoid occlusion of branch ducts which is more likely with a plastic stent. Although few data is available for hilar tumors, the current evidence favors the placement of SEMSs as they provide a superior palliation in comparison to plastic stents in terms of early and late complications.[6,55] The initial higher cost is offset by lower incidence of reintervention and hospitalization for complications.[52] However, a major limiting factor of SEMSs is that they cannot be removed other than surgically.[22] So plastic stent placement for the palliative therapy can be recommended if diagnosis is clinically ambiguous or SEMSs placement is impossible. Covered metal stents are not appropriate for hilar strictures as intrahepatic side branches can be inadvertently obstructed.[56] Covered stents may lead to the inadvertent occlusion of intrahepatic side branches, but cystic or pancreatic duct obstruction by covered stents does not usually result in cholecystitis or pancreatitis.

2. Percutaneous Palliation

Percutaneous palliation in patients with unresectable hilar tumors is usually performed when appropriate ERCP expertise is not available. However, some biliary specialists still favor the percutaneous approach over the endoscopic approach for the palliation of unresectable hilar tumors, particularly Bismuth type III and IV strictures in which endoscopic stent placement is problematic.[9,10,57] Percutaneous biliary drainage and stenting in these patients has evolved into a safe and effective technique, and is equally effective for the treatment of hilar obstruction as compared with distal biliary obstruction. SEMSs have proved to be superior to plastic stents in percutaneous radiological intervention and should therefore be used.[58]

1) Percutaneous drainage

Percutaneous biliary drainage in hilar tumors is usually performed in Europe and the USA, when experts for endoscopic procedures are unavailable. In addition, it may be necessary in the following situations, in which endoscopic biliary drainage may not be feasible: papilla inaccessible via peroral route during ERCP due to obstructing luminal tumors or alternated anatomy by reconstructive surgery, tight strictures to be passed through with a guidewire, and the existence of contaminated segments unable to be endoscopically drained.[10,31,41,47] Performing PTBD has no additional benefits on patients with complex hilar obstruction whose jaundice has not responded properly to targeted endoscopic stenting, because the jaundice is usually caused by advanced intrahepatic tumor.[50] The percutaneous biliary drainage is technically simple and provides better demonstration of the proximal extent of the tumor, when compared to endoscopic drainage. Percutaneous biliary drainage can be performed externally or internally.

2) Percutaneous stenting

SEMSs are generally prefered to plastic stents for percutaneous biliary drainage for the palliation of unresectable hilar tumors. Dilatation of the stricture prior to stent deployment may be helpful. This allows easier passage of the stent delivery catheter and accelerates full expansion of the metal stent. The studies for the percutaneous biliary metal stenting in hilar tumors revealed a technical success rate of 93-100% and procedure-related mortality of less than 5%.[10,52,59,60] Reintervention for recurrent jaundice was required in 30~38% of patients during long-term follow up.[52,60]

If the contralateral duct system is not opacified during PTC, drainage of a single lobe is sufficient, especially if CT or MRI imaging reveals atrophy of the non-opacified lobe of the liver. However, if the patient's jaundice fails to be resolved, or if there is cholangitis of the contralateral lobe, bilateral drainage should be carried out. The shortest survival rate has been observed in those with cholangiographic opacification of both lobes but drainage of only one.[48,61,62] Deployment of two stents can be achieved either through a single transhepatic tract or by using two separate punctures to gain access to each lobe (Fig. 12). Planned percutaneous metal stenting, which results in drainage of almost all of the hepatic segments, can be undertaken in accordance with the anatomic types of strictures described under the Bismuth classification.[32] It can be performed either with a single stent or multiple stents in a Y, T, or chi-configuration (X

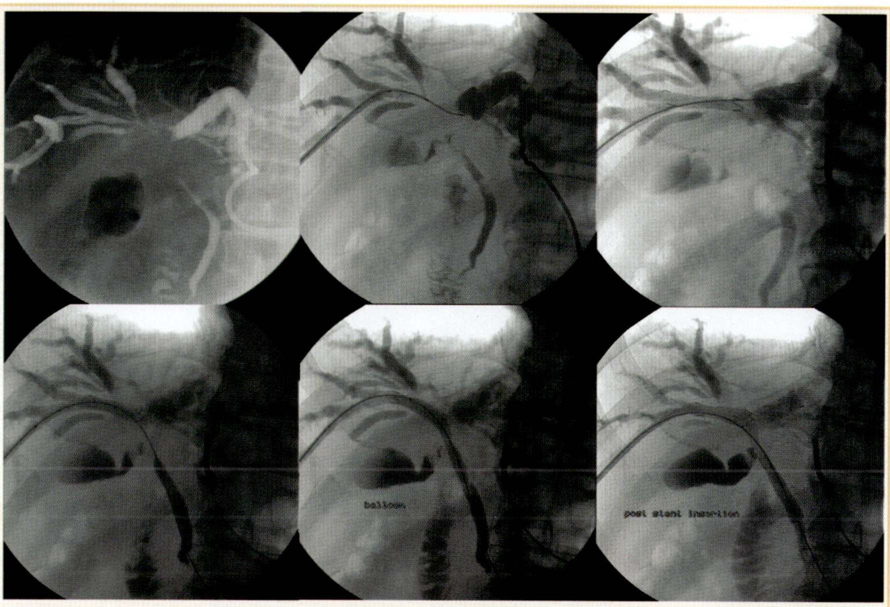

Fig. 13 Percutaneous placement of bilateral stenting in a T-configuration in patients with Bismuth type II malignant hilar obstruction

T-configuration stenting was performed via the right side PTBD route, as the first metal stent, being a Y-stent, was percutaneously inserted through the hilar stricture into the left hepatic duct, thereafter a second metal stent, being a conventional biliary stent, was inserted following the same percutaneous route through the wide-mesh portion of the center of the first inserted stent into the common bile duct after balloon dilatation of the central portion of the first stent.

shape). In Bismuth type I, unilateral PTBD and subsequent unilateral stenting could be considered sufficient. In Bismuth type II, T-configuration stenting can be performed through a unilateral PTBD route, but Y-configuration stenting through the bilateral PTBD routes are a more common practice (Fig. 13). If bilateral PTBDs are undertaken in Bismuth III or more, Y- or chi-configuration stenting are recommended choices, even if T-configuration stenting is also available. In chi-configuration stenting, one stent extends from the left duct through the hilar stricture into either the right anterior or right posterior intrahepatic bile duct, the other stent is placed into one of right intrahepatic ducts whichever has not been occupied yet, extending past the hilar stricture and finally reaching the common bile duct or transpapillary duodenum. Therefore it allows drainage of the entire major segmental ducts (Fig. 14).[32]

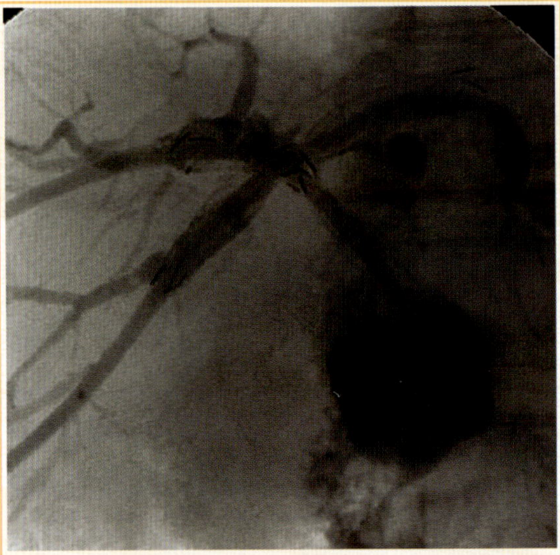

Fig. 14 Percutaneous placement of bilateral stenting in a Chi-configuration in patients with Bismuth type IIIa malignant hilar obstruction

One stent extended from the right posterior intrahepatic bile duct through the hilar stricture into the left hepatic duct via the PTBD route of the right posterior intrahepatic bile duct, and the other stent was placed into the right anterior intrahepatic duct through the central portion of the first stent into the common bile duct via the PTBD route of the right anterior intrahepatic bile duct, resulting in its X-shaped configuration.

Conclusion

Cholangiocarcinoma is a relatively rare neoplasm of the bile ducts which is increasing in incidence. Surgical resection is the best available therapy but, unfortunately, the majority of patients present with unresectable disease at the time of diagnosis. This has led to the emergence of several non-surgical palliative managements, usually by means of endoscopic or percutaneous radiological techniques. Such palliative management of these patients is challenging for all biliary specialists, because there is no single correct approach for it and there are several controversies in choice of therapies according to the location and extension of cholangiocarcinoma. For palliation of distal lesions, an endoscopic approach should be initially used with percutaneous radiological intervention reserved for its failures. For palliation of hilar lesions, either an endoscopic or percutaneous approach can be the procedure of choice depending on the institutions, because outcomes of them are influenced by the operators' skill and experience. There is still a lack of clear consensus on the use of covered versus uncovered metal stents in distal cholangiocarcinoma and plastic versus metal stents and unilateral versus bilateral drainage in hilar cholangiocarcinoma. This decision should be made on an individual basis, till acceptable results are acquired in randomized, controlled trials to further evaluate these therapies.

Reference

1. Bismuth H, Castaing D, Traynor O. Resection or palliation: priority of surgery in the treatment of hilar cancer. World J Surg 1988;12:39-47.
2. Ahrendt SA, Nakeeb A, Pitt HA. Cholangiocarcinoma. Clin Liver Dis 2001;5:191-218.
3. Lazaridis KN, Gores GJ. Cholangiocarcinoma. Gastroenterology 2005;128:1655-67.
4. Farley DR, Weaver AL, Nagorney DM. "Natural history" of unresected cholangiocarcinoma: patient outcome after noncurative intervention. Mayo Clin Proc 1995;70:425-9.
5. Berr F. Photodynamic therapy for cholangiocarcinoma. Semin Liver Dis 2004;24:177-87.
6. Chang WH, Kortan P, Haber GB. Outcome in patients with bifurcation tumors who undergo unilateral versus bilateral hepatic duct drainage. Gastrointest Endosc 1998;47:354-62.
7. Chahal P, Baron TH. Endoscopic palliation of cholangiocarcinoma. Curr Opin Gastroenterol 2006;22:551-60.
8. Speer AG, Cotton PB, Russell RC, Mason RR, Hatfield AR, Leung JW, MacRae KD, Houghton J, Lennon CA. Randomised trial of endoscopic versus percutaneous stent insertion in malignant obstructive jaundice. Lancet 1987;2:57-62.
9. Cowling MG, Adam AN. Internal stenting in malignant biliary obstruction. World J Surg 2001;25:355-9; discussion 359-61.
10. England RE, Martin DF. Endoscopic and percutaneous intervention in malignant obstructive jaundice. Cardiovasc Intervent Radiol 1996;19:381-7.
11. Levy MJ, Baron TH, Gostout CJ, Petersen BT, Farnell MB. Palliation of malignant extrahepatic biliary obstruction with plastic versus expandable metal stents: An evidence-based approach. Clin Gastroenterol Hepatol 2004;2:273-85.
12. Raijman I. Biliary and pancreatic stents. Gastrointest Endosc Clin N Am 2003;13:561-92, vii-viii.
13. Speer AG, Cotton PB, MacRae KD. Endoscopic management of malignant biliary obstruction: stents of 10 French gauge are preferable to stents of 8 French gauge. Gastrointest Endosc 1988;34:412-7.

14. Prat F, Chapat O, Ducot B, Ponchon T, Pelletier G, Fritsch J, Choury AD, Buffet C. A randomized trial of endoscopic drainage methods for inoperable malignant strictures of the common bile duct. Gastrointest Endosc 1998;47:1-7.
15. Khan SA, Davidson BR, Goldin R, Pereira SP, Rosenberg WM, Taylor-Robinson SD, Thillainayagam AV, Thomas HC, Thursz MR, Wasan H. Guidelines for the diagnosis and treatment of cholangiocarcinoma: consensus document. Gut 2002;51 Suppl 6:VI1-9.
16. Kaassis M, Boyer J, Dumas R, Ponchon T, Coumaros D, Delcenserie R, Canard JM, Fritsch J, Rey JF, Burtin P. Plastic or metal stents for malignant stricture of the common bile duct? Results of a randomized prospective study. Gastrointest Endosc 2003;57:178-82.
17. Davids PH, Groen AK, Rauws EA, Tytgat GN, Huibregtse K. Randomised trial of self-expanding metal stents versus polyethylene stents for distal malignant biliary obstruction. Lancet 1992;340:1488-92.
18. Soderlund C, Linder S. Covered metal versus plastic stents for malignant common bile duct stenosis: a prospective, randomized, controlled trial. Gastrointest Endosc 2006;63: 986-95.
19. O'Brien S, Hatfield AR, Craig PI, Williams SP. A three year follow up of self expanding metal stents in the endoscopic palliation of longterm survivors with malignant biliary obstruction. Gut 1995;36:618-21.
20. Knyrim K, Wagner HJ, Pausch J, Vakil N. A prospective, randomized, controlled trial of metal stents for malignant obstruction of the common bile duct. Endoscopy 1993;25: 207-12.
21. Stern N, Sturgess R. Endoscopic therapy in the management of malignant biliary obstruction. Eur J Surg Oncol 2008;34:313-7.
22. Khan SA, Thomas HC, Davidson BR, Taylor-Robinson SD. Cholangiocarcinoma. Lancet 2005;366:1303-14.
23. Kanasaki S, Furukawa A, Kane T, Murata K. Polyurethane-covered Nitinol Strecker stents as primary palliative treatment of malignant biliary obstruction. Cardiovasc Intervent Radiol 2000;23:114-20.
24. Park DH, Kim MH, Choi JS, Lee SS, Seo DW, Kim JH, Han J, Kim JC, Choi EK, Lee SK. Covered versus uncovered wallstent for malignant extrahepatic biliary obstruction: a cohort comparative analysis. Clin Gastroenterol Hepatol 2006;4:790-6.
25. Suk KT, Kim HS, Kim JW, Baik SK, Kwon SO, Kim HG, Lee DH, Yoo BM, Kim JH, Moon YS, Lee DK. Risk factors for cholecystitis after metal stent placement in malignant biliary obstruction. Gastrointest Endosc 2006;64:522-9.
26. Isayama H, Kawabe T, Nakai Y, Tsujino T, Sasahira N, Yamamoto N, Arizumi T, Togawa O, Matsubara S, Ito Y, Sasaki T, Hirano K, Toda N, Komatsu Y, Tada M, Yoshida H, Omata M. Cholecystitis after metallic stent placement in patients with malignant distal biliary obstruction. Clin Gastroenterol Hepatol 2006;4:1148-53.

27. Nakai Y, Isayama H, Komatsu Y, Tsujino T, Toda N, Sasahira N, Yamamoto N, Hirano K, Tada M, Yoshida H, Kawabe T, Omata M. Efficacy and safety of the covered Wallstent in patients with distal malignant biliary obstruction. Gastrointest Endosc 2005;62:742-8.

28. Kahaleh M, Tokar J, Conaway MR, Brock A, Le T, Adams RB, Yeaton P. Efficacy and complications of covered Wallstents in malignant distal biliary obstruction. Gastrointest Endosc 2005;61:528-33.

29. Bezzi M, Zolovkins A, Cantisani V, Salvatori FM, Rossi M, Fanelli F, Rossi P. New ePTFE/FEP-covered stent in the palliative treatment of malignant biliary obstruction. J Vasc Interv Radiol 2002;13:581-9.

30. Yoon WJ, Lee JK, Lee KH, Lee WJ, Ryu JK, Kim YT, Yoon YB. A comparison of covered and uncovered Wallstents for the management of distal malignant biliary obstruction. Gastrointest Endosc 2006;63:996-1000.

31. Hatzidakis A, Adam A. The interventional radiological management of cholangiocarcinoma. Clin Radiol 2003;58:91-6.

32. Lee KH, Lee DY, Kim KW. Biliary intervention for cholangiocarcinoma. Abdom Imaging 2004;29:581-9.

33. Pinol V, Castells A, Bordas JM, Real MI, Llach J, Montana X, Feu F, Navarro S. Percutaneous self-expanding metal stents versus endoscopic polyethylene endoprostheses for treating malignant biliary obstruction: randomized clinical trial. Radiology 2002; 225:27-34.

34. Naggar E, Krag E, Matzen P. Endoscopically inserted biliary endoprosthesis in malignant obstructive jaundice. A survey of the literature. Liver 1990;10:321-4.

35. Dowsett JF, Vaira D, Hatfield AR, Cairns SR, Polydorou A, Frost R, Croker J, Cotton PB, Russell RC, Mason RR. Endoscopic biliary therapy using the combined percutaneous and endoscopic technique. Gastroenterology 1989;96:1180-6.

36. Kaufman SL. Percutaneous palliation of unresectable pancreatic cancer. Surg Clin North Am 1995;75:989-99.

37. Jarnagin WR, Fong Y, DeMatteo RP, Gonen M, Burke EC, Bodniewicz BJ, Youssef BM, Klimstra D, Blumgart LH. Staging, resectability, and outcome in 225 patients with hilar cholangiocarcinoma. Ann Surg 2001;234:507-17; discussion 517-9.

38. Pichlmayr R, Weimann A, Klempnauer J, Oldhafer KJ, Maschek H, Tusch G, Ringe B. Surgical treatment in proximal bile duct cancer. A single-center experience. Ann Surg 1996;224:628-38.

39. Liu CL, Lo CM, Lai EC, Fan ST. Endoscopic retrograde cholangiopancreatography and endoscopic endoprosthesis insertion in patients with Klatskin tumors. Arch Surg 1998;133:293-6.

40. Singhal D, van Gulik TM, Gouma DJ. Palliative management of hilar cholangiocarcinoma. Surg Oncol 2005;14:59-74.

41. Schima W, Prokesch R, Osterreicher C, Thurnher S, Fugger R, Schofl R, Havelec L, Lammer J. Biliary Wallstent endoprosthesis in malignant hilar obstruction: long-term results with regard to the type of obstruction. Clin Radiol 1997;52:213-9.
42. Silverman W, Slivka A. New technique for bilateral metal mesh stent insertion to treat hilar cholangiocarcinoma. Gastrointest Endosc 1996;43:61-3.
43. Baer HU, Rhyner M, Stain SC, Glauser PW, Dennison AR, Maddern GJ, Blumgart LH. The effect of communication between the right and left liver on the outcome of surgical drainage for jaundice due to malignant obstruction at the hilus of the liver. HPB Surg 1994;8:27-31.
44. De Palma GD, Galloro G, Siciliano S, Iovino P, Catanzano C. Unilateral versus bilateral endoscopic hepatic duct drainage in patients with malignant hilar biliary obstruction: results of a prospective, randomized, and controlled study. Gastrointest Endosc 2001;53:547-53.
45. De Palma GD, Pezzullo A, Rega M, Persico M, Patrone F, Mastantuono L, Persico G. Unilateral placement of metallic stents for malignant hilar obstruction: a prospective study. Gastrointest Endosc 2003;58:50-3.
46. Polydorou AA, Chisholm EM, Romanos AA, Dowsett JF, Cotton PB, Hatfield AR, Russell RC. A comparison of right versus left hepatic duct endoprosthesis insertion in malignant hilar biliary obstruction. Endoscopy 1989;21:266-71.
47. Freeman ML, Sielaff TD. A modern approach to malignant hilar biliary obstruction. Rev Gastroenterol Disord 2003;3:187-201.
48. Deviere J, Baize M, de Toeuf J, Cremer M. Long-term follow-up of patients with hilar malignant stricture treated by endoscopic internal biliary drainage. Gastrointest Endosc 1988;34:95-101.
49. Hintze RE, Abou-Rebyeh H, Adler A, Veltzke-Schlieker W, Felix R, Wiedenmann B. Magnetic resonance cholangiopancreatography-guided unilateral endoscopic stent placement for Klatskin tumors. Gastrointest Endosc 2001;53:40-6.
50. Freeman ML, Overby C. Selective MRCP and CT-targeted drainage of malignant hilar biliary obstruction with self-expanding metallic stents. Gastrointest Endosc 2003;58:41-9.
51. Abu-Hamda EM, Baron TH. Endoscopic management of cholangiocarcinoma. Semin Liver Dis 2004;24:165-75.
52. Wagner HJ, Knyrim K, Vakil N, Klose KJ. Plastic endoprostheses versus metal stents in the palliative treatment of malignant hilar biliary obstruction. A prospective and randomized trial. Endoscopy 1993;25:213-8.
53. Anderson CD, Pinson CW, Berlin J, Chari RS. Diagnosis and treatment of cholangiocarcinoma. Oncologist 2004;9:43-57.
54. Dumas R, Demuth N, Buckley M, Peten EP, Manos T, Demarquay JF, Hastier P, Caroli-Bosc FX, Rampal P, Delmont JP. Endoscopic bilateral metal stent placement for malignant hilar stenoses: identification of optimal technique. Gastrointest Endosc 2000;51:334-8.

55. Peters RA, Williams SG, Lombard M, Karani J, Westaby D. The management of high-grade hilar strictures by endoscopic insertion of self-expanding metal endoprostheses. Endoscopy 1997;29:10-6.

56. Sung J. Are covered stents superior to uncovered stents in the management of malignant biliary obstruction? Nat Clin Pract Gastroenterol Hepatol 2004;1:20-1.

57. Nelsen KM, Kastan DJ, Shetty PC, Burke MW, Sharma RP, Venugopal C. Utilization pattern and efficacy of nonsurgical techniques to establish drainage for high biliary obstruction. J Vasc Interv Radiol 1996;7:751-6.

58. van Delden OM, Lameris JS. Percutaneous drainage and stenting for palliation of malignant bile duct obstruction. Eur Radiol 2008;18:448-56.

59. LaBerge JM, Doherty M, Gordon RL, Ring EJ. Hilar malignancy: treatment with an expandable metallic transhepatic biliary stent. Radiology 1990;177:793-7.

60. Stoker J, Lameris JS, van Blankenstein M. Percutaneous metallic self-expandable endoprostheses in malignant hilar biliary obstruction. Gastrointest Endosc 1993;39:43-9.

61. Hwang MH, Tsai CC, Chou CY, Mo LR, Yang CT, Lin RC, Yueh SK. Percutaneous cholangiofiberscopic endoluminal forceps biopsy of intrabile duct diseases. Hepato-gastroenterology 1998;45:2073-8.

62. Motte S, Deviere J, Dumonceau JM, Serruys E, Thys JP, Cremer M. Risk factors for septicemia following endoscopic biliary stenting. Gastroenterology 1991;101:1374-81.

XI · Special Types of Biliary Cancers

XI·I
Mucin-hypersecreting Cholangiocarcinoma and Biliary Papillomatosis

1. Mucin-hypersecreting Cholangiocarcinoma

1) Clinical findings

This type of tumor showes unique clinical, radiologic, and pathologic features, distinct from those of ordinary bile duct carcinomas. Clinically, it secretes large quantities of viscous mucin into the duct lumen, leading to intermittent blockage of the bile duct system and thereby causing ductal dilatation and various biliary symptoms. In a study, most patients presented with biliary pain and acute cholangitis at admission, or had suffered from episodic attacks of biliary pain and recurrent cholangitis before admission. These symptoms are unusual for "common" bile duct tumors, and may be considered as the characteristic clinical features in which this particular tumor differs from more usual bile duct tumors.[1,2]

2) Radiologic findings

In cases of this tumor, bile duct dilatation can occur not only in the bile duct distal to the main pathologic lesion, but also in the bile duct proximal to the lesion, because of partial obstruction by mucin. In addition, it is often unclear whether an intraductal filling defect is caused by mucin or neoplastic mass. Therefore, the actual extent of the pathologic lesion cannot be surmised exactly on the basis of conventional raiologic study. When generalized biliary dilatation is evident on images that also show disproportionately more severe or aneurysmal dilatation in part of the biliary tree and excessive mucin in the bile duct, a diagnosis of intraductal papillary mucinous tumor of the bile duct should be considered. US, CT, and MR images should be carefully scrutinized for evidence of mucin-producing papillary tumor depicted at US, CT, ERCP or tube cholangiography, or MR cholangiography, one can make a diagnosis of intraductal papillary mucinous tumors of the bile ducts.[3] Mucin hypersecreting bile duct cancer is a rarely encountered entity and is similar to intraductal papillary mucinous neoplasm (IPMN) of the pancreas. The fundamental similarity is mucin over-producing property and this overproduced mucin is relatively viscous, and causes ductal obstruction and upstream duct dilatation. Mucin hypersecreting bile duct cancer shows diffuse bile duct dilatation and mucinous ductal ectasia just similar to pancreatic duct ectasia in the patient with intraductal papillary mucinous tumor. Another similarity is pathologic findings. Mucin hypersecreting bile duct cancer shows villous or papillary mucosal projections on histologic examination, as if mucinous ductal ectasia shows papillary or villous mucosal tumors. Mucin hypersecreting bile duct cancer causes frequent attacks of obstructive cholangitis by mucus plugging, while IPMN of the pancreas frequently induces an obstructive pancreatitis.[4]

3) Endoscopic findings

Patulous ampullary orifice with mucin excretion is a characteristic duodenoscopic finding. Cholangioscopic examination was able to provide detailed information on the extent of disease, and the surgical treatment appropriate to individual patients could be decided. Preoperative direct observation of the bile duct may be indispensable for determining the best management plan.[1]

The determination of exact extent of tumor by cholangiography or pancreatogaphy is quite difficult in both entities because mucin also is a cause of filling defects on cholangiography or pancreatography obsecuring the extent of true tumor. During cholangioscopic examination of mucin hypersecreting bile duct cancer, the cholangioscopist should be cautious not to overlook minute mucosal tumor. The bile duct is usually dilated and as the intraductal mucin absorbs some fraction of the light

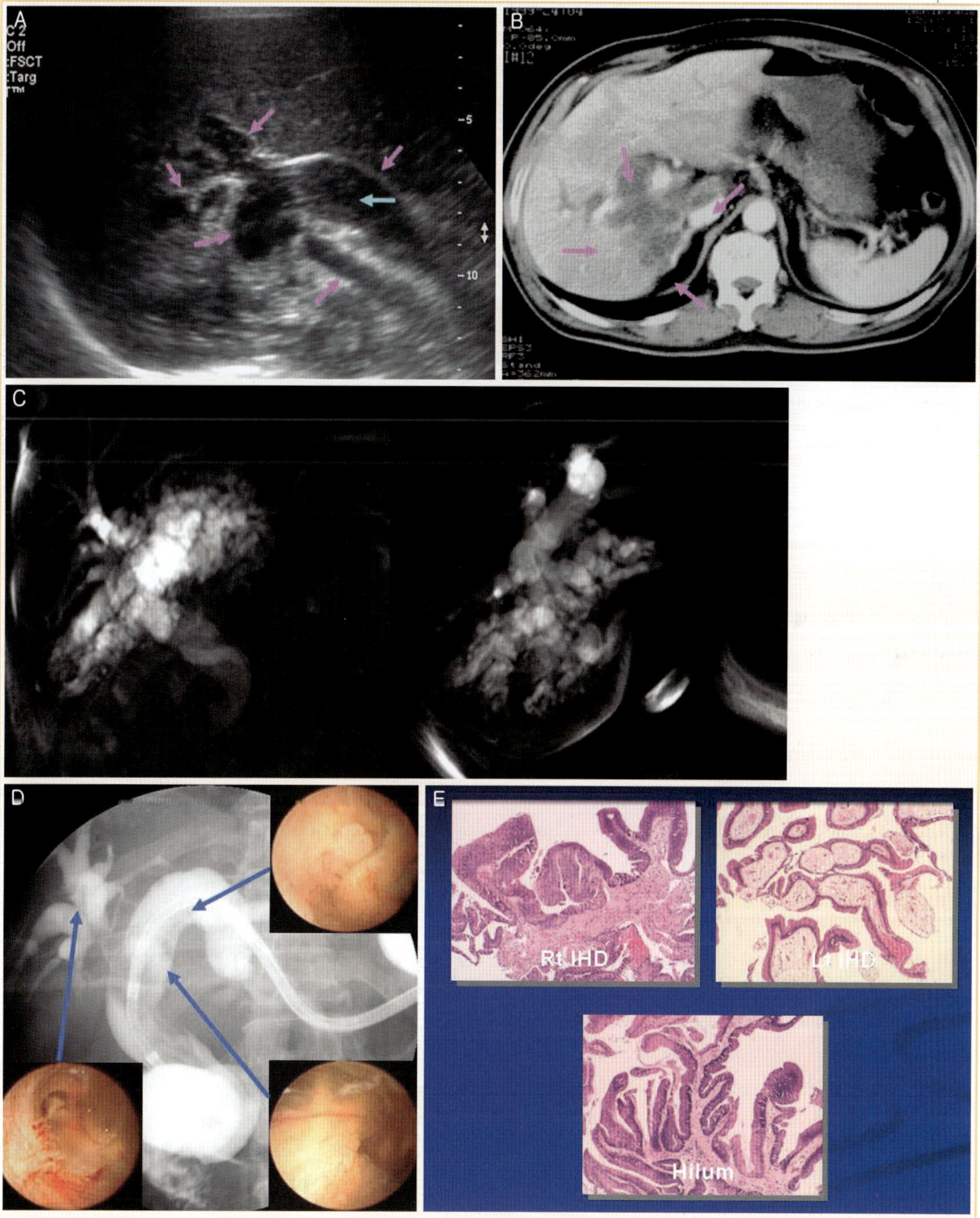

Fig. 1A~E Findings of mucin-hypersecreting cholangiocarcinoma

A: Dilatation of the intrahepatic duct is seen on ultrasonography. B: Abdominal CT shows dilatation of the intrahepatic and extrahepatic bile ducts. C: MRCP shows dilatation of the bile duct with irregularity. D: PTCS and cholangiography show mucin like material and papillary lesions at the hilar and both intrahepatic ducts. E: Biopsy reveals papillary adenoma and adenocarcinoma.

which is emitted from the tip of cholangioscope resulting in dark visual field. Therefore it is not easy to detect tiny tumor and determine the extent of tumor in the markedly dilated duct with full of mucin. Sometimes even tiny villous or papillary mucosal tumor can produce massive amount of mucin. Mucin has variable viscosity and thick mucin tends to cause round filling defect in cholangiogram, while thin mucin does thread-like linear filling defects. The cholangioscopic finding of mucin hypersecreting bile duct cancer can be either villous tiny mucosal projections or papillary tumors in the wall of bile duct. These mucosal lesions are usually highly friable and easily removed by biopsy forceps.[4] Under cholangioscopic examination, the majority of patients showed a distinct papillary mass. Minute frogspawn-like mucosal changes were also observed. Such endoscopic findings closely resembled those associated with IPMT of the pancreas.[5,6] Under microscopic examination, the tumor was often seen to be accompanied by a wide range of histologic findings, such as hyperplasia, adenoma, carcinoma in situ, and invasive carcinomas. This suggests that the pathogenesis of this tumor is in the sequence hyperplasia-adenoma-carcinoma.[7]

4) Clinical course

The high resectability and long-term survival may be attributed to early detection of the tumor due to the acute biliary symptoms caused by the mucin, in addition to the slow-growing biological behavior of the tumor. The mucin-hypersecreting bile duct tumor may be characterized by a striking homology with IPMT of the pancreas in clinical, radiologic, and pathologic features. If mucin from the ampulla is observed during ERCP, a thorough evaluation should be made for the early detection of mucin-hypersecreting bile duct tumor.[1]

2. Biliary Papillomatosis

Biliary papillomatosis (BP)[8] is a disease characterized by multiple papillary tumors of variable distribution and extent in the intrahepatic and/or extrahepatic biliary tree.

Although BP is basically a collection of benign papillary adenomas, papillary adenocarcinoma can develop within these lesions[1,9] and has a tendency to spread superficially along the bile duct mucosa.[10,11] Because BP is a scarce entity, the clinical features and outcome are not well known, and few reports to date have described the clinical characteristics and prognosis of this biliary papillary neoplasm[12-15] BP is classified as either mucin-hypersecreting type (MBP) or nonmucin-producing type (NMBP) because both disease types have similar macroscopic and microscopic findings, except for mucin hypersecretion.

1) Pathogenesis

Although there have been several studies on BP published to date,[12,16] to our knowledge the pathogenesis of this disease has not been well characterized. Most authors suggest that bile stasis and recurrent infection induced by chronic biliary diseases such as hepatolithiasis or clonorchiasis may lead to the development of periductal inflammation, mucosal hyperplasia, dysplasia (low and high grade), CIS, and adenocarcinoma.[17,18] The investigations regarding BP are mainly of patients in Far Eastern countries such as Korea, Taiwan, and Japan.[12,17-20] These countries are endemic areas of hepatolithiasis and clonorchiasis, which are risk factors for BP. In the current study, approximately half of the patients were diagnosed with biliary stones or clonorchiasis. These findings suggest that BP is associated strongly with these biliary diseases. BP has been considered to be a benign disease with low malignant potential.[21,22] Some series have reported only anecdotal cases that progressed to malignancy.[10,12-14,23-25] However, in a study, 48 (83%) of 58 patients were diagnosed with BP that revealed papillary carcinoma (42 patients with adenocarcinoma and 6 patients with mucinous carcinoma) in the background of adenoma on cholangioscopic biopsy or surgically resected specimens. Most of the patients in the study were diagnosed with cancer after a thorough examination of the entire biliary tree by PTCS and cholangioscopic-targeted multiple biopsies for all of the lesions. Therefore, BP is not a benign disease with low malignant potential as previously believed. Rather, it is a premalignant disease with high malignant potential. Moreover, the findings of mixed pathologic types in each case as well as papillary adenocarcinoma in the background of papillary adenoma suggest that BP represents a continuous histologic spectrum of neoplastic biliary disease from dysplasia to carcinoma with papillary configuration.The tissue specimens in the current study demonstrated lining epithelia of biliary type. Goblet cell metaplasia was found to be more predominant in patients with MBP.[8]

However, there was no significant difference noted in the frequency of colonic and foveolar metaplasia between the two groups, which is somewhat different from the results provided by Chen et al.[19]

2) Diagnosis of BP Using Imaging Studies

The most common abnormal finding of US and CT scans in these patients was IHD and/or common bile duct dilatation. When intraductal masses were not detected on US or CT scan, they were diagnosed as biliary stones, clonorchiasis, and benign biliary strictures. ERCP may be useful in making the diagnosis of BP. The characteristic ERCP findings of BP are multiple small filling defects and the serrated irregularity of the bile duct wall. In patients with MBP, hypersecreted mucin is drained through the ampulla and a patulous ampulla is the characteristic duodenoscopic finding. On cholangiography, diffuse bile duct dilatation and amorphous filling defects in the bile duct are characteristic. However, a large amount of mucin secretion and obstruction by the tumor prevent complete opacification of the entire biliary tract. As a result, precise evaluation of ductal extent by ERCP is often suboptimal.[12,26]

3) Endoscopic findings

Biliary papillomatosis is characterized by multicentric papillary tumors in the biliary tract. Diagnosis of this entity can be made on the following histological criteria; macroscopically, multifocal papillary growing tumors in the extrahepatic bile duct with or without intrahepatic bile duct involvements and microscopically, branching papillary fronds covered by columnar epithelium and supported by delicate fibrovascular stalks. Biliary papillomatosis is basically a collection of benign papillary adenomas, however, these lesions can be transformed into papillary adenocarcinoma.

Radiologic findings and cholangioscopic findings reflects these histological characteristics. Cholangioscopic examination of biliary papillomatosis shows multiple or numerous papillary masses in the biliary tree. The masses are soft and friable and the surface color is usually bright yellow or pinkish. Since papillary lesions are multifocal in biliary papillomatosis, the normal intervening mucosa can be seen between lesions. Histologically this normal looking area shows mild inflammatory changes. In the patient with biliary papillomatosis, main papillary masses are usually located in the extrahepatic bile duct. However, cholangioscopist should be careful about intrahepatic small or minute papillary lesions which are remote from main extrahepatic tumors. Careful cholangioscopic examination is indispensable for the determination of exact extent of tumor and type of surgery.[4]

Cholangioscopic evaluation provided detailed information regarding the extent of disease, which enabled the appropriate surgical treatment to be provided to patients. PTCS evaluation has some advantages over conventional radiologic imaging. First, it may visualize the bile duct mucosa directly and detect small or subtle mucosal lesions that are not evident by direct cholangiogram. The recurrence rate of BP after surgery is reported to be high.[24] Incomplete preoperative evaluation of the extent of BP might be an important contributing factor for the high disease recurrence rate. Because small papillomas may not be detected by conventional radiologic methods,[12,26,27] these undetected lesions, usually remote from the main tumor, may be the foci of recurrence.[28,29]

In 6 of the 21 patients in a study in whom the disease was confined to the EHD by radiologic images including ERCP and MRCP, a Whipple procedure was planned initially. However, as cholangioscopy revealed additional IHD lesions, the surgical procedure was changed to a more aggressive one. Therefore, the patients underwent partial hepatectomy in addition to pancreaticoduodenectomy and all tumors were resected. Another advantage of cholangioscopy is to confirm the histology of the lesions shown by conventional radiologic imaging. We prefer PTCS to peroral cholangioscopy because peroral cholangioscopic examination may be inferior to PTCS for complete evaluation of the IHD due to the difficulty in using the remote control of the babyscope. Therefore, PTCS examination is an indispensable preoperative procedure for determining treatment modalities and the appropriate extent of resection in BP. It is more useful in patients with MBP because mucin is observed as filling defects on direct cholangiography.

After curative surgery, the prognosis of patients with BP was excellent and was similar to that reported in previous studies.[8,12,20,30-34]

4) Clinical course

24 (41%) of 58 patients underwent surgical resection. None of these patients had regional lymph node metastasis or vascular invasion and tumors were confined to the mucosa in nine patients. Twenty of 24 patients underwent curative surgical resection and the 5-year survival rate of these patients was 81%.[8] Thirty-four of 58 patients underwent only palliative drainage. Their mean survival was 37 months, which is significantly longer than that of patients with usual cholangiocarcinoma.[35-37] The reason is that BP is less invasive and grows slowly. In a study, there was no significant survival difference noted based on the histologic class.[8] Moreover, two of seven patients with a Class 2 histologic diagnosis category of benign adenoma as determined by cholangioscopic biopsy died of disease progression. Although these patients were classified only as having high-grade dysplasia, they showed clinicoradiologic features of malignancy on follow-up. One patient had portal vein encasement on magnetic resonance angiography. The other patient, who underwent only PTBD because of the involvement of both lobes by the tumor, showed disease progression on follow-up CT scans. This discrepancy between pathologic class by biopsy and clinical diagnosis may reflect the difficulty in excluding a carcinoma with a limited biopsy specimen. BP should not be regarded as a benign disease with low malignant potential but, rather, as a premalignant lesion with high malignant potential. The pathogenesis of progression from benign to malignant disease may follow the adenomacarcinoma sequence. Although clinical presentations and gastroenteric metaplasia were somewhat different, the long-term survival rate was not found to be significantly different between patients with NMBP and MBP. Because patients with BP have a better prognosis than patients with usual cholangiocarcinoma, surgical resection can be curative. Therefore, early and accurate diagnosis is important in this disease (Fig. 2A~C, Fig. 3A, B, Fig. 4A, B).

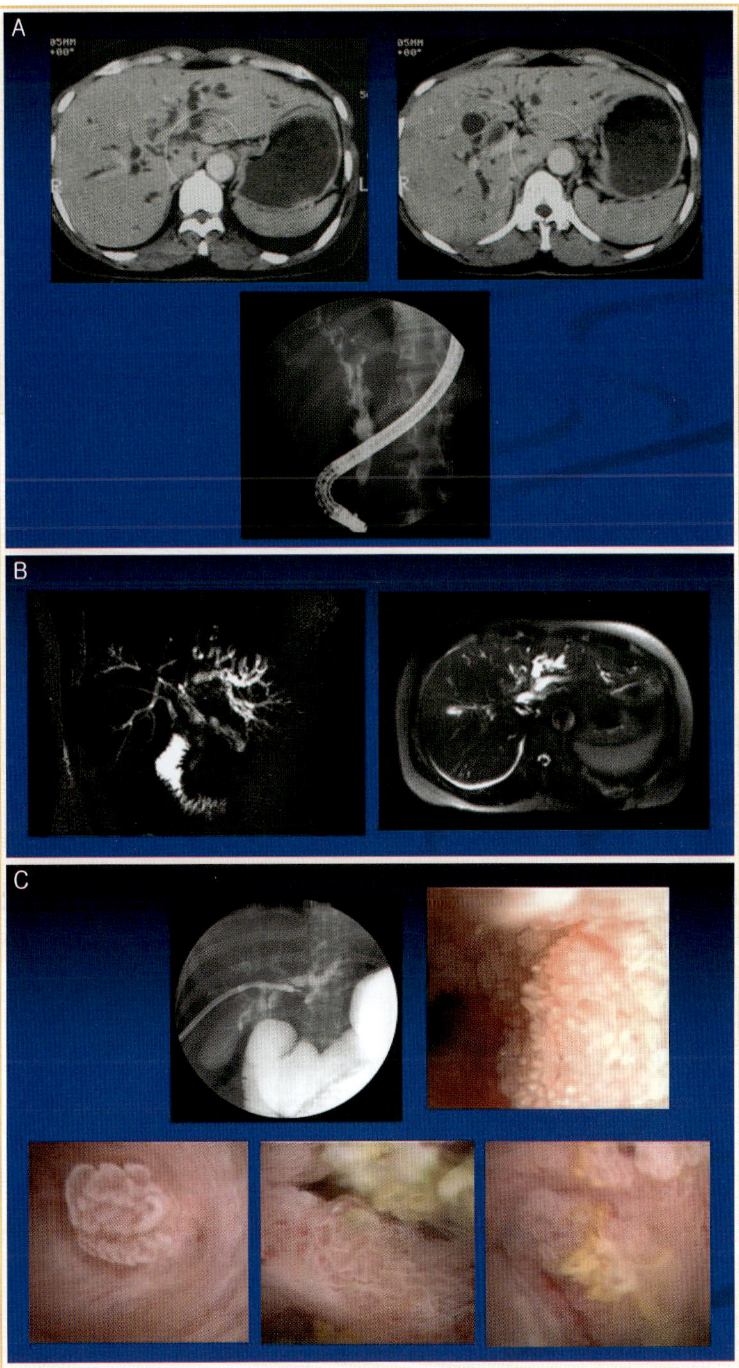

Fig. 2A~C Findings of biliary papillomatosis

A: Dilatation of bile ducts and irregular ragged bile duct wall on cholangiography, involving the hilum. B: These are the findings of MR with hilar involvement. C: On PTCS, type IV papillary tumor was diagnosed.

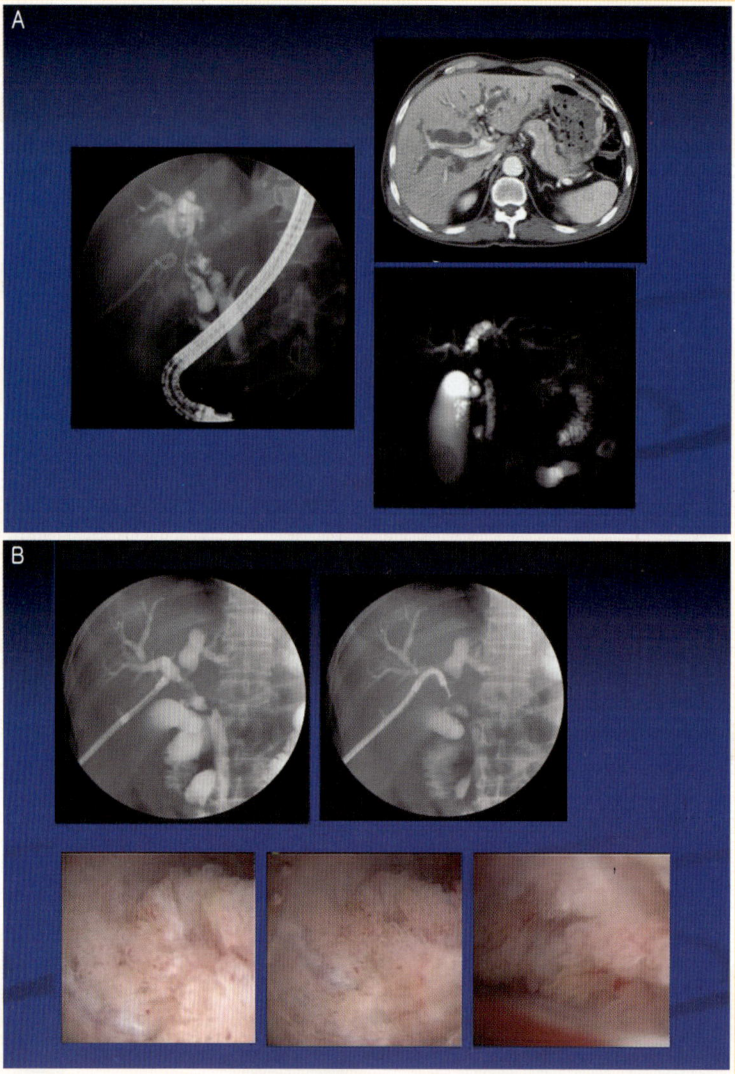

Fig. 3A, B Findings of biliary papillomatosis

A: Findings of type II lesion on imaging studies are seen. B: On PTCS, type IIIA biliary papillomatosis with malignant change was diagnosed.

Reference

1. Kim HJ, Kim MH, Lee SK, et al. Mucin-hypersecreting bile duct tumor characterized by a striking homology with an intraductal papillary mucinous tumor (IPMT) of the pancreas. Endoscopy 2000;32: 389-393.

2. Kukubo T, Itai Y, Ohtomo K, et al. Mucin hypersecreting intrahepatic biliary neoplasm. Radiology 1988;168:609-614.

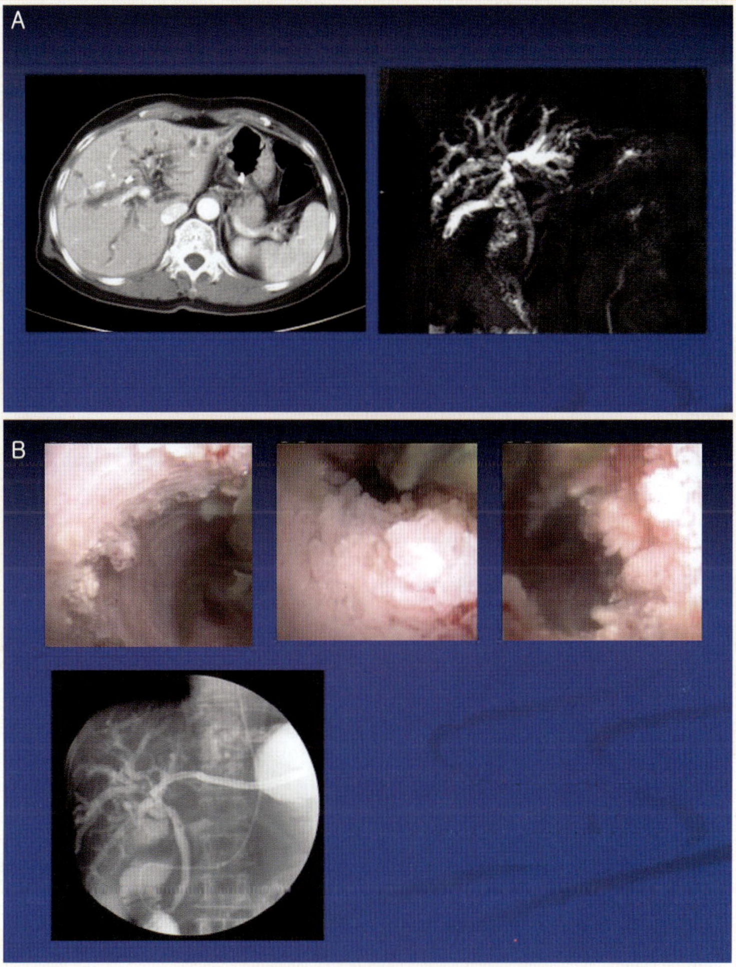

Fig. 4A, B Findings of biliary papillomatosis

A: This is a type IIIa lesion with imaging studies. B: On PTCS, the lesions was diagnosed as a type IV lesion.

3. Lim JH, Yoon KH, Kim SH, et al. Intraductal papillary mucinous tumors of the bile ducts. RadioGraphics 2004;24:53-67.

4. Seo DW, Lee SK, Kim MH, Min YI. Neoplasms of the biliary tree. In: Cholangioscopy. Seoul, Korea: Koonja, Inc., 2002: 95-98.

5. Seo DW, Kim MH, Lee SK, et al. The value of pancreatoscopy in patients with mucinous ductal ectasia. Endoscopy 1997;29:315-318.

6. Myung SJ, Kim MH, Kim HJ, Lee SK, Min YI. Magnetic resonance cholangiopancreatography is insufficient for the detection of flat lesions in mucinous ductal ectasia: pancreatoscopy may be needed additionally. Am J Gastroenterol 1998;93:1189.

7. Obara T, Maguchi H, Saitoh Y, et al. Mucin producing tumor of the pancreas: natural history and serial pancreatogram changes. Am J Gastroenterol 1993;88:564-569.
8. Lee SS, Kim MH, Lee SK, et al. Clinicopathologic review of 58 patients with biliary papillomatosis. Cancer 2004;100:783-793.
9. Okulski EG, Dolin BJ, Kandawalla NM. Intrahepatic biliary papillomatosis. Arch Pathol Lab Med 1979;103:647-649.
10. Neumann RD, LiVolsi VA, Rosenthal NS, Burrell M, Ball TJ. Adenocarcinoma in biliary papillomatosis. Gastroenterology 1976;70:779-782.
11. Terada T, Mitsui T, Nakanuma Y, Miura S, Toya D. Intrahepatic biliary papillomatosis arising in nonobstructive intrahepatic biliary dilatations confined to the hepatic left lobe. Am J Gastroenterol 1991;86:1523-1526.
12. Kim YS, Myung SJ, Kim SY, et al. Biliary papillomatosis: clinical, cholangiographic and cholangioscopic findings. Endoscopy 1998;30:763-767.
13. Romano C, Wilson MS. Biliary tumors of the liver. Semin Liver Dis 1995;15:405-407.
14. Holtkamp W, Reis HE. Papillomatosis of the bile ducts: papilloma-carcinoma sequence. Am J Gastroenterol 1994;89:2253-2255.
15. Lam CM, Yuen ST, Yuen WK, Fan ST. Biliary papillomatosis. Br J Surg 1996;83:1715-1716.
16. Amaya S, Sasaki M, Watanabe Y, et al. Expression of MUC1 and MUC2 and carbohydrate antigen Tn change during malignant transformation of biliary papillomatosis. Histopathology 2001;38:550-560.
17. Nakanuma Y, Sasaki M, Ishikawa A, Tsui W, Chen TC, Huang SF. Biliary papillary neoplasm of the liver. Histol Histopathol 2002;17:851-861.
18. Kim YI, Yu ES, Kim ST. Intraductal variant of peripheral cholangiocarcinoma of the liver with clonorchis sinensis infection. Cancer 1989;63:1562-1566.
19. Chen TC, Nakanuma Y, Zen Y, et al. Intraductal papillary neoplasia of the liver associated with hepatolithiasis. Hepatology 2001;34:651-658.
20. Suh KS, Roh HR, Koh YT, Lee KU, Park YH, Kim SW. Clinicopathologic features of the intraductal growth type of peripheral cholangiocarcinoma. Hepatology 2000;31:12-17.
21. Nakanuma Y, Sripa B, Vantanasapt V, Leong AS-Y, Ponchon T, Ishak KG. Intrahepatic cholangicarcinoma. In: Hamilton SR , Aaltonen LA , editors. World Health Organization classification of tumours. Pathology and genetics. Tumors of the digestive system. Lyon: IARC Press, 2000:173-180.
22. Padfield CJ, Ansell ID, Furness PN. Mucinous biliary papillomatosis: a tumour in need of wider recognition. Histopathology 1988;13:687-694.
23. Helpap B. Malignant papillomatosis of the intrahepatic bile ducts. Acta Hepatogastroenterol. 1977;24: 419-425.

24. Ohta H, Yamaguchi Y, Yamakawa O, et al. Biliary papillomatosis with the point mutation of K-ras gene arising in congenital choledochal cyst. Gastroenterology 1993;105:1209-1212.

25. Tireli M, Uslu A. Multiple biliary papillomatosis. HPB Surg 1992;6:125-127.

26. Lee SS, Kim MH, Lee SK, et al. MR cholangiography versus cholangioscopy for evaluation of longitudinal extension of hilar cholangiocarcinoma. Gastrointest Endosc 2002;56:25-32.

27. Kawakatsu M, Vilgrain V, Zins M, Vullierme M, Belghiti J, Menu Y. Radiologic features of papillary adenoma and papillomatosis of the biliary tract. Abdom Imaging 1997;22:87-90.

28. Gouma DJ, Mutum SS, Benjamin IS, Blumgart LH. Intrahepatic biliary papillomatosis. Br J Surg 1984;71:72-74.

29. Taguchi J, Yasunaga M, Kojiro M, Arita T, Nakayama T, Simokobe T. Intrahepatic and extrahepatic biliary papillomatosis. Arch Pathol Lab Med 1993;117:944-947.

30. Garg PK, Tandon RK. Preoperative assessment of cholangiocarcinoma: meeting the challenge. J Gastroenterol Hepatol 1999;14:615-617.

31. Tamada K, Yasuda Y, Nagai H, et al. Limitation of cholangiography in assessing longitudinal spread of extrahepatic bile duct carcinoma to the hepatic side. J Gastroenterol Hepatol 1999; 14:691-698.

32. Kim MH. Percutaneous transhepatic cholangioscopic examination: a necessity for the biliary endoscopist (perspectives). Gastrointest Endosc 2001;53:695-697.

33. Sato M, Inoue H, Ogawa S, et al. Limitations of percutaneous transhepatic cholangioscopy for the diagnosis of the intramural extension of bile duct carcinoma. Endoscopy 1998;30:281-288.

34. Nimura Y, Hayakawa N, Kamiya J, Kondo S, Shionoya S. Hepatic segmentectomy with caudate lobe resection for bile duct carcinoma of the hepatic hilus. World J Surg 1990;14:535-544.

35. Chen MF, Jan YY, Chen TC. Clinical studies of mucin-producing cholangiocellular carcinoma: a study of 22 histopathology-proven cases. Ann Surg 1998;227:63-69.

36. Shimonishi T, Zen Y, Chen TC, et al. Increasing expression of gastrointestinal phenotypes and p53 along with histologic progression of intraductal papillary neoplasia of the liver. Hum Pathol 2002;33: 503-511.

37. Lai EC, Tompkins RK, Mann LL, Roslyn JJ. Proximal bile duct cancer. Quality of survival. Ann Surg 1987;205:111-118.

XI·II
Klatskin Tumor

Hilar biliary malignancy refers to any neoplastic biliary obstruction involving the hepatic hilus. Clinically, this includes all tumors involving the proximal 2 cm of the common hepatic duct and/or the left and right hepatic ducts and their branches.[1] Hilar cholangiocarcinom was described to be a particular entity of biliary carcinmas by G. Klatskin in 1965.[2] After that, Klatskin tumors were defined as an adenocarcinma of the hepatic duct at the bifurcation within the porta hepatis. They now, usually include upper-third cancers of the common bile duct down to the jucntion with the cystic duct. They are also known as: proximal cancer of the confluence of biliary tract, cancer of superior biliary confluence, and malignant stricuter of biliary confluence. They must be differentiated from cholangiocarcinmas, which are adenocarcinomas involving intrahepatic ducts.

The first hilar resection for cholangiocarcinoma was undertaken only 40 years ago[3] and it was only 30 years ago that Klatskin reported a series of 13 patients with resected biliary adenocarcinoma at the hepatic duct confluence.[2] His report was the beginning of a focused approach to these tumors, now commonly referred to as "Klatskin tumors."

1. Incidence

Cancer of the bile duct, cholangiocarcinoma, is an uncommon malignancy comprising less than 2% of all cancer diagnoses.[4] The overall rate of occurrence of cholangiocarcinoma is 1.2/100,000 individuals, with two-thirds of all cases occuring in patients more than 65 years old, and a near 10-fold increase in patients over 80 years of age.[5] Each year, there are approximately 2,500 new cases of hilar cholangicarcinoma and 1,000 cases of distal cholangicarcinom in the United States alone.[6] Worldwide, cholangiocarcinoma accounts for 3% of all gastrointestinal cancers[7] and is the second most common primary hepatic tumor.[7,8] Tumors at the biliary confluence at the hilum of the liver are the most common and comprise of 40% to 60% of the total bile duct cancer.[9-11] A small percentage of patients (<10%) may present diffuse tumors involving the entire extrahepatic bile duct; and in these cases, operation is almost never curative, and the survival rate is unfavorable.[12,13]

2. Pathogenesis and Tumor Biology

Although no clear causal agent for cholangiocarcinoma has been identified. Certain pathological conditions that result in either acute or chronic biliary epithelial injury appear to predispose to its development. Occult cholangiocarcinoma has been identified in up to 40% of autopsy specimens and in 9% to 36% of liver specimen after liver transplantation in patients with primary sclerosing cholangitis (PSC).[4,12,14,15] It is now evident that pericholangitis, PSC, and cholangiocarcinoma may represent a spectrum of the same disease process. Cholangiocarcinoma in such patients tends to occur earlier, in 30~50 year age-groups[12,16], than in sporadic cases. About a third of patients with PSC who develop cholangiocarcinoma do so within 2 years of diagnosis and the risk of cholangiocarcinogenesis seems unrelated to the duration of the inflammatory disease.[12,17] A second group of patients, carrying a significant rate of occurrence of cholangiocarcimoma, are those with congenital abnormalities of the biliary tree associated with Caroli's dsyndrome, congenital hepatic fibrosis, and choledochal cysts. A 2.5% to 28% rate of occurrence of malignant transformation of congenital cyst epithelium has been documented and may be related to chronic biliary inflammation caused by an associated anomalous pancreaticobiliary duct junction.[12,14] The overall incidence of cholangiocarcinoma in patients with untreated cysts is up to 28%.[18,19]

Additional risk factors for the development of cholangiocarcinoma include biliary tract infection with liver fluke endemic to Southeast and far east Asia, namely, Clonorchis sinensis and Opisthorchis viverrin. Human beings are infected by eating undercooked fish with adult worms inhabiting and laying eggs in the biliary system.[12-14,20] Hepatolithiasis is associated with a 5% to 12% lifetime rate of occurrence of cholangiocarcinoma.[12-14,21] However, hepatolithiasis is associated with peripheral intrahepatic cholangiocarcinoma. Cirrhosis, of any cause including hepatitis B and C virus, has also been associated with intrahepatic cholangiocarcinoma.[22,23] However the relationship between Klatskin tumor and hepatolithiasis and viral hepatitis is still unclear.

In general, hematogenous spread of Klatskin tumor is rare, whereas nodal metastases may be present in up to one-third of patients.[4,24,25] The histomorphological features of the Klatskin tumor are identical with other extra- and intrahepatic bile duct carcinomas. Extensive subepithelial tumor spread beyond the gross tumor margin is common (Fig. 1), and longitudinal spread may extend 15 to 20 mm proximally and 5 to 10 mm distally, depending on tumor type.[26,27] Therefore, after curative resection surgery the local recurrence rate of the tumor is still high . Proximal tumors have been shown to invade both veins and nerves in 20% and 80% of cases respectively.[14]

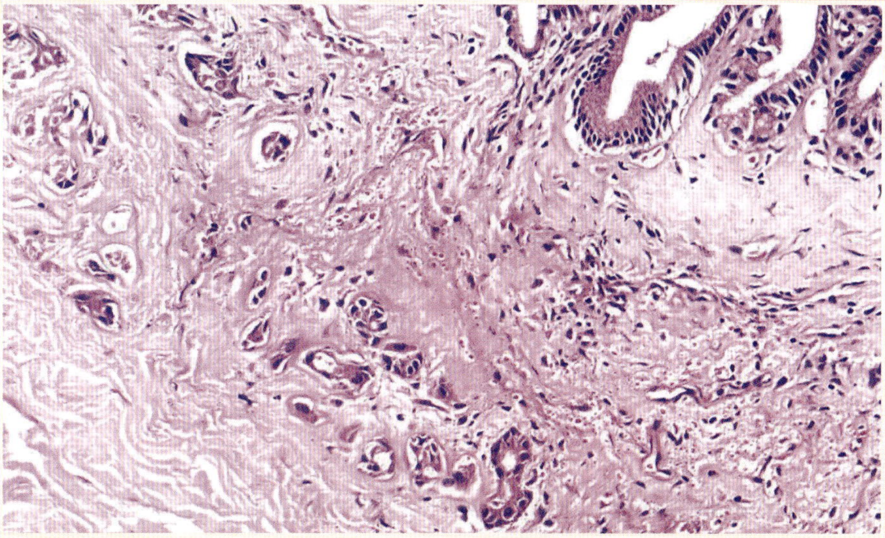

Fig. 1 The infiltrating type tumor frequently spread along the submucosa

3. Classification

Bismuth and Corlette developed a classification system for stricutres caused by hilar biliary malignancy according to the degree of the proxiamal tumor extension within the intrahepatic biliary radicles (Table 1).[28,29] Bismuth I strictures involve the hepatic confluence, but not the primary bifurcation. Bismuth II strictures involve and occlude the primary bifurcation. Bismuth III strictures occlude the primary bifurcation and extend to involve the secondary confluence on either the left or right side. Bismuth IV strictures involve the both secondary confluence on the left and right side (Fig. 2). In an analysis of database registries of the Surveillance Epidemiology and End Results (SEER) 1975~99, 92% of Klatskin tumors were classified as intrahepatic cholangiocarcinoma.[30]

The Hilar tumor is also classified into three types on the basis of the macrosopic appearance resulting from their growth pattern. This classification system is adapted from classification of primary liver cancer proposed by the Liver Cancer Study Group of Japan.[31] The *intraductal-growing type* comprises 10% of all cholangiocarcinomas and grows primarily as an intraluminal soft, polypoid tumor with a limited propensity for transmural growth. Tumor multicentricity occurs more frequently with the papillary variant and may be reflective of a field change in the biliary epithelium.[25,32,33] This type of cholangiocarcinma carries a more favorable prognosis and is most common in the mid to distal bile duct, however it can also occur in the hilar and intrahepatic bile duct. The *mass-forming type* occurs most commonly in the upper and mid bile duct and generally presents as a fibrotic mass with intraductal projection. The *periductal-infiltrating type* comprises 70% of all tumors at the hilum and histologically appears as an annular thickening of the bile duct with both

Table 1. Modified Bismuth-Corlette classification for hilar cholangiocarcinoma.

Type I	Below the confluence
Type II	Confined to confluence
Type IIIa	Extension into right hepatic duct
IIIb	Extension into left hepatic duct
Type IV	Extension into right and left hepatic ducts

[a] Other modifications of the Bismuth-Corlette classification system have been suggested but have not been widely accepted.

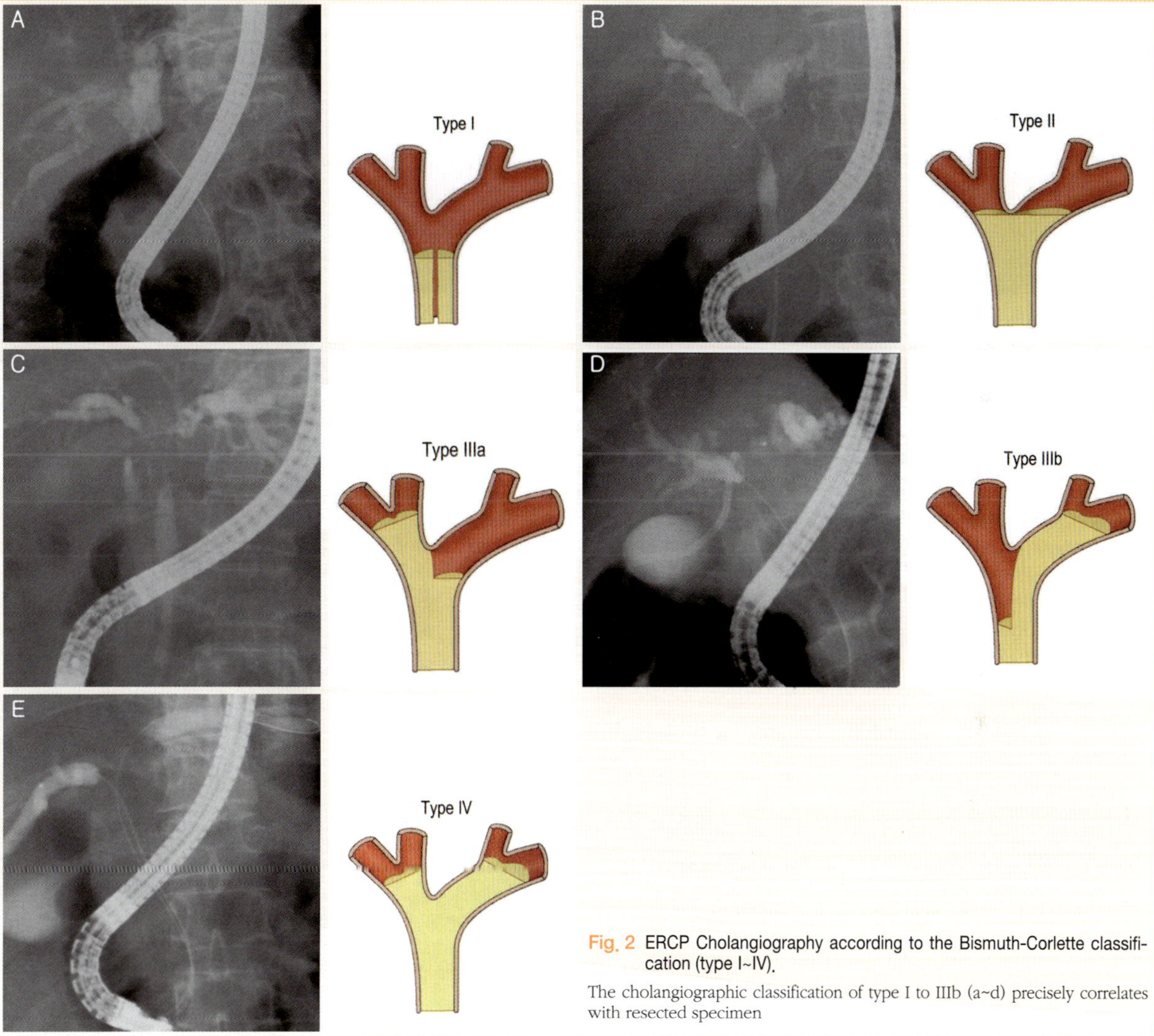

Fig. 2 ERCP Cholangiography according to the Bismuth-Corlette classification (type I~IV).

The cholangiographic classification of type I to IIIb (a~d) precisely correlates with resected specimen

longitudinal and radial tumor infiltrations, a definite mass is rarely seen on sonogram. Knowledge of these growth patterns of hilar cancer should be taken into consideration when selecting appropriate operative and other therapeutic methods.

4. Staging

There are currently two primary staging system used for hilar tumor. The first is that of the American Joint Committee on Cancer (AJCC),[34] which incorporates the extent

Table 2. AJCC staging systems for cholangiocarcinoma.

Stage 0	Tis	N0	M0
Stage I	T1	N0	M0
Stage II	T2	N0	M0
Stage III	T1, 2	N1, 2	M0
Stage IVA	T3	Any	M0
Stage IVB	Any	Any	M1

AJCC, American Joint Committee on Cancer; Tis, carcinoma in situ; T1, tumor invades subepithelial connective tissue (T1a) or fibromuscular layer (T1b); T2, tumor invades perifibromuscular connective tissue; T3, tumor invades adjacent structures, i.e., liver, pancreas, duodenum, stomach, gallbladder, colon, or stomach; N1, metastasis in the cystic duct, pericholedochal, and/or hilar lymph nodes; N2, metastasis in the peripancreatic (head only), paraduodenal, periportal, celiac, superior mesenteric, and/or posterior pancreaticoduodenal lymph nodes; M0, no distant metastases; M1, distant metastases.

of tumor invasion into the wall of the bile duct, as well as nodal metastasis, and finally, distant metastasis (Table 2). This staging system is used for all cholangiocarcinoma, and therefore may not accurately differentiate between the different patterns of the growth of hilar tumor versus distal cholangiocarcinomas. This system is helpful in identifying prognostic subsets, but is applicable only to the minority of patients who undergo surgical resections, because the T staging requires transmural histopathologic evaluation of the tumor. The modified Bismuth-Corlette classification system[28] for hilar tumor is a more anatomic description of the location of the tumor. That is, it groups those tumors based upon their extension into the hepatic ductal system. Although this system provides an anatomic classification that can guide therapy, it does little to describe those patients who are surgical candidates, or to provide prognostic information about each subset.

The memorial Sloan-Kettering Group[35] has proposed a modification to the AJCC system that takes into account biological factors related to hilar cholangiocarcinoma. This is directed at alterations in the T stage and includes a variety of factors that are identified on preoperative imaging. The goal of this modification is to allow categorization of those patients who are appropriate candidates for exploration with attempted surgical resection, as well as to provide anatomic information as to the local extent of the tumor. The modification of the T staging is as follows (Table 3): T1, tumor confined to the right, left, or confluence without portal vein involvement or liver atrophy; T2, same as T1, but with ipsilateral liver atrophy; T3, same as T1, but

Table 3. Proposed modified T-stage criteria for hilar cholangiocarcinoma.

T1	Tumor confined to the confluence and/or right or left hepatic duct without portal vein involvement or liver atrophy
T2	Tumor confined to the confluence and/or right or left hepatic duct with ipsilateral liver atrophy; no portal vein involvement demonstrated
T3	Tumor confined to the confluence and/or right or left hepatic duct with ipsilateral portal vein branch involvement with/without associated ipsilateral lobar liver atrophy; no main portal vein involvement (occlusion, invasion, or encasement)
T4	Any of the following: 1) Tumor involving both right and left hepatic ducts up to secondary biliary radicals bilaterally 2) Main portal vein encasement

with ipsilateral portal vein atrophy without main portal vein involvement; and T4, tumor involving both right and left hepatic ducts to secondary radicles bilaterally. or main portal vein encasement. This staging system provides data that is helpful during preoperative evaluation, such as defining the T stage based on the likelihood of survival. The limitations of this system are its absolute dependence on accurate preoperative identification of the extent of the tumor and on correct interpretation of preoperative radiologic imaging.

5. Clinical Features

Over 90% of patients with hilar malignancy present obstructive jaundice.[36] Patients without jaundice usually have either incomplete obstruction or very high lesions causing only lobar or segmental obstruction.[2,37] Not all patients with hilar tumor will present with jaundice, as obstruction of one hepatic duct without complete obstruction of the CHD may allow for sufficient bile excretion to prevent its development. Therefore, Klatskin's tumor patients with deep jaundice shows advanced bile duct infiltration by the tumor. Most of these patients have atrophied liver parenchyme caused by hepatic artery occlusion and controlateral compensatory hypertrophied liver parenchyme. If the tumor spreads to involve the portal vein, ipsilateral hepatic lobal atrophy can develop, in which case an isolated alkaline phosphatase elevation may be the only clinical finding.[35]

Although patients with either partial or complete obstruction of the bile duct may harbor bacteria in the obstructed biliary tree, cholangitis is rarely part of the initial presentation. However, the rate of occurrence of both cholangitis and bactobilia increases markedly with either endoscopic or percutaneous biliary tract instrumentation.[6]

Depending on the severity of jaundice, patients may also experience pruritus, which usually appear if the serum level of bilirubin more than 10 mg/dl. Additional complaints are generally nonspecific and include weight loss, abdominal pain , and occasionally fever.[12-14] Itching is the most commonly reported symptom, occuring in up to 30% of patients, and may precede the development of jaundice.[6] Patients with metastatic disease can harbor associated symptoms such as fatigue, lethargy, and weight loss.

Examination findings are consistent with obstructive jaundice with few specific features. Tender hepatomegaly (up to 75%), liver failure and occasionally a palpable or tender gallbladder might also be noted.[2,38]

6. Natural History

The prognosis of untreated proximal biliary malignancy is poor even compared with other malignancies. Although hilar cholangiocarcinoma has been characterized as a slow-growing and late metastasizing tumor, post-therapeutic prognosis has remained poor. Median reported survival time for unresectable tumors is between 3 and 12 months.[39-43] Without treatment, survival of patients with Klatskin tumor ranges between 4 and 8 months. Palliative biliary drainage by stents or prostheses appears to confer a survival benefit of only a few months.[44-51] In rare cases, some patients survive more than 1 year if adequate biliary drainage is provided without any other cancer treatment. The most common causes of death are liver failure and sepsis due to chronic biliary obstruction.

7. Diagnosis

1) Biochemical investigations

Obstructive jaundice typically results in a non-specific rise in serum bilirubin and the liver enzymes alkaline phosphatase and gamma-glutamyl transpeptidase, but it is common for the transaminase concentrations to also increase.[52] There are no tumor markers specific for cholangiocarcinoma. However, several are useful as a diagnostic guide. The most commonly used are carbohydrate antigen (CA) 19-9 and carcinoembryonic antigen (CEA). However CA 19-9 have low sensitivity and specificity.[53-55] Therefore, this is not suitable as a screening tool for the diagnosis of malignant bile duct cancer. CEA alone, has also unsatisfactory sensitivity and specificity for diagnosis of cholangiocarcinoma.[56] Several new and potentially useful tumor markers are currently being studied, with no clear data as of yet.[57]

2) Diagnostic radiology

The role of radiological evaluation in malignant jaundice is to delineate anatomy, identify a cause, demonstrate the level of obstruction, and determine resectability and decompression options. Radiological evaluation that excludes patients in whom surgery would provide no added benefit helps reduce surgical mortality and morbidity and helps select patients for endoscopic and radiological palliation.

(1) Ultrasonography

Ultrasonography is usually the first investigation in obstructive jaundice. Tumor of the biliary hilus are particularly amenable to US, as the liver provides an excellent acoustic window. Therefore, sonography is accurate in visualizing the biliary obstruction at the level of the hepatic hilus. Although accurate in determining the level of obstruction, the cause was often missed as tumor visualization was difficult.[58,59] Overall, sonography detects about 21% of these tumors. However, later studies have reported improved detection rates of 87~90%.[60-63] Detection rate is dependent on tumor type. Although intraductal polypoid tumor is seen as a well-defined isoechoic mass in contrast to the surrounding anechoic bile, the detection of the infiltrative or exophytic type tumor is difficult. Tumors of the biliary hilus are particularly amenable to US, as the liver provides an excellent accoustic window compared with the lower biliary tree where the are is often obscured by intestinal gas.

(2) Computed Tomography

Although it is difficult to diagnose hilar cholangiocarcinoma with conventional CT because of its small size. Dynamic contrast enhanced CT used in assessment showed a sensitivity rate of 40~63% in tumor detection.[60,64,65] The main role is with preoperative assessment. CT showed 40~42% accuracy in determination of resectability.[59,64,66] CT is able to demonstrate the actual tumor mass, the presence of lobar atrophy, and the relationship between the tumor and caudate lobe: which are important surgical considerations.[36]

Spiral CT with contrast enhancement and multiphasic scanning has improved visualization of the tumor, its spread, as well as demonstration of the status of the hepatic arterial or portal venous circulation. Studies found hepatic arterial dominant phase scans able to demonstrate 91~100% of tumor masses.[64,67,68]

On contrast-enhanced CT, infiltrating tumors are seen as a focally thickened ductal wall obliterating the lumen. About 80% of these tumors are hyperattenuating relative to the liver on arterial or portal phase or both.[62,69] Nonunion of the right and left hepatic ducts with or without a visibly thickened wall is a typical finding of infiltrating hilar cholangiocarcinoma.[70] Mass-forming exophytic type lesion manifests as a low-attenuation mass with peripheral rim enhancement in the arterial dominant phase and homogenous hypoattenuation in the portal dominant phase similar to the finding of peripheral cholangiocarcinoma. It can be difficult or even impossible to ascertain whether the carcinoma arises at the main hepatic junction or represents a peripheral cjolangiocarcinoma that secondarily obliterates the hilar area.[70] Intraductal polypoid lesion is hypoattenuating relative to the hepatic parenchyme.[68,71]

Identification of the proximal extent of the tumor is important for planning surgical treatment. In a study with thin-section spiral CT, the investigators correctly predicted intraductal tumor extent in 63% of cases.[68] Careful tracing of the bile duct from the periphery of the liver enabled identification of segmental bile ducts and the presence of the secondary confluence proximal to the tumor. However, CT was ineffective in detecting superficially spreading tumor that extended above the level of biliary obstruction because of the preserved lumen in the tumor; this extent of intraductal tumor spread tends to be underestimated with CT.[70] In an equivocal case, the combined assessment of CT and cholangiography or choledochoscopy through the percutaneous tract and biopsy are needed to evaluate exact tumor extent.[71]

Angiography including hepatic arteriography and indirect portal venography may be helpful in determining vascular involvement. Vascular involvement such as focal or segmental narrowing (encasement) of the involved vessel can be depicted by angiography. However, angiography cannot determine vascular invasion that does not change the diameter of the involved vessel.[70] With thin-sectional spiral CT, obliteration of the fat plane between the biliary tumor and the hepatic artery or portal vein can be used as a criterion for vascular invasion.[68] In addition, because the liver has a dual blood supply, obstruction or significant stricture of one vessel causes compensatory hyperperfusion of the other.[72] Using this criterion, vascular invasion of ther portal vein and hepatic artery can be correctly diagnosed in 87% and 62% respectively.[68] With rapid advancements in multi-detector CT and three-dimensional display techniques, the accuracy of CT in predicting non-resectability is expected to improve (Fig. 3).

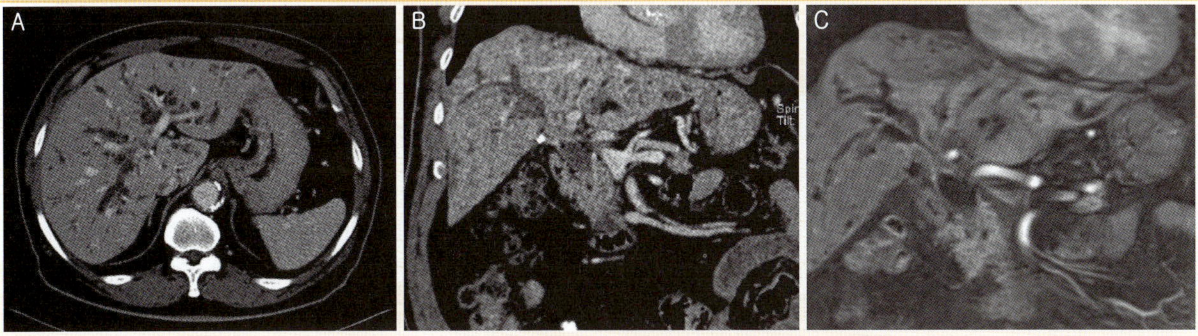

Fig. 3 CT (A, B) and MRCP (C) imaging of Klatskin tumor

A, B: Axial and coronal CT of hilar stticture involving confluence of both main intrahepatic and proximal extrahepatic bile duct. C: Contrast-enhanced T-1 weighted coronal image of the same patient, suggesting Bismuth type IV cholangiocarcinoma.

(3) Magnetic resonance imaging

Magnetic resonance cholangiopancreatiography provides a non-invasive alternative that can be as sensitive and specific as endoscopic cholangiography (ERC) in depicting tumors, in addition to allowing full demonstration of relevant biliary anatomy without introducing contrast media above the stricture which can be a cause of lethal cholangitis.[73] Therefore there are strong assertions that MRCP should replace diagnostic ERC and percutaneous transhepatic cholangiography (PTC) because of the higher risks of these invasive procedures. Owing to intrinsically high tissue contrast and multiplanar capability, MRCP is probably superior to ERCP for defining the anatomy of tumors and assessing resectibility, and is increasingly becoming the imaging modality of choice.[73,74] However, it should be noted that the correlation between MRCP findings and the extent of cholangiocarcinoma suggests that MRCP understages disease in up to 20% of malignant hilar strictures.[75]

The morphology of bile duct stricture detectable on MR cholangiography closely reflects the gross morphologic changes occurring along the biliary ductal walls. On cross-sectional MR images, the periductal-infiltration and intraductal polypoid lesions appear hypointense to the liver on T1-weighted images and moderately hyperintense with a high signal on T2-weighted images. A diffusely infiltrating cancer may be seen as a stretch of narrowed lumen and designated as the periductal infiltrating type and a intraductal polypoid cholangiocarcinoma may be visualized as a protuberant end morphology of the bile duct. In addition, combined use of MR cholangiopancreato-graphy and dynamic MRI can display the overall extent of biliary tree involvement and the correct diagnosis of biliary malignancies (Fig. 3).[72]

(4) Direct cholangiography

Delineation of bile duct using direct cholangiography has long been regarded the definitive investigation for hilar tumors.[59,76] Proximal extension has important therapeutic connotations and direct cholangiography allows complete evaluation of the entire biliary tree.[36] However, the major drawback of ERCP and PTC have been procedure-related risks. Therefore these direct cholangiogrphy is now used more as a therapeutic purpose rather than a diagnostic tool. The choice between ERCP and PTC is largely dependent on local expertise, availability, and failure of one or other technique, usually ERCP. Anatomical characteristics are also important. If the obstructions located in high level of intrahepatic duct and complicated, PTC and following PTBD is rational than performing ERCP.

The high resection rates currently performed seems to directly correlate with the extent and quality of the diagnostic work-up. In this work-up, PTC still plays a central role.[77-79] A German group also reported that PTC is crucial for the proper pre-operative evaluation of peripheral tumor extension.[80,81] However, as previously mentioned, non-invasive diagnostic modalities have replaced direct cholangiography in many institute.

(5) PET scanning

PET scanning with the focal accumulation of nucleotid tracer 18-fluorodeoxyglucose (FDG) is an emerging staging technique for many cancers. The technique can detect nodular cholangiocarcinomas as small as 1 cm, but is less helpful for infiltrating tumors.[82] A study of 30 cases with extrahepatic cholangiocarcinoma compared FDG-PET scan with CT for initial staging. Tumors were interpreted as malignant on the basis of CT in 24(80%) patients, while PET revealed increased FDG uptake in 18 (60%) patients.[83] With respect to lymphadenopathy, there was no difference in sensitivity between the two techniques, but PET had a specificity of 100% compared with 59% for CT.[83] A retrospective study assessed FDG-PET scans in 21 patients with intraheatic cholangiocarcinoma (both hilar and peripheral) who had undergone CT and MRI.[84] For the detection of lymph node metastasis, FDG-PET and CT and MRI were concordant in 16 patients and discordant in five. FDG-PET identified unsuspected distant metastases in four patients, all of whom had peripheral cholangiocarcinoma. The ability of PET to detect distant metastases could alter the surgical management plan in up to 30% of cases.[82,85]

(6) Tissue diagnosis and differential diagnosis

Methods used to obtain material for cytology include bile aspiration at percutaneous drainage (positive in up to 34%); preoperative fine-needle aspiration (sensitivity 50-77%) and endoscopic biopsy or brush cytology.[36] Unfortunately, adequate histological specimens are difficult to obtain because of the character of these tumors. More importantly the diagnostic yield in sclerotic type is low. Abundant fibrous tissue and submucosal tumor spreading prevent effective tissue acquisition. Therefore, result of biopsy with direct visualization of the lesion through cholangioscopy is also not satisfactory. Preoperative histological confirmation of an hilar cancer can be difficult to obtain. Percutaneous needle biopsies and endoscopic brush biopsies are reliable only if they identify a malignancy, and excessive reliance on negative results may miss the opportunity to operate an early lesion.[86,87] Whereas the vast majority of extrahepatic strictures, particularly hilar strictures, are the result of an hilar cancer, histological diagnosis is not mandatory before exploration. The resection has to be performed even if the results of a biopsy or of a cytological test are negative. The general rule has to be applied that malignant growth can never be excluded by a negative test.[6] As a consequence, as many as 10% of isolated bile strictures are benign,[36] the rate of benign strictures in patients resected for suspicious hilar obstruction is around 15%.[88] Alternative diagnoses include metastatic diseases, gallbladder cancer, Mirizzi's syndrome, lesions masquerading as malignant such as focal biliary sclerosis, and other benign causes such as stricture caused by cholangitis.

(7) Choledochoscopy

Bile duct tumors exhibit characteristic cholangioscopic findings and cholangioscopy seems to be useful for differential diagnosis.[89] Most importantly the presence of tumor vessel may be a valuable cholangioscopic finding that indicates the presence of a malignant biliary stricture. The combination of the irregularly dilated and tortuous vessel, the tumor vessel, observation and PTCS-guided biopsy may improve the preoperative diagnosis of malignancy and reduce the result of a false negative (Fig. 4).[90] PTCS in patients with focal stricture of the intrahepatic duct unrelated to stone disease is useful for diagnosis including detection of early bile duct cancer.[91] Therefore PTCS is also applicable to hilar

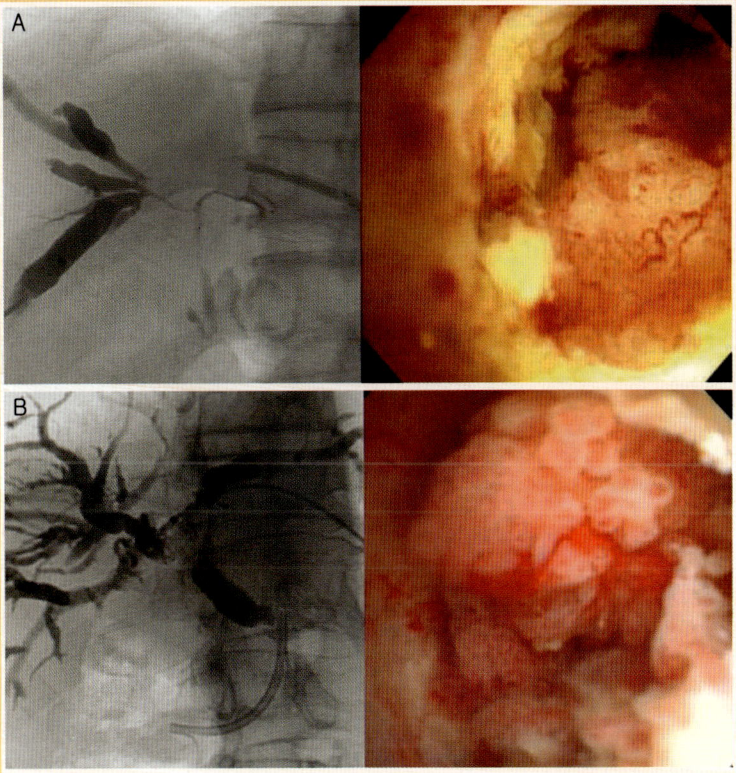

Fig. 4 Choledoscopic findings of Klatskin tumor

A: tumor vessel on the mass. B: papillary mass resembling that of frog eggs.

stricture with unknown causes.

There was good overall agreement between MRC and PTCS with respect to longitudinal extension of hilar cholangiocarcinoma. For stenotic hilar cholangiocarcinoma, as determined by selective cholangiography, MRC may replace PTCS for determination of longitudinal tumor extension. For polypoid types of hilar cholahgiocarcinoma, however, the accuracy of MRC was significantly lower compared with the stenotic type, and therefore in such cases PTCS is necessary for accurate preoperative assessment of longitudinal tumor extension.[92]

New imaging modality, PTCS through the use of Narrow-band imaging (NBI) has been introduced. This may be helpful for the observation of both fine mucosal structures and tumor vessels.[93] And thin peroral cholangiopancreatoscopy system, with 4-way deflected steering and dedicated irrigation channels, is designed and commercially available for the diagnosis and therapy of bile duct stricture.[94] These new systems are now being further characterized in prospective multicenter clinical trials.

(8) Laparoscopy

Staging laparoscopy is playing a larger role in the evaluation of patients to reduce the number of unnecessary open procedures. In a series of 56 patients with hilar cholangiocarcinoma, staging laparoscopy was found to have a 51% accuracy in detecting unresectable disease in patients with stage II-III disease that was potentially resectable, laparoscopy identified 36% of patients as unresectable.[95] Therefore, laparoscopy is proving to be a useful staging procedure in selected patients. With the improvement of MD-CT and MRI imaging, the need for preoperative laparoscopy is diminishing.

8. Treatment

1) Operation

(1) Resectability

Resectability is defined by the surgical possibilities of resection for Klatskin tumors according to the preoperative criteria established by the surgeon with respect to the surgical techniques. Hilar cholangiocarcinoma usually demonstrates a tendency of intramural growth, perineural, and perifocal lymphatic infiltration. Moreover, the adjacent liver parenchyma may be infiltrated. On the other hand, lymph nodes are involved in only 30 to 40% and distant metastases are observed in only 10% of the patients at the time of surgery. Due to the particular localization of this tumor and its propensity to infiltrate the hilar region, hilar cholangiocarcinoma remains a challenge for surgeons.[96-101]

CT scan is essential, as unilateral atrophy is an indicator of arterial involvement. CT or MRI angiography can be as precise as arteriography, and have the added advantage of being noninvasive. Cholangiography is necessary in order to define the type of stricture (Bismuth classification) and the degree of dilatation of the bile ducts. Furthermore, it provides a map of the intrahepatic biliary tract to assess the tumoral extent and, in case of nonresectability, which ducts should be drained. ERCP and PTC were previously used for these purposes. Both techniques have been condemned by surgeon, if there is extension into the portal vein.[102] All invasive investigations can now be replaced by CT and MRCP.

Despite aggressive resection involving both the extra- and intrahepatic biliary tree, patients are frequently left with positive margins because it can be impossible to predict the proximal extent of microscopic disease based on preoperative imaging studies.[103,104] Further resection in these cases may be impossible owing to encroachment on the remaining lobe or vital structures necessary for the normal function of that lobe.

The dismal prognosis of this tumor encourages resection by whatever means possible, The absence of effective chemotherapy, coupled with profound symptoms at presentation, further encourages surgical intervention even when extension of the biliary cancer necessitates morbid and potentially fatal in-continuity hepatic resection. Clinical study documents that even with cancer-positive margins, patients undergoing resection for hilar cholangiocarcinoma showed a survival advantage.[105]

According to publications from Asian countries, a comprehensive preoperative diagnostic work-up and more aggressive attitude toward resection have contributed to reaching high resection rate.[46,77,103,106-108] The difference in surgical approach is impressively demonstrated in a published comparison of a American and a Japanese center.[79] Surgery was performed in 80% of the Japan patients, while in comparison, only 25% of the patients in the American hospital were considered to be resectable. In this comparison, it is clear that patient selection did not play a big role. The attitude toward resection led to a higher resection rate, because the surgical specimens in Japan demonstrated more advanced tumors than in the US.

Although there is some disagreement about the criteria for resectability among surgeons, non-resectability of hilar cholangiocarcinoma is suggested by (a) hepatic duct involvement up to secondary biliary radicals, bilaterally, (b)

Table 4. Criteria for unresectability.

1. Hepatic duct involvement up to secondary biliary radicals bilaterally
2. Encasement or occlusion of the main portal vein proximal to its bifurcationa
3. Atrophy of one hepatic lobe with encasement of contralateral portal vein branch
4. Atrophy of one hepatic lobe with contralateral involvement of secondary biliary radicals
5. Distant metastases (peritoneum, liver, lung)

[a] Relative criterion. Portal vein resection and reconstruction may be possible.

encasement or occlusion of the main portal vein proximal to its bifurcation (relative criterion. portal vein resection and reconstruction may be possible[78,109,110], (c) atrophy of one hepatic lobe with encasement of contralateral portal vein branch, (d) atrophy of one hepatic lobe with contralateral involvement of secondary biliary radicals, (e) distant metastases (peritoneum, liver, lung).[111] Unilateral involvement of the hepatic artery, portal vein, or both vessels is compatible with resection. Involvement of the main hepatic artery or portal vein is the most common contraindication to resection although some centers support en bloc resection with vascular reconstruction (Table 4).[109-111] Other local factors that affect resectability include lobar atrophy. Peritoneal and superficial liver metastases are rarely detected with current imaging and laparoscopy has identified additional disease in up to a third of cases in some series.[95]

(2) Preoperative preparation

a. Preoperative biliary drainage

In order to decrease the operative risk of hepatectomy in jaundiced patients, Japanese authors emphasize the value of routine preoperative biliary drainage by PTBD. However, this is very controversial. Five randomized trials failed to show any significant benefit of this drainage[112-116] and postoperative infectious complications are more frequent.[117]

However, serious complications are sometimes encountered after resection of the cholestatic liver with or without cholangitis. Therefore, biliary decompression is mandatory before cholestatic liver resection, although some surgeons have reported disadvantages of preoperative biliary decompression.[112,115,116] Furthermore, cholangiits should be noticed as a very serious condition that should be resolved before liver surgery,[118,119] and segmental cholangitis is a specific preoperative complication of advanced hilar cholangiocarcinoma which must be treated by selective PTBD.[120] Multiple PTBD for hilar cholangiocarcinma offers some advantages in both preoperative management of cholestatic liver with or without cholangitis and preoperative precise diagnosis of the extent of tumor along the separated intrahepatic bile duct.[78] Impaired mitochondrial and microsomal function of the liver should be resolved before hepatectomy, preferably using bilateral PTBD, which has an advantage over unilateral PTBD.[121-124] Resectional surgery after the serum bilirubin level has fallen to 2 mg/dL or less provides excellent long-term outcome.[125] Even with remained controversies among the surgeons, preoperative biliary drainage is preferred in patients with cholestasis who are planed for liver resection.)

b. Portal vein (or arterial) embolization

Extended hepatectomy with extrahepatic biliary resection and lymphadenectomy has been proposed, but this procedure has an increased operation related complications. The extensive nature of these right side resections often leaves only 20~30% of the liver parenchyma with potentially high rate of liver insufficiency and attendant mortality.[126] The liver failure is due to reduction of hepatic functional volume, but this complication does not occur if preoperative thrombosis of the portal vein exists. For this reason, preoperative embolization of the portal vein have been proposed to initiate a compensatory hypertrophy on the other side of the liver and avoid a sudden increase of portal pressure after hepatectomy.[127]

After right embolization, the volume of the left part of the liver ranges from 36% to 49% of the liver volume. Surgery is performed 2~4 weeks after embolization. After embolization, the functional benefit in the remaining liver is reached rapidly and is greater than the volume increase.[128] The volume of the liver remnant should be approximately 40% of the initial volume to safely perform a liver resection.[129] Portal vein embolization has allowed an increasing number of patients to be offered extended resections who would otherwise have been poor candidates for treatment based on inadequate liver size or function.[126,130]

With same rationale, embolization of the homolateral hepatic artery with biliary drainage of the liver remnant was proposed. With this technique, volumetric measurement, using a helical CT scan, has shown an increase of the left liver lobe volume from 11% to 68% with median 35%.[100]

(3) Surgical strategy and results

Surgical therapy have a dual objective. The First is removal of the obstruction and, with it, the jaundice. And secondly, treatment of the cancer of the biliary tract, which is often given a too pessimistic prognosis. Surgery remains as the only life-prolonging and potentially lifesaving approach. Even patients with palliative resection benefit from surgery compared to those without resection.[105] The surgical experience differs considerably from the results of radiological and medical studies. The problem is reflected by an astounding number of patients who are deemed unresectable due to misleading preoperative information. Remarkably, high resection rates seem to correlate with the extent and quality of the diagnostic work-up.[101] Overestimation of the tumor extent was the most common mistake during diagnostic work-up (Fig. 5). R0 resection and survival, however, were not significantly worse in patients with overestimated lesions

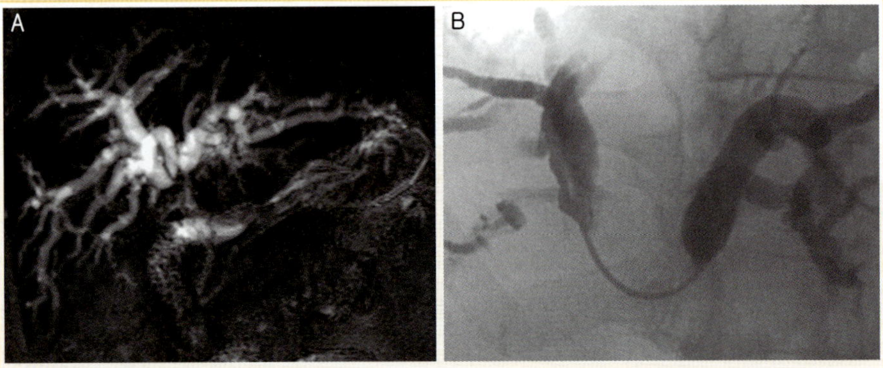

Fig. 5

Resectable case where (A) MR and (B) direct cholangiography regarded it as unresectable (Bismuth type IV) compared to correctly assessed tumors. It would have been fatal if overinterpretation of the real situation had led to the exclusion of these patients from surgery. It is obvious that tumor infiltration may be mimicked by benign conditions, which leads to the over-interpretation of tumor extent.

During the past two decades, the outcome of surgical treatment has improved considerably, mainly owing to the application of wider resections. En bloc resection of tumor and liver results in superior survival compared to hilar resection.[103,106,131] Whereas the 5-year survival of patients with hilar resection ranges between 0 and 10%, it reaches 25 to 30% after en bloc resection. This difference is particularly evident in type I and type II tumors (0 vs 55%).[132] Most data suggest that the hospital mortality after en bloc resection is not higher compared to hilar resection.

It is well recognized that R0 resections with margins more than 5 mm, en bloc partial hepatectomy and lymphatic invasion remain important factors that affect survival.[125] the Japanese were first to stress the importance of en bloc hepatic resection, including caudate lobectomy, in order to obtain negative margins. Today, extended right or left hepatectomy with caudate lobectomy, and excision of all neural and lymphatic tissue within the hepatoduodenal ligament, is the standard of surgery.[126] Occasionally, portal vein resection and en bloc pancreatoduodenectomy may be needed to obtain negative margins. Even with curative resections local recurrence is common and the 5 year survival rate varies between 15 and 35 per cent but, when these procedures are performed with minimum mortality, the 5 year survival rates can reach up to 40 per cent in an intension-to-treat analysis.[125]

Morphological studies of the surgical anatomy of the hepatic hilus and segmental anatomy of the intarahepatic bile ducts demonstrated the necessity for caudate lobe resection which has been emphasized by Japanese surgeons.[133-136] The Bismuth classification system takes into account extension of tumor into the right and left biliary system, with segment 4 lying anterior to the tumor. Hilar tumors, however, equally extend in posterior direction, involving the usually short bile ducts of the caudate lobe (segment 1). Resection of the caudate lobe along with all or part of segment 4, is therefore mandatory to remove all tumor. Nimura et al. found microscopic cancer involvement in the bile ducts of the caudate lobe in the resected specimens from 44 of the 46 patients who underwent curative caudate lobe resection.[137] An R0 resection without removal of the caudate lobe is virtually impossible.[101]

Portal vein embolization has the potential benefit for patients with advanced biliary cancer who are to undergo extended, complex hepatectomy. The Nagoya group studied 240 consecutive patients with biliary cancer (150 cholangiocarcinoma and 90 gallbladder cancer) who underwent portal vein embolization before an extended hepatectomy (right or left trisectionectomy or right hepatectomy).[130] The 3- and 5-year survival rate after hepatectomy was 41.7% and 26.8% in cholangiocarcinoma. The overall postoperative mortality was 4.5% in patients with cholangiocarcinoma. The clinical application of portal vein embolization has contributed to the improvement of the postoperative outcome of hilar cholangiocarcinoma.

Currently, owing to the improvement of diagnostic and therapeutic technique, the resectability of hilar cholangiocarcinoma is amazingly increased with acceptable morbidity and mortality. Therefore, curative resection after aggressive preoperative management is recommended as a reasonable surgical approach to hilar cholangiocarcinoma.

Orthotopic liver transplantation has been performed for both resectable and unresectable cholangiocarcinoma. In most centers, however, the high mortality and morbidity, high recurrence and short survival rates in addition to organ shortage prevent this practice form becoming widely accepted.138,139? In pilot studies, OLT following preooperative chemoirradiation for unresectable cholangicarcinoma has resulted in long-term survival of carefully selected patients and may be appropriate within clinical trials.[140]

2) Palliative therapy

Many patients diagnosed with Klatskin tumor are not candidates for surgical resection. The palliation of obstructive jaundice becomes the first priority. Palliation of obstructive jaundice can be achieved successfully through three major routes:

surgically, by the creation of a hepaticojejunostomy; percutaneously, via percutaneous transhepatic biliary drainage (PTBD); and endoscopically, via ERCP and stent placement. Before the introduction of endoscopic and percutaneous therapy, surgical biliary bypass was the only way to achieve palliation of malignant biliary obstruction. This is associated with high success but at the expense of high operative mortality, morbidity and cost, as well as long recovery time. Studies comparing surgical and nonsurgical (endoscopic and percutaneous) palliation showed equal results of jaundice and survival. However, nonsurgical palliation offers a significantly lower morbidity, mortality and cost. Therefore, surgical bypass is usually performed only when an attempt at curative resection is unsuccessful because of evidence of unresetable disease at laparotomy.

(1) Endoscopic palliation

Plastic stent made of polyethylene or teflon and self-expandable metal stent (SEMS) made of various alloys, such as titanium alloy, are used. SEMS allows for a much longer duration of stent patency because of the larger diameter up to 30 Fr.. Plastic stents become occluded by a biofilm of bacteria and proteinaceous material that is especially problematic in the smaller caliber stent (7Fr.) compared with the larger caliber one (10 Fr.). Many endoscopiest prefer to insert SEMS as the initial palliative method depending on the condition and life expectancy of the patient. SEMS are more cost effective in patients who survive at least 3 to 6 months.[141] Owing to the superior stent patency, the need for repeat endoscopic intervention to manage recurrent jaundice is decreased. Even though the superiority of the stent has not been proven in randomized controlled trials in the palliation of obstructive jaundice in Klatskin tumor, several nonrandomized studies have proven the superior efficacy of SEMS in managing malignant hilar strictures.[142,143]

The decision whether to place a single biliary stent or multiple stents depends initially on the location of the stricture in the biliary tract. It is known that only 25 to 30% of the liver needs to be drained to achieve adequate palliation of obstructive jaundice.[144] Therefore, a single stent into one lobe of the liver should provide adequate palliation of jaundice, assuming the drained lobe is free of disease. Several studies have attempted to address whether unilateral or bilateral drainage is the preferred for palliation of obstructive jaundice in patients with hilar tumor. In many studies, unilateral drainage is sufficient palliative therapy for the relief of obstruction in Klatskin tumor.[142,145-147] In addition, prolonged efforts to place a second stent have no survival benefits and may lead to an increase in early complications due to the contamination of bacteria of the undrained lobe caused during contrast injection, which can lead to cholangitis or/and sepsis.[146] Close collaboration with interventional radiologiest is essential during ERCP, because the undrained bile duct should be drained immediately after the procedure to avoid complication.[142,145]

Regardless of the number of stent inserted, it is more important to select the intact, unatrophied lobe for drainage for stent insertion. It is still not clear whether bilateral stenting leads to improved survival, however failed attempts at placing bilateral stents have shown to decrease survival. This evidence has led to the use of selective and planned endoscopic drainage via MRCP guidance. MRCP provides a road map for the biliary endoscopist to define the biliary anatomy, allowing them to determine the optimal hepatic lobe and biliary segments for drainage prior to ERCP. This allows the avoidance of atrophied segments and minimizes the need to inject contrast agent into multiple segments of the liver during ERCP.[147,148] About 10~15% of metal stents eventually become occluded due to tumor ingrowth through the wire mesh or tumor overgrowth above or below the stent. This can be solved by inserting another stent, either plastic or metal, through the occluded stent.

Current designs of Y-type and T-type bare metal stents are applied to hilar malignant obstruction by means of peroral and percutaneous methods[149,150] respectively, in order to allow easy insertion of a second stent through the wide opening in the middle portion of the first stent. Overlapping of the two endoprostheses is considered effective in preventing displacement of the metal stents. It is worth noting that parallel bilateral positioning of two metal stents in patients with tight hilar stricture due to advanced cholangiocarcinoma is unfeasible and may even cause severe discomfort to patients. These newly designed Y- or T-type stent have yielded a high success rate of 80% to 100%

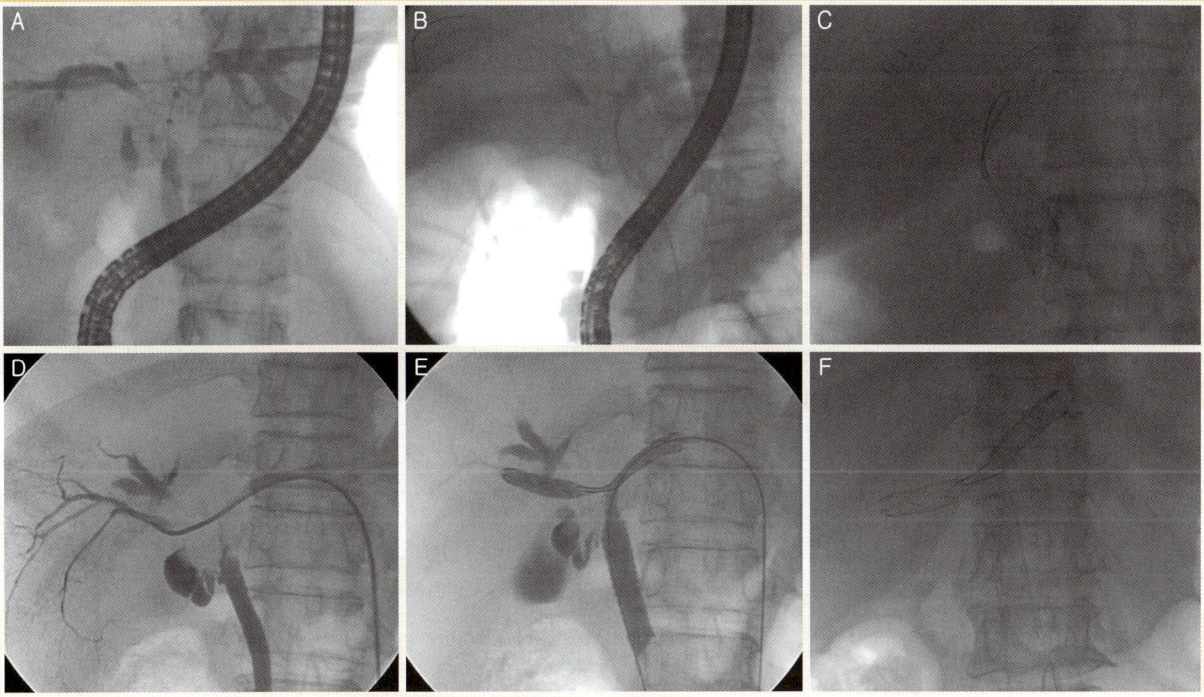

Fig. 5 Y-type (A-C) and T-type (D-F) metal stent insertion for Klatskin tumor.
Second metal stent insertion through the mid-portion with wide opening of first stent (B and E)

without inducing severe discomfort to the patient after stent deployment (Fig. 6). The main drawback of these type of stents is the difficulty of re-intervention when stent occlusion occur due to tumor ingrowth or overgrowth. Further studies will be needed to determine the ideal endoscopic management of Klatskin tumor.

(2) Percutaneous treatment

External biliary drainage was the first non-surgical technique used for decompression in malignant jaundice,[151,152] but recent advances in other forms of palliation limit its current use. However, there are still instances in which external biliary drainage is preferred. - preoperative cholangiography evaluation and drainage, - in the presence of cholangitis if internal drainage cannot be established, - for temporary drainage to minimize infection if stent insertion has failed, - for the establishment of percutaneous access for brachytherapy, - for postoperative decompression for management of complications.[152,153]

The disadvantage include risk of spontaneous dislodgement, inflammation and pain at the insertion site, bile leaks and loss of fluid and electrolytes.[153,154] Patients also report additional discomfort and difficulty with regular flushing and dressing, and problems with the required frequent catheter exchanges, which serves as a constant reminder of the patient's disease.[154,155]

Percutaneous insertion of semi-permanent endoprostheses is a well established palliative modality. This method is a very useful rescue procedure when peroral approach fails. Much clinical experience has been reported in this area. Technical success and the successful drainage rate is very high for both plastic and metal stents, and procedure-related and 30-day mortality compare favorably with surgical and endoscopic procedures.[156] The T-type metal stent insertion is very effective for the palliation of advanced Klatskin's tumor. The overall technical success is very high even in cases of unsuccessful stent insertion with ERCP. The foremost/primary advantage of this technique is its ability to drain both biliary systems from a single transhepatic access by means of arranging the stents in a T-configuration.[149,159,160]

(3) Chemotherapy

At present, chemotherapy and/or radiation therapies for cholangiocarcinoma have not been evaluated in the context of randomized controlled trials, and, therefore, their efficacy remains dubious, including the use of adjuvant chemotherapy after surgical resection to diminish the risk of cancer recurrence.[6]

Chemotherapy for cholangiocarcinoma is administered to patients who are not operative candidates, and the results are largely disappointing. Most studies encompass the bile duct cancer and gallbladder cancer together, However, it is very rare to find studies confined specifically on hilar cholangiocarcinoma.[161] Two review articles on non-operative management of cholangiocarcinoma have found no overall mortality benefit. Among those patients who have responded, a key prognostic factor is performance status. Most of the studies to date have used systemic 5-fluorouracil (5-FU)-based regimens.[74] More recently, it was shown that gemcitabine as a single agent had a partial response rate of 30%.[162] The combination of gemcitabine and capecitabine have shown to have some benefit in patients with advanced biliary cancer.[163] Oxalliplatin is also a promising agent with a combination of 5 FU and leucovorine in the treatment of pancreatic cancer.[164] This combination can be applied to bile duct cancer. Nonetheless, the best available chemotherapeutic treatment for advanced biliary tract cancer remains to be determined. Accumulating data from recently reported phase II trials, however, suggest that single agent gemcitabine represents an active and well tolerated treatment option. Gemcitabine may also be combined safely with other agents, and further improvements in the efficacy response and survival warrant confirmation in future randomized studies in the treatment of biliary tract carcinoma.[74]

(4) Radiation therapy

Intraluminal brachytherapy (ILBT) for the palliation of unresectable cholangiocarcinoma has been evaluated in various uncontrolled retrospective studies with mixed results.[165-167] The procedure can be performed endoscopically or percutaneously. Iridium-192 seeds mounted on a catheter are placed directly across the stricture in the bile ducts. Some studies have shown improved survival in patients with inoperable cholangiocarcinoma,[165,166] whereas others have not yielded any benefit or have even shown an increased incidence of complications due to cholangitis.[167] Moreover, without any definite prolongation of survival in patients with a high complication rate, brachytherapy is not accepted as established therapy for initial palliative and postoperative adjuvant purposes.[168]

The potential radiosensitising effect of 5-FU suggests that combination of radiation and chemotherapy would be more effective than either alone. This approach has been used in some early studies with encouraging results.[169] However, there are no prospective trials of this combined treatment and a retrospective case study showed no benefit with adjuvant chemoradiation therapy.[170]

(5) Photodynamic therapy

The current use of photodynamic therapy in palliative management of extrahepatic cholangiocarcinoma has yielded promising results. PDT involves light activation of a photosensitizer that is preferentially retained with some degree of selectivity in neoplastic cells. Tumor selectivity of PDT results in the accumulation of the photosensitizer in tumor tissue and is characterized by the concentration ratio between tumor cells and normal tissue. PDT has been shown to induce local regression of malignant tumors.[171]

In non-randomized studies of small groups of patients with unresectable cholangiocarcinoma, PDT induced a decrease in serum bilirubin levels, improved quality of life with a nominal increase in survival. Other non-randomized trials have failed to show clinical benefits. The first prospective, randomized controlled study with PDT in the PDT-randomized patients was so impressive that it was considered to be unethical to continue randomized trial. PDT resulted in prolongation of survival (median 493 days vs. 98 days; $p<0.0001$) and also improved biliary drainage and quality of life.51 However, further studies are expected in unselected patients with unresectable cholangiocarcinoma before PDT, which may be considered as the standard adjuvant therapy. Palliative PDT and subsequent stenting resulted in longer survival than stenting alone and has a similar survival time compared with incomplete R1 and R2 resection.[172] However, these improvements in palliative treatment by PDT will not change the concept of an aggressive resectional approach.

Reference

1. Hii MWJ, Gibson RN. Role of radiology in the treatment of malignant hilar biliary strictures 1:Review of the literature. Australian Radiol 2004;48:3-13.
2. Klatskin G. Adenocarcinoma of the hepatic duct at its bifurcation within the porta hepatis. Am J Med 38;341-356.
3. Brwon G. surgical removal of tumors of the hepatic ducts. Postgrad Med 1954;16:79.
4. Kirschbaum JD, Kozoll DC. Carcinoma of the gallbladder and extrahepatic bile ducts, SGO 1941;73:740-753.
5. Carriaga MT, Henseon DE. Liver, gallbaldder, extrahepatic bile ducts, and pancreas. Cancer 1995;75:171-190.
6. Chamberlain RS, Blumgart LH. Hilar cholangiocarcinoma: A review and commentary. Ann Surg Oncol 2000;7:55-66.

7. Vauthey JN, Blumgart LH. Recent advances in the management of cholangiocarcinomas. Semin Liver Dis 1994;14:109-114.

8. Khan SA, Taylor-Robinson SD, Toledano MB, Beck A, Elliott P, Thomas HC. Changing international trends in mortality rates for liver, biliary and pancreatic tumours. J Hepatol 2002;37:806-813.

9. Nakeeb A, Pitt HA, Sohn TA, et al. Cholangiocarcinoma: a spectrum of intrahepatic, perihilar, and distal tumors. Ann Surg 1996;224:463-475.

10. Tompkins RK, Thomas D, Wile A, et al. Prognostic factors in bile duct carcinoma. Ann Surg 1981;194:447-455.

11. Reding R, Buard JL, Lebeau G, Launois B. Surgical management of 552 carcinomas of the bile duct (gallbladder and periampullary excluded). Ann Surg 1991;213:236-241.

12. Pitt HA, Dooley WC, Yeo CJ, Cameron JL. Malignancies of the biliary tree. Curr Prob Surg 1995;32:1-90.

13. Thuluvath PJ, Rai R, Vembrux AC, Yeo CJ. Cholangiocarcinoma: a review. Gastroenterologist 1997;5:306-315.

14. Blumgart LH, Benjamin IS. Cancer of the bile ducts. In: Blumgart LH, ed. Surgery of the liver and biliary tract. 2nd ed. London: Churchill Livingstone, 1994:1051-1067.

15. Shaked A, Colonna JO, Goldstein L, Busuttil RW. The interrelation between sclerosing cholangitis and ulcerative colitis in patients undergoing liver transplantation. Ann Surg 1992;215:598-605.

16. Broome U, Olssson R, Loof L, et al. Natural history and prognostic factors in 305 Swedish patients with primary sclerosing cholangitis. Gut 1996;38:610-615.

17. Berquist A, Glaumann H, Persson B, Broome U. Risk factors and clinical presentation of hepatobiliary carcinoma in patients with primary sclerosing cholangitis: a case-control study. Hepatology 1998;27:311-316.

18. Lipsett PA, Pitt HA, Colombani PM, Boitnott JK, Cameron JL. Choledochal cyst disease: a changing pattern of presentation. Ann Surg 1994;220:644-652.

19. Ohtsuka T, Inoue K, Ohuchida J, et al. Carcinoma arising in choledochocele. Endoscopy 2001;3:614-619.

20. Watanapa P, Watanapa WB. Liver fluke-associated cholangiocarcinoma. Br J Surg 2002; 89:962-970.

21. Kubo S, Kinoshita H, Hirohashi K, Hamba H. Hepatoliyhiasis associatied with cholangiocarcinoma. World J Surg 1995;19:637-641.

22. Shaib YH, El-Serag HB, Davila JA, Norgan R, McGlynn KA. Risk factors of intrahepatic cholangiocarcinoma in the United States: a case-control study. Gastroenterology 2005;128: 620-626.

23. Sorensen HT, Friis S, Olsen JH, et al. Risk of liver and other types of cancer in patients with cirrhosis: a nationwide cohort study in Denmark. Hepatology 1998;28:921-925.

24. Kuwayti K, Baggenstoss AH, Stauffer MH, Preistley JI. Carcinoma of the major intrahepatic and extrahepatic bile ducts exclusive of the papilla of Vater. Surg Gynecol Obstet 1957;104:357-366.
25. Weinbren K, Mutumm SS. Pathological aspects of cholangiocarcinoma. J Pathol 1983;139:217-238.
26. Shimada H, Nimoto S, Matsuba A, et al. The infiltration of the bile duct carcinoma along the bile duct wall. Int Surg 1988;73:87-90.
27. Skamoto E, Nimura Y, Hayakawa N, et al. The pattern of infiltration at the proximal border of hilar bile duct cancer: a histological analysis of 62 resected cases. Ann Surg 1998; 227; 405-411.
28. Bismuth H, Corlette MB. Intrahepaticcholangioenteric anastomosis in carcinoma of the hilus of the liver. Surg Gynecol Obstet 1975;140:170-178.
29. Bismuth H, Nakache R, Diamond T. Management strategies in resection for hilar cholangiocarcinoma. Ann Surg 1992;215:31-38.
30. Shaib Y, El-Serag HB. The epidemiology of cholangiocarcinoma. Semin Liver Dis 2004; 24:115-125.
31. Liver Cancer Study Group of Japan (2000) The general rules for the clinical and pathological study of primary liver cancer, 4th ed. Kanehara, Tokyo.
32. Sako K, Seitzinger GL, Garside E. Carcinoma of the extra-hepatic bile ducts: review of the literature and report of six cases. Surgery 1957;41:416-437.
33. Gertsch P, Thomas P, Baer H, Lerut J, Zimmermann A, Blumgart LH. Multiple tumors of the biliary tract. Am J Surg 1990;159:386-388.
34. American Joint Commission on Cancer, editors. AJCC cancer staging manual. 5th edition. Philadelphia: Lipincott-Raven; 1997.
35. Burke EC, Jarnagin WR, Hochwald SN, Pisters PW, Fong Y, Blumgart LH. Hilar cholangicarcinoma: pattern of spread, the importance of hepatic resection for curative operation, and a presurgical clinical staging system. Ann Surg 1998;228:385-394.
36. Stain SC, Baer HU, Dennison AR, Blumgart LH. Current management of hilar cholangiocarcinoma. Surg Gynecol Obstet 1992;175:579-588.
37. Farley DR, Weaver AL, Nagorney DM. 'Natural history' of unresected cholangiocarcinoma: patient outcome after non-curative intervention. Mayo Clin Proc 1995;70:425-429.
38. Altaee MY, Johnson PJ, Farrant JM, Williams R. Etiologic and clinical characteristics of peripheral and hilar cholangiocarcinoma. Cancer 1991;68:2051-2055.
39. Lee MJ, Dawson SL, Mueller PR et al. Failed metallic biliary stents: causes and management of delayed complications. Clin Radiol 1994;49:857-862.
40. Lameris JS, Stoker J, Nijs HGT, et al. Malignant biliary obstruction: percutaneous use of self expandable stents. Radiology 1991;179:703-707.

41. Gordon RL, Ring EJ, LaBerge JM, Doherty MM. Malignant biliary obstruction: treatment with expandable metallic stents - follow up of 50 consecutive patients. Radiology 1992; 182: 697-701.

42. Gilliams A, Dick R, Dooley JS, Wallstent H, El-Din A. Self-expandable stainless steel braided endoprosthesis for biliary strictures. Radiology 1990;174:137-140.

43. Nicholson DA, Cjetty D, Jackson JE, Roddie ME, Adam A. Patency of side branches after peripheral placement of metallic biliary endoprosthesis. J. Vasc Intervent Radiol 1992;3: 127-130.

44. Cheng JL, Bruno MJ, Bergman JJ, Rauws EA, Tytgat GN, Huibregtse K. Endoscopic palliation of patients with biliary obstruction caused by nonresectable hilar cholangiocarcinoma: efficacy of self-expandable metallic Wallstents. Gastrointest Endosc 2002;56:33-39.

45. Gerhards MF, den Hartog D, Rauws EA, et al. Palliative treatment in patients with unresectable hilar cholangiocarcinoma: results of endoscopic drainage in patients with type III and IV hilar cholangiocarcinoma. Eur J Surg 2001;167:274-280.

46. Golfieri R, Giampalma E, Muzzi C, et al. Unresectable hilar cholangiocarcinoma: combined percutaneous and radiotherapeutic treatment. Radiol Med(Torino) 2001;101:495-502.

47. Figueras J, Llado L, Valls C, et al. Changing strategies in diagnosis and management of hilar cholangiocarcinoma. Liver Transpl. 2000;6:786-794.

48. Kaiho T, Miyazaki M, Ito H, et al. Treatment of unresectable hepatic hilar malignancies with self-expanding metallic stents. Hepatogastroenterology 1999;46:2781-2790.

49. Schima W, Prokesch R, Osterreicher C, et al. Biliary Wallstent endoprosthesis in malignant hilar obstruction: long-term results with regard to the type of obstruction. Clin Radiol 1997; 52:213-219.

50. Wiedmann MW, Berr R, Schiefke I, et al. Photodynamic therapy in patients with non-resectable hilar cholangiocarcinoma: 5-year follow-up of a prospective phase II study. Gastrointest Endosc 2004; 60:68-75.

51. Ortner ME, Caca K, Berr F, et al. Successful Photodynamic therapy for nonresectable cholangiocarcinoma: a randomized prospective study. Gastroenterology 2003;125: 1355-1363.

52. Khan SA, Thomas HC, Davidson BR, Taylor-Robinson SD. Cholangiocaarcinoma. Lancet 2005;366:1303-1314.

53. Patel AH, Harnois DM, Klee GG, Larusso NF, Gores GJ. The utility of CA19-9 in the diagnoses of cholangiocarcinoma in paatients without primary sclerosing cholangitis. Am J Gastroenterol 2000;95:204-207.

54. Lamerz R. Role of tumour markers, cytogenetics. Ann Oncol 1999;10(suppl 4):145-149.

55. Albert MB, Steinberg WM, Henry JP. Elevated serum levels of tumor marker CA19-9 in acute cholangitis. Dig Dis Sci 1988;33:1223-1225.

56. Siqueira E, Schoen RE, Silverman W, et al. Detecting cholangiocarcinoma in atients with primary sclerosing cholangitis. Gastrointest Endosc 2002;56:40-47.
57. Nehls O, Gregor M, Klump B. Serum and bile markers for cholangiocarcinoma. Semin Liver Dis 2004;24:139-154.
58. Soyer P, Bluemke DA, Reiche R, et al. Imaging of intrahepatic cholangiocarcinoma: 2. Hilar cholangiocarcinoma. AJR 1995;165:1433-1436.
59. Nesbit GM, Johnson CD, James EM, MacCarty RL, Nagorney DM, Bender CE. Cholangiocarcinoma: diagnosis and evaluation of resectability by CT and sonography as procedures complementary to cholangiography. AJR 1988;151:933-938.
60. Gibson RN, Yeung E, Thompson JN, et al. Bile duct obstruction: Radiologic evaluation of level, cause, and tumour resectability. Radiology 1986;160:43-47.
61. Hann LE, Fong Y, Shriver CD, et al. Malignant hepatic hilar tumors: can ultrasonography be used as an alternative to angiography with CT arterial portography for determination of resectability? J Ultrasound Med 1996;15:37-45.
62. Hann LE, Greatrex KV, Bach AM, Fong Y, Blumgart LH. Cholangiocarcinoma at the hepatic hilus: sonographic findings. AJR 1997;168:985-989.
63. Robledo R, Muro A, Prieto ML. Extrahepatic bile duct carcinoma: US characteristics and accuracy in demonstration of tumors. Radiology 1996;198:869-873.
64. Tillch M, Mischinger JJ, Preisegger KH, Rabi H, Szolar DH. Multiphasic helical CT in diagnosis and staging of hilar cholangiocarcinoma. AJR 1998;171:651-658.
65. Choi BI, Lee JH, Han MC, Kim SH, Yi JG, Kim C-W. Hilar cholangiocarcinoma: comparative study with sonography and CT. Radiology 1989;172:689-692.
66. Baer HU, Stain SC, Dennison AR, Eggers B, Blumgart LH. Improvements in survival by aggressive resections of hilar cholangiocarcinoma. Ann Surg 1993;217:20-27.
67. Feydy A, Vilgrain V, Denys A, et al. Helical CT assessment in hilar cholangiocarcinoma: Correlation with surgical and pathological findings. AJR 1999;172:73-77.
68. Han JK, Choi BI, Kim TK, et al. Hilar cholangiocarcinoma: thin-section spiral CT findings with cholangiographic correlation. Radiographics 1997;17:1475-1485.
69. Ferrucci. Liver tumor imaging: current concepts. Radiol Clin North Am 1994;32:39-54.
70. Choi BI, Lee JM, Han JK. Imaging of intrahepatic and hilar cholangiocarcinoma. Abdom Imaging 2004;29:548-557.
71. Lim JH, Kim MH, Kim TK, et al. Papillary neoplasm of the bile duct that mimic biliary stone disease. Radiographics 2003;23:447-455.
72. Choi BI, Han JK, Kim TD. Diagnosis and staging of cholangiocarcinoma by computed tomography. In: Meyers MA edi. Neoplasm of the digestive tract: imaging, staging and management. Lippincott-Raven, Philadelphia, pp503-516.
73. Manfredi R, Barbaro B, Masselli G, Vecchioli A, Marano P. Magnetic resonance imaging of cholagiocarcinoma. Semin Liver Dis 2004;24:155-164.

74. Khan SA, Davidson BR, Goldin R, et al. Guideline for the diagnosis and management of cholangiocarcinoma. Gut 2002;51,SVI:V11-V19.

75. Zidi SH, Prat F, Le Fuen O, Rondeau Y, Pelletier G. Performance characteristics of magnetic resonance cholangiography in the staging of malignant hilar strictures. Gut 2000;46:103-106.

76. Yamashita Y, Takahashi M, Kanazawa S, Charnsangavej C, Wallace S. Hilar cholangiocarcinoma. An evaluation of subtypes with CT and angiography. Acta Radiologica 1991;33:351-355.

77. Nimura Y, Kamiya J, Kondo S, Nagino M, Kanai M. Technique of inserting multiple biliary drains and management. Hepatogastroenterology 1995;42:323-331.

78. Nimura Y, Kamiya J, Kondo S, et al. Aggressive preoperative management and extended surgery for hilar cholangiocarcinoma: Nagoya experience. J Hep Bil Pancr Surg 2000;7: 155-162.

79. Tsao JI, Nimura Y, Kamiya J, et al. Management of hilar cholangiocarcinoma: comparison of an American and Japanese experience. Ann Surg 2000;232:166-174.

80. Otto G, Romaneehsen B, Bittinger F, et al. Preoperative imaging of hilar cholangiocarcinoma: surgical evaluation of standard practices. Z Gastroenterol 2004;42:9-14.

81. Otto G, Romaneehsen B, Hoppe Lotichius M, Bittinger F. Hilar cholangiocarcinoma: resectability and radicality after routine diagnostic imaging. J Hep Bil Pancr Surg 2004; 11: 310-318.

82. Anderson CD, Rice MH, Pinson CW, Chapman WC, Chari RS, Delbeke D. Fluorodeoxyglucose PET imaging in the evaluation of gallbladder carcinoma and cholangiocarcinoma. J Gastrointest Surg 2004;8:90-97.

83. Kato T, Tsukamoto E, Kuge Y, et al. Clinical role of (18)F-FDG PET for initial staging of patients with extrahepatic bile duct cancer. Eur J Nucl Med Mol Imaging 2002;29: 1047-1054.

84. Kim YJ, Yun M, Lee WJ, Kim KS, Lee JD. Usefulness of 18F-FDG PET in intrahepatic cholangiocarcinoma. Eur J Nucl Med Mol Imaging 2003;30:1467-1472.

85. Fritscher-Ravens A, Bohuslavizki KH, Boering DC, et al. FDG PET in the diagnosis of hilar cholangiocarcinoma. Nucl Med Commun 2001;22:1277-1285.

86. Wetter LA, Ring EJ, Pellegrini CA, Way LW. Diferential diagnosis of sclerosing cholangiocarcinomas of the common hepatic duct (Klatskin tumors). Am J Surg 1991; 161: 57-62.

87. Ryan ME. Cytologic brushings of ductal lesions during ERCP. Gstointest Endosc 1991; 37: 139-142.

88. Gerhards MF, Vos P, Van Gulik TM, Rauws EAJ, Bosma A, Gouma DJ. Incidence of benign lesions in patients resected for suspicious hilar obstruction. Br J Surg 2001;88:48-51.

89. Seo DW, Lee SK, You KS, et al. Cholangioscopic findings in bile duct tumors. Gastrointest Endosc 2000;52:630-634.

90. Kim H-J, Kim M-H, Lee S-K, et al. Tumor vessel: a valuable cholangioscopic clue of malignant biliary stricutre. Gastrointest Endosc 2000;52:635-638.

91. Seo DW, Kim M H, Lee SK, et al. Usefulness of cholangioscopy in patients with focal stricuture of the intrahepatic duct unrelated to intrahepatic stones. Gastrointest Endosc 1999;49:204-209.

92. Lee SS, Kim M-H, Lee SK, et al. MR cholangiography versus cholangioscopy for evaluation of longitudinal extension of hilar cholangiocarcinoma. Gastrointest Endosc 2002; 56:25-32.

93. Itoi T, Sofuni A, Itokawa F, et al. Peroral cholangioscopic diagnosis of biliary-tract diseases by using narrow-band imaging. Gastrointest Endosc 2007;66:730-736.

94. Chen YK, Pleskow DK. SpyGlass single-operator peroral cholangiopancreatoscopy system for the diagnosis and therapy of bile-duct disorders: a clinical feasibility study. Gastrointest Endosc 2007;65:832-841.

95. Weber SM, DeMatteo RP, Fong Y, Blumgart LHm Jarnagin WR. Staging laparoscopy in patients with extrahepatic biliary carcinoma. Analysis of 100 patients. Ann Surg 2002; 235: 392-399.

96. Klempnauer J, Werner M, Weimann A, Pichlmayr R. Resectional surgery of hilar cholangiocarcinoma: a multivariate analysis of prognostic factors. J Clin Oncol 1997;15: 947-954.

97. Nakajima T, Kondo Y, Miyazaki M, Okui K. A histopathologic study of 102 cases of intrahepatic cholangiocarcinoma: histologic classification and modes of spreading. Hum Pathol 1988;19:1228-1234.

98. Kosuge T, Yamamoto J, Shimada K, Yamasaki S, Makuuchi M. Improved surgical results for hilar cholangiocarcinoma with procedures including major hepatic resection. Ann Surg 1999;230:663-671.

99. Lillemoe KD, Cameron JL. Surgery for hilar cholangiocarcinoma: the Jphns Hopkins approach. J Hep Bily Pancr Surg 2000;7:115-121.

100. Neuhaus P, Jonas S, Bechstein WO, et al. Extended resections for hilar cholangiocarcinoma. Ann Surg 1999;230:808-819.

101. Otto Gerd. Doagnostic and surgical approaches in hilar cholangiocarcinoma. Int J Colorectal Dis 1007;22:101-108.

102. Nimura Y, Hayakawa K, Kamiya J, et al. Combined portal vein and liver resection for carcinoma of the biliary tract. Br J Surg 1991;78:727-731.

103. Lee SG, Lee JY, Park KM, et al. One hundred and eleven liver resections for hilar bile duct cancer. J Hep Bil Pancr Surg 2000;7:135-141.

104. Bismuth H, Castaing D, Traynor O. Resection or palliation: priority of surgery in the treatment of hilar cancer. World J Surg 1988;12:39-47.

105. Zervos EZ, Pearson H, Durkin AJ, et al. In-continuity hepatic resection for advanced hilar cholangiocarcinoma. Am J Surg 2004;188:584-588.

106. Miyazaki M, Ito H, Nakagawa K, et al. Parenchyma-preserving hepatectomy in the surgical tretment of hilar cholangiocarcinoma. J Am Coll Surg 1999;189:575-583.

107. Nagino M, Nimura Y, Kamiya J, et al. Segmental liver resections of hilar cholangiocarcinoma. Hepatogastroenterology 1998;45:7-13.

108. Nagino M, Nimura Y, Kamiya J, et al. Preoperative management of hilar cholangiocarcinoma. J Hepatobiliary Pancreat Surg 1995;2:215-223.

109. Blumgart LH, Benjamin IS, Hadjis NS, Beazley R. Surgical approaches to cholangiocarcinoma at confluence of hepatic ducts. Lancet 1984;1:66-70.

110. Ebata T, Nagino M, Kamiya J, Uesaka K, Nagasaka T, Nimura Y. Hepatectomy with portal vein resection for hilar cholangiocarcinoma: audit of 52 consecutive cases. Ann Surg 2003; 5:720-727.

111. D'Angelica MI, Jarnagin WR, Blumgart LH. Resectable hilar cholangiocarcinoma: Surgical treatment and long-term outcome. Surg Today 2004;34:885-890.

112. Hatfied AR, Tobias R, Terblanche J, et al. Preoperative external biliary drainage in obstructive jaundice. Lancet 1982;2:896-899.

113. Lai EC, Mok Ep, Fan ST. Preoperative endoscopic drainage for malignant obstructive jaundice. Br J Surg 1994;81:1195-1198.

114. Lygidakis NJ, van der Heyde MN, Lubbers MJ. Evaluation of preoperative biliary drainage in the surgical management of pancreatic head carcinoma. Acta Chir Scand. 1987;153: 665-668.

115. McPherson GAP, Benjamin IS, Hodgsons JF, et al. Preoperative percutaneous transhepatic biliary drainage: the results of a controlled trial. Br J Surg 1984;71:371-375.

116. Pitt HA, Gomes AS, Lois JF, et al. Does preoperative percutaneous biliary drainage reduce operative risk or increase hospital cost. Ann Surg 1985;201:545-553.

117. Brennan M. Periampullary and pancreatic cancer. In:Blumgart LH, Fong Y(eds). Surgery of the liver and biliary tract. WB Saunders, London, 2000, pp1059-1073.

118. Kato S, Nagano I, Nimura Y, Wakabayashi T. Hepatic recovery after biliary drainage in experimental obstructive jaundice complicated by biliary infection. Hepatogastroenterology 1994;41:217-221.

119. Nagano I, Kato S, Nimura Y, Wakabayashi T. Hepatic mitochondrial changes in experimental obstructive jaundice complicated by biliary infection. Hepatogastroenterology 1994;41:432-437.

120. Kanai M, Nimura Y, Kamiya J, et al. Preoperative intrahepatic segmental cholangitis in patients with advanced carcinoma involving the hepatic hilus. Surgery 1996;119:498-504.

121. Koyama K, Takagi Y, Ito K, Sato T. Experimental and clinical studies on the effect of biliary drainage in obstructive jaundice. Am J Surg 1981;142:293-239.

122. Miyata K. Delayed recovery of mitochondrial function in rat liver after releasing biliary obstruction. Nagoya J Med Sci 1983;45:97-105.

123. Miyazaki Y, Nimura Y, Tanaka M, Ozawa T. Delayed recovery of rat liver microsomal function after relief of biliary obstruction. J Clin Biochem Nutr 1989;6:127-134.

124. Kanai M, Tanaka M, Nimura Y, Nagino M, Katoh T, Ozawa T. Mitochondrial dysfunction in the non-obstructed lobe of rat liver after selective biliary obstruction. Hepato-gastroenterology 1992;39:385-391.

125. Seyama Y, Kubota K, Sano K, et al. Long-term outcome of extended hemihepatectomy for hilar bile duct cancer with no mortality and high survival rate. Ann Surg 2003;238:73-83.

126. Khan AZ, Makuuchi M. Trends in the surgical management of Klatskin tumours. Br J surg 2007;94:393-394.

127. Makuuchi M, Thai B, Takayasu K, et al. Preoperative portal embolization to increase safety of major hepatectomy for bile duct carcinoma: a preliminary report. Surgery 1990;107: 521-527.

128. Uesaka K, Nimura Y, Nagino M, et al. Changes in hepatic lobar function after right portal vein embolization: and appraisal by biliary indocyanine green excretion. Ann Surg 1996;223:77-83.

129. Launois B Wemyss-Holden S, Maddern GJ. Current and future trends in management and treatment of Klatskin tumour. Int J Clin Oncol 2002;7:91-102.

130. Nagino M, Kamiya J, Nishio H, Ebata T, Arai T, Nimura Y. Two hundred forty consecutive portal vein embolizations before extended hepatectomy for biliary cancer: surgical outcome and long-term follow-up. Ann Surg 2006;243:364-372.

131. Capussotti L, Muratore A, Polastri R, Ferrero A, Massucco P. Liver resection for hilar cholangiocarcinoma: in-hospital mortality and longterm survival. J Am Coll Surg 2002; 195: 641-647.

132. Launois B, Reding R, Lebeau G, Buard JL. Surgery for hilar cholangiocarcinoma: French experience in a collective survey of 552 extraheatic bile duct cancers. J Hepatobiliary Pancreat Surg 2000;7:128-134.

133. Mizumoto R, Suzuki H. Surgical anatomy of the hepatic hilum with special reference to the caudate lobe. world J Surg 1988;12:2-10.

134. Kamiya J, Nimura Y, Hayakawa N, Kondo S, Nagino M, Kanai M. Preoperative cholangiography of the caudate lobe: surgical anatomy and staging for biliary carcinoma. J Hep Bil Pancr Surg 1994;1:385-389.

135. Nimura Y, Hayakawa N, Kamiya J, Kondo S, Nagino M, Kanai M. Hilar cholangiocarcinoma-surgical anatomy and curative resection. J Hep Bil Pancr Surg 1995;2:239-248.

136. Nimura Y. Surgical anatomy of the biliary ducts. In: Rossi P, ed. Biliary tract radiology. Berlin Heidlberg: Springer, 1996:21-30.

137. Nimura Y, Hayakawa N, Kamiya J, Kondo S, Shionaya S. Hepatic segmentectomy with caudate lobe resection for bile duct carcinoma of the hepatic hilus. World J Surg 1990; 14: 535-544.

138. Iwatsuki S, Todo S, Marsh JW, et al. Treatment of hilar cholangiocarcinoma with hepatic resection or transplantation. J Am Coll Surg 1998;187:358-364.

139. Jeyarajah DR, Klintmalm GB. Is liver transplantation indicated for cholangiocarcinoma. J Hep Bil Pancr Surg 1998;5:493-496.

140. Rea DJ, Heimbach JK, Bosen CB, et al. Liver transplantation with neoadjuvant chemoradiation is more effective than resection for hilar cholangiocarcinoma. Ann Surg 2005;242:451-461.

141. Kaassis M, Boyer J, Dumas R, et al. Plastic or metal stents for malignant stricture of the common bile duct? Results of a randomized prospective study. Gastrointest Endosc 2003;57:178-182.

142. Chang WH, Kortan P, Haber GB. Outcome in patients with bifurcation tumors who undergo unilateral versus bilateral hepatic duct drainage. Gastrointest Endosc 1998;47: 354-362.

143. Peters RA, Williams SG, Lombard M, et al. The management of high-grade hilar strictures by endoscopic insertion of self-expanding metal endoprostheses. Endoscopy 1997;29:10-16.

144. Dowsett JF, Vaira D, Hatfield AR, et al. Endoscopic biliary therapy using the combined percutaneous and endoscopic technique. Gastroenterology 1989;96:1180-1186.

145. Deviere J, Baize M, de Toeuf J, Cremer M. Long-term follow-up of patients with hilar malignant stricture treated by endoscopic internal biliary drainage. Gastrointest Endosc 1988;34:95-101.

146. De Palma GD, Galloro G, Siciliano S, et al. Unilateral versus bilateral endoscopic hepatic duct drainage in patients with malignant hilar biliary obstruction: results of a prospective, randomized, and controlled study. Gastrointest Endosc 2001;53:547-553.

147. De Palma GE, Pezzullo A, Rega M, et al. Unilateral placement of metallic stents for malignant hilar obstruction: a prospective study. Gastrointest Endosc 2003;58:50-53.

148. Hintze RE, Abou-Rebyeh H, Adler A, et al. Magnetic resonance cholangiopancreatography-guided unilateral endoscopic stent placement for Klatskin tumors. Gastrointest Endosc 2001;53:40-46.

149. Kim CW, Park AW, Won JW, Kim S, Lee JW, Lee SH. T-configurated ductal stent placement in malignant biliary hilar duct obstructions with a newly designed stent. J Vasc Inter Radiol 2004;15:713-717.

150. Lee JH, Kang DW, Kim JY, et al. Endoscopic bilateral metal stent placement for advanced hilar cholangiocarcinoma: a pilot study of a newly designed Y stent. Gastrointest Endosc 2007;66:364-369.

151. Molnar W, Stockum AE. Relief of obstructive jaundice through percutaneous transhepatic catheter-a new therapeutic method. AJR 1974;122:356-367.

152. Barth KH. Percutaneous biliary drainage for high obstruction. Radiol Clin North Am 1990;28:1223-1235.

153. Gunther RW, Schild H, Thelen M. Review article: Percutaneous transhepatic biliary drainage: experience with 311 patients. Cardiovasc Intervent Radiol 1988;11:65-71.

154. Speer A, Cotton PB, Russel RCG et al. Randomized trial of endoscopic versus percutaneous stent insertion in malignant obstructive jaundice. Lancet 1987;2:57-70.

155. Lammer J. Biliary endoprosthesis; plastic versus metal stents. Radiol Clin North Am 1990; 28:1223-1235.

156. Kuvshinoff BW, Armstrong JG, Fong Y, et al. Palliation of irresectable hilar cholangiocarcinoma with biliary drainage and radiotherapy. Br J Surg 1995;82:1522-1555.

157. Eschelman DJ, Shapiro MJ, Bonn J, et al. Malignant biliary duct obstruction: long term experience with Giantruco stents and combined modality radiation therapy. Radiology 1996;200:717-724.

158. Hii MWJ, Gibson RN. Role of radiology in the treatment of malignant hilar biliary strictures:Review of the literature. Australian Radiol 2004;48:3-13.

159. Lee KH, Kim KW. Biliary intervention for cholangiocarcinoma. Abdom Imaging 2004; 29: 581-589.

160. Inal M, Akgul E, Aksungur E, Seydaoglu G. Percutaneous placement of biliary metallic stents in patients with malignant hilar obstruction: Unilobar versus bilobar drainage. J Vasc Interv Radiol 2003;14:1409-1416.

161. Mulholland MW, Yahanda A, Teo CJ. Multidisciplinary management of perihilar bile duct cancer. J Am Coll Surg 2001;193:440-447.

162. Schleithauer W. Review of gemcitabine in biliary tract carcinoma. Semin Oncol 1002; 29 (suppl 20):40-45.

163. Knox JJ, Hedley D, Oza A, et al. Combining gemcitabine and capecitabine in patients with advanced biliary cancer: A phase II trial. J Clin Oncol 2005;23:2332-2338.

164. Airoldi M, Cattel L, Passera R, Pedani F, Milla P, Zanon C. Gemcitabine and oxaliplatin in patients with pancreatic adenocarcinoma. Pancreas 2006;32:44-50.

165. Bruha R, Petryl J, Kubecova M, et al. Intraluminal brachytherapy and self expandable stents in nonresectable biliay malignancies-the question of long-term palliation. Hepatogastroenterology 2001;48:631-637.

166. Montemaggi P, Costamagna G, Dobelbower RR, et al. Intraluminal brachytherapy in treatment of pancreas and bile duct carcinoma. Int Radiat Oncol Biol Phys 1995;32:437-443.

167. Gerhards MF, vanGulik TM, Gonzalez GD, Rauws EA, Gouma DJ. Results of postoperative radiotherapy for resectable hilar cholangiocarcinoma. World J Surg 2003; 27: 173-179.

168. Pitt HA, Nakeeb A, Abrams RA, et al. Perihilar cholangiocarcinoma. Postoperative radiotherapy does not improve survival. Ann Surg 1995;221:788-797.

169. Anderson CD, Pinson CW, Berlin J, Chari RS. Diagnosis and treatment of cholangiocarcinoma. Oncologist 2004;9:43-57.

170. Figueras J, Llado L, Valls C, et al. Changing strategies in diagnosis and management of hilar cholangiocarcinoma. Liver Transpl 2000;6:786-794.

171. Rauws EAJ. Photodynamic therapy and Klatskin tumour: An overview. Scan J Gastroenterol 2006;41(Suppl 243):135-138.

172. Witzigmann H, Berr F, Ringel U, et al. Surgical and palliative management and outcome in 184 patients with hilar cholangiocarcinoma: palliative photodynamic therapy plus stenting is comparable to R1/R2 resection. Ann Surg 2006;244:230-239.

XII • Early Bile Duct Cancer

XII Early Bile Duct Cancer

Myung-Hwan Kim, M.D., Jae Myung Cha, M.D.

XII
Early Bile Duct Cancer

Even with recent advances in diagnostic modalities, an early diagnosis of bile duct cancer remains notoriously difficult because of its late clinical presentation until the tumor has grown to an advanced stage. Advanced bile duct cancer is usually fatal and over half of the cases present with unresectable malignancies. Surgery still remains the only curative treatment for bile duct cancer and there is no effective nonsurgical therapeutic modalities.[1] Therefore, early detection is a prerequisite for the curative resection, and there has been a need to diagnose bile duct cancer at its early stage.[2,3] However, the definition and concept of early bile duct cancer has not been broadly accepted at the present time, in contrast with the established concept of early cancer in the hollow viscus.

The aim of differentiating early bile duct cancer from advanced bile duct cancer is to predict a better prognosis based on a high rate of curative resections through early diagnosis. Since the reported papers on early bile duct caner have been scarce and mainly originate from Japan and Korea,[2-11] physicians from other countries may have overlooked cases of early bile duct cancer due to a lack of recognition and the rarity of this disease. In this chapter, the definition, clinicopathological features, and long-term survival rate of early bile duct cancer will be covered based on recent studies. This chapter will assist in understanding the concept of early bile duct cancer and ultimately serve to identify more of such cases.

1. Anatomy of the Bile Duct

Bile ducts are anatomically classified as either an intrahepatic or extrahepatic bile duct. Extrahepatic bile ducts are classified as perihilar or distal bile ducts,[12,13] and intrahepatic bile ducts are classified as either intrahepatic large bile ducts or intrahepatic small bile ducts.[14,15] Intrahepatic large bile ducts are grossly visible and characterized by the presence of a fibrous ductal wall, while intrahepatic small bile ducts are recognizable using only a microscope and are characterized by the absence of a fibrous ductal wall.[14,15] Microscopically, the layer of bile duct wall is different from that of hollow viscus, as the layers of muscular mucosa, submucosa, and muscular propria are absent in the bile duct wall. The bile duct is lined by a single layer of columnar cells and its walls consist of intermixed dense fibrous tissue and muscle fibers, the fibromuscular layer.[16,17] Biliary epithelial cells lining the extrahepatic bile duct and intrahepatic large bile ducts have a different embryologic origin and phenotype from biliary epithelial cells lining intrahepatic small bile ducts.[18] Defining the layer of the bile duct wall is often not easy in intrahepatic large bile ducts and impossible in intrahepatic small bile ducts, as the fibromuscular layer is very scant or absent.[16,17] For such reasons, the articles dealing with early bile duct cancer, which requires the histologic determination on the extent of bile duct wall invasion, have been mainly limited to extrahepatic bile duct cancers.

2. Definition

The concept of early bile duct cancer was initially raised by the Japan Biliary Association in 1983,[19] and there have been a few articles regarding early bile duct cancer since then (Table 1).[3-10] The need for such a concept was based on the observation that bile duct cancer of this type had a more favorable prognosis. In the literature review, the reported 5 year survival rates for early bile duct cancer ranged from 80% to 100%. Mizumoto *et al*[6] reported a 5 year survival rate for patients with cancer invasion within the fibromuscular layer of 100%, on the other hand, rates for patients with cancer invasion to serosa was 15%. Kurosaki *et al*[8] reported a 5-year

Table 1. Publications on Early Bile Duct Cancers

Author	Year	5 year survival rate	Number of early cancer	Total number of cholangiocarcinoma
Tsunoda *et al*[4]	1989	NM	8 (6%)	146
Yamaguchi[5]	1992	NM	7	NM
Mizumoto *et al*[6]	1993	100%	14 (8%)	171
Bhuiya *et al*[7]	1993	NM	7 (10%)	70
Kurosaki *et al*[8]	1998	86%	7 (8%)	90
Tamada *et al*[9]	2001	NM	10 (18%)	55
Lim *et al*[10]	2006	NM	23 (3%)	742
Cha *et al*[3]	2006	80%	61 (10%)	614

NM: not mentioned

survival rate for 7 patients with extrahepatic pT1 bile duct cancer of 86%. Recently, we also demonstrated a 5-year survival rate of 80% for patients with bile duct cancers confined within the fibromuscular layer.[3] Based on these observations, bile duct cancer which invasion is confined within the fibromuscular layer of extrahepatic bile duct was termed 'early bile duct cancer' (Fig. 1), while invasion beyond the fibromuscular layer was termed 'advanced bile duct cancer'.

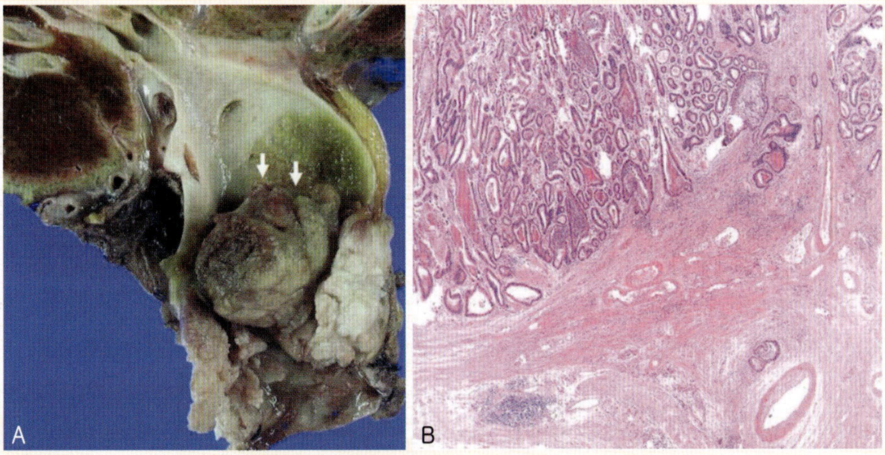

Fig. 1 Macroscopic and microscopic findings of an extrahepatic early bile duct cancer

A: A papillary mass (arrows) protruding into the common bile duct lumen is noted. B: Although it is fairly large, its invasion is confined within the fibromuscular layer (HE x 100). (Reprint permission from World J Gastroenterol 2007;13:3409-3416).

On the other hand, attempts to define intrahepatic early bile duct cancer have been much less productive because the fibromuscular layer, which is the histologic boundary to define early cancer, is very scant or totally absent in the intrahepatic bile ducts.[16,17] Recently, we suggested that intrahepatic early bile duct cancer arising from intrahepatic large bile duct may be defined using the same criteria for extrahepatic early bile duct cancer (Fig. 2),[3] because the histology of intrahepatic large bile duct does not differ from that of extrahepatic bile duct.[16] In contrast, defining the layer of the bile duct wall is impossible for intrahepatic small bile ducts,[16,17] and mass-forming cholangiocarcinoma arising from intrahepatic small bile ducts differ clinicopathologically from bile duct cancer arising from extrahepatic bile duct or intrahepatic large bile duct.[20] Therefore, mass-forming cholangiocarcinoma, so called "peripheral cholangiocarcinoma", should be differentiated, and excluded from the concept of early bile duct cancer.[2,3] For the concept of early cancer in mass-forming peripheral cholangiocarcinoma, a different criterion such as solitary cholangiocarcinoma without vascular invasion may be developed in the further studies.[21]

In summary, early bile duct cancer may be defined as a bile duct cancer whose invasion is confined within the fibromuscular layer of the extrahepatic bile duct or intrahepatic large bile duct without distant metastasis irrespective of lymph node involvement.[2,3] However, an internationally agreed concept of early bile duct cancer for extrahepatic and intrahepatic bile duct lesion is necessary and should be defined

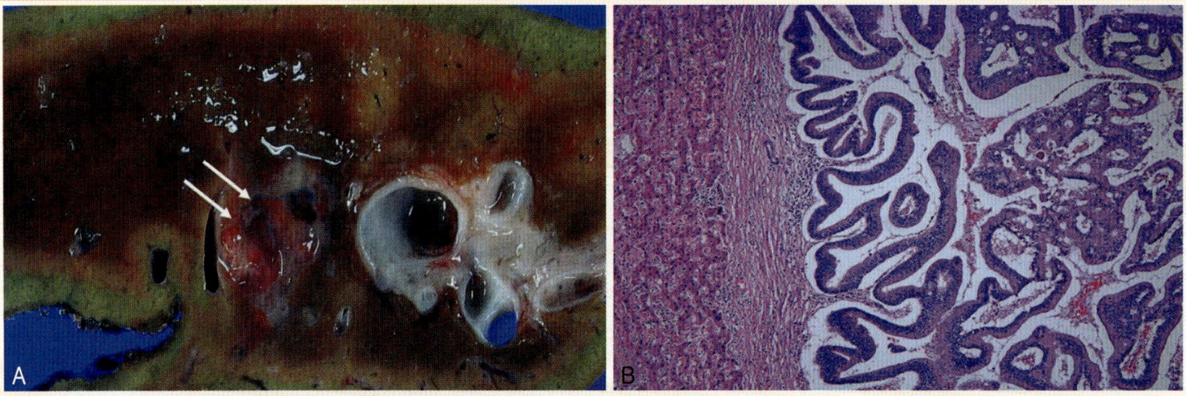

Fig. 2 Macroscopic and microscopic findings of an intrahepatic early bile duct cancer

A: Gross specimen of resected liver in a patient with papillary mass (white arrows) within the intrahepatic large bile duct. B: Tumor invasion is confined within the fibromuscular layer without hepatic parenchymal invasion (H & E stain, ×100).

at worldwide meeting of experts, including gastroenterologists, pathologists, radiologists and surgeons.

The T classification for extrahepatic bile duct cancer was refined in the new 6th edition of the American Joint Committee on Cancer (AJCC) staging system.[22] The previous T1 classification on 5th edition of AJCC staging,[23] was defined as "tumors invading subepithelial connective tissue (T1a) and the fibromuscular layer (T1b)", however, it was refined as "tumors confined to the bile duct histologically" in the AJCC 6th edition. Because the current T1 classification is defined using vague terms as "confined to the bile duct" without the mention about a precise histological layer such as a fibromuscular layer,[24] it may be difficult to discriminate extrahepatic early bile duct cancer from T1 extrahepatic bile duct cancer exactly in this new staging system. Intrahepatic early bile duct cancer, which is staged similarly to hepatocellular carcinoma by vascular invasion and tumor size, is also differentiated from T1 intrahepatic bile duct cancer.[21]

3. Prevalence

Bile duct cancer is more prevalent in Asian countries than in the United States and Europe. Although there is a significant geographic variation in the incidence of bile duct cancer, the worldwide incidence of bile duct cancer has risen over the past three decades.[25-27] The exact prevalence of early bile duct cancer among overall bile duct cancer is unknown. Around 3~21% of resected bile duct cancers are classified as early cancers in the literature (Table 1).[3-10] We previously reported that 10% of 614 patients with histologically confirmed primary bile duct cancer after resection were found to be early bile duct cancers.[3] In this report, 11% of overall intrahepatic bile duct cancers and 9% of total extrahepatic bile duct cancers were early bile duct cancers, respectively. However, worldwide epidemiologic studies regarding the prevalence of early bile duct cancer are necessary, since articles on early bile duct cancer have originated mainly from the geographically adjacent Japan and Korea.[3-11] The more frequent occurrence of early bile duct cancer in Japan and Korea might be explained by two reasons: (1) known risk factors for bile duct cancer such as hepatolithiasis or liver-fluke infestation, are endemic in the East Asia,[25-27] and (2) higher chances to detect early bile duct cancers incidentally from more frequent performance of percutaneous transhepatic cholangioscopy (PTCS) for other biliary diseases in these countries.[28] While an early bile duct cancer is not a common disease, it may not be a very rare entity either.

4. Clinical Characteristics

Little has been known about the clinical characteristics and risk factors of early bile duct cancer. The peak age for patients with early bile duct cancer is the seventh decade and the gender incidence shows a slight male preponderance.[3-11] Presenting symptoms of patients with early bile duct cancer are characteristic, in that they rarely complain of abdominal pain or jaundice typically associated with advanced bile duct cancer patients. We reported that 39% of patients with early bile duct cancer were asymptomatic and 84% of patients were non-jaundiced.[3] Among known risk factors for bile duct cancer,[25-27,29] hepatolithiasis, liver-fluke infestation, biliary papillomatosis and choledochal cyst with or without anomalous union of pancreaticobiliary ducts are also associated with early bile duct cancers.[2,3] Since articles on early bile duct cancer have originated mainly from Asian countries,[3-11] its association with primary sclerosing cholangitis, which is a main risk factor for bile duct cancer in the Western countries,[30-32] should be elucidated from the future studies. Close association with papillomatosis and early bile duct cancer is no wonder, and it is consistent with the fact that biliary papillomatosis has recently been shown to be a highly premalignant condition.[33] These chronic biliary diseases may lead to long-term irritation and inflammation of the bile duct epithelium with resultant fibrosis and dysplasia.[26,33]

Most of patients with early bile duct cancer showed a cholestatic profile on liver function tests. Elevated levels of bile duct origin enzyme (serum alkaline phosphatase and gamma glutamyltransferase) are the most frequent abnormal biochemical results linked to patients with early bile duct cancer.[3] Serum CA 19-9 screening may have a limited value in the diagnosis of early bile duct cancer because its levels were significantly elevated in only 15% of patients with early bile duct cancer.[3]

The Liver Cancer Study Group of Japan has recently proposed that bile duct cancers could be classified as one of three types based on gross morphology: mass-forming, periductal-infiltrating or intraductal-growing types.[34] The periductal-infiltrating type was reported to be the most common gross type of overall extrahepatic bile duct cancer,[25,35] whereas the most common gross type of early bile duct cancer is intraductal-growing type, which are observed in 47~100% of patients.[2,3-6,9,36] Occasionally, it may be difficult to classify gross type of early bile duct cancers due to its subtle gross changes.[3] Early bile duct cancers may cause large and fairly extensive tumors despite early stages in some patients (Fig. 1), because it grew mainly intraluminally without deep invasion into the bile duct wall.[2,3]

For histological classification, adenocarcinoma has been found to comprise greater than 90% of overall bile duct cancers,[25-27,29] while it comprises only 10~67% of early bile duct cancers.[2,3,5,6,9,10,36] On the other hand, papillary carcinoma is more common in early bile duct cancers, comprising up to 31~90%.[2-4,7-9,33,37] Frequent occurrence of intraductal-growing type or papillary carcinoma in patients with early bile duct cancer may be explained by the fact that these tumor types grow and spread superficially along the bile duct mucosa and do not invade deeply into the bile duct wall.[38] Limited locoregional extensions in patients with early bile duct cancer also support the concept of early bile duct cancer. Early bile duct cancer without venous or perineural invasions and lymph node metastasis were reported as 71~100% in previous studies.[3,5,6,9]

5. Diagnosis

Comprehensive approaches using noninvasive and invasive modalities are necessary for the diagnosis of early bile duct cancer. Early bile duct cancers, when they are small, may not be depicted using abdominal ultrasound (US) or computed tomography (CT).[10] We failed to identify an evident mass using abdominal US in approximately half of patients with early bile duct cancer.[3] Focal biliary stricture or suspicious intraductal polypoid mass with proximal ductal dilatation detected on these tests raises high suspicion for the existence of early bile duct cancer. The most valuable finding of early bile duct cancer on conventional imaging studies is a demonstration of the bile duct wall and its integrity.[10] Because bile duct dilatation on imaging study was coupled with a high level of bile duct origin enzyme in 93% of patients with early bile duct cancer,[3] this combination warrants further evaluation for early bile duct cancer despite non-visualization of masses with conventional imaging studies. Magnetic resonance cholangiography (MRC) can facilitate overviews of longitudinal cancer spread by assessing bile ducts upstream and downstream of the tumor simultaneously and permits assessment of the vessels.[39,40] The noninvasive nature of MRC may play a more important role in detecting patients with early bile duct cancer because many of these patients were asymptomatic.[3]

Asymptomatic patients may be reluctant to undergo major operations without the certainty of a malignancy, as a radiographic findings alone may not distinguish reliably between malignant and benign lesions.[41-43] If the suspected lesion is extrahepatic in location, histopathologic sampling is possible without any difficulty by brush cytology and/or biopsy through endoscopic retrograde cholangiopancreatography (ERCP). Transpapillary peroral cholangioscopy (POCS) with or without narrow-band imaging (NBI) can also be attempted, if available.[44,45] POCS with NBI may be helpful for the detection of early bile duct cancer by observation of both fine mucosal structure and tumor vessels, however its value in identifying early bile duct cancer has not been addressed. Endoscopic ultrasound (EUS) appears to be an emerging technique for evaluating asymptomatic dilatation of the extraheptic bile duct,[46] and EUS-guided fine needle aspiration (FNA) was reported with a greater sensitivity for detecting malignancy than ERCP with brush cytology in cases with extrahepatic bile duct wall thickening.[47] The PTCS is useful for the histological diagnosis of intrahepatic bile duct lesions.[28] Cholangioscopic findings in patients with early bile duct cancer were diverse from subtle mucosal changes to evident papillary masses of the bile duct,[2,3,33] and identification of these changes may allow targeted biopsy for accurate diagnosis.

New molecular and imaging diagnostic modalities may emerge as a promising tool in the diagnosis of early bile duct cancer. Recently, digitized image analysis and fluorescence *in situ* hybridization may offer greater promise to evaluate bile duct cancers for cellular aneuploidy and chromosomal aberrations.[48-50] These molecular methods may become valuable tools for the detection of early bile duct cancer in the future as recent reports[49,50] have demonstrated that their sensitivities are superior to and specificities are similar to standard cytology for the diagnosis of bile duct cancer. For imaging modalities, positron emission tomography (PET) is an emerging diagnostic technique for the detection of bile duct cancer,[51] which can be utilized to ascertain malignancy by finding hot uptake at the suspected site when histological sampling is difficult. As this technique has become widely available recently, additional information on its use for the diagnosis of early bile duct cancer will be forthcoming.

6. Algorithm for Detecting Early Bile Duct Cancer

In clinical practice, there are largely two clinical settings that early bile duct cancer can be diagnosed prospectively (Fig. 3). The first starts off from detection of bile duct dilatation on conventional radiologic imaging.[2,10] This could be from asymptomatic patients undergoing health screening, from the workup of vague or nonspecific abdominal discomfort or incidentally detected abnormalities in the enzyme of bile duct origin. If the suspected lesion is extrahepatic in location, histopathologic sampling is possible without difficulty by brush cytology and/or biopsy through ERCP. If available, POCS with or without NBI[45] or EUS-guided FNA[47] can also be attempted. If the suspected lesion is intrahepatic in location, PET can be utilized to ascertain its malignant nature by finding hot uptake at the suspected site. For PET-negative intrahepatic lesions, PTCS with biopsy may be helpful to confirm the histological diagnosis. Although some do not recommend percutaneous biopsy for potentially resectable bile duct cancer due to the risk of tumor seeding,[52] confirmating of a malignancy in equivocal cases greatly increases both the compliance of patients without symptoms and the confidence of the physician planning a major operation such as hepatic resection.[2]

The second clinical pathway that early bile duct cancer can be diagnosed is during the follow up of patients with known risk factors for bile duct cancer. Detection of progressive increase of bile duct origin enzyme and tumor marker or progression of bile duct dilatation during surveillance suggests change in their clinical status and

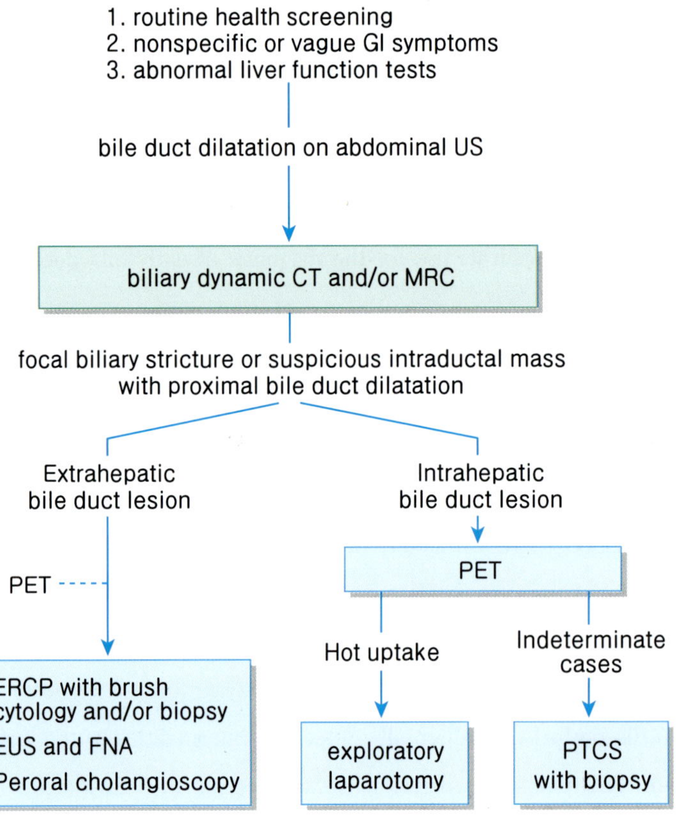

Fig. 3 Proposed algorithm for detecting an early bile duct cancer

GI, gastrointestinal; US, ultrasound; CT, computed tomography; MRC, magnetic resonance cholangiography; PET, positron emission tomography; ERCP, endoscopic retrograde cholangiopancreatography; EUS, endoscopic ultrasound; FNA, fine needle aspiration; PTCS, percutaneous transhepatic cholangioscopy. (Reprint permission from World J Gastroenterol 2007;13:3409-3416).

warrant further evaluation. Finding of newly appeared or aggravated ductal stricture and/or mass suggests development of a bile duct cancer, and the subsequent workup follows the clinical pathway previously mentioned.

7. Prognosis and Disease Recurrence

As the prognosis of overall bile duct cancer remains disappointing and no recent breakthrough has been achieved, it is encouraging to see a dramatic improvement in the prognosis of a subset of bile duct cancer identified as an early stage. As previously mentioned, a reported 5 year survival rates for extrahepatic early bile duct cancer ranged from 80% to 100% (Table 1). Recently, we also reported a 5-year survival rate of 80% for patients with early bile duct cancer including extrahepatic and intrahepatic lesions.[3] Therefore, detection of early bile duct cancer may provide the better prognosis in patients with bile duct cancer.

Disease recurrence in early bile duct cancer have been very low by 0~14%.[3-6] Disease recurrences despite its early stage was explained by the frequent occurrence of intraductal-growing types or papillary carcinomas in early bile duct cancers, which may remain undetected by conventional imaging studies due to their tendency to spread superficially along the mucosa. It suggests that more thorough pre-operative evaluation of disease extent should be emphasized in patients with early bile duct cancer.

Major prognostic determinant may be the detection of early cancer rather than histological tumor types, as a longer survival was linked with early detection regardless of gross or histological types in patients with early bile duct cancer.[3] Papillary carcinomas have been believed to have a more favorable outcome than other histological types in bile duct cancers,[53] however, Kurosaki *et al*[8] found that patients with pT1 papillary carcinoma showed relatively prolonged survival, whereas patients with pT2 or pT3 papillary carcinoma did not show such a long survival rate.

Conclusion

Early bile duct cancer may be defined as a carcinoma, whose invasion is confined within the fibromuscular layer of the extrahepatic bile duct or intrahepatic large bile duct without distant metastasis irrespective of lymph node involvement. Approximately 3~10% of resected bile duct cancers have been reported to be early cancers in the literature. The clinicopathological features of patients with early bile duct cancer differ from those of patients with advanced bile duct cancer, with more frequent asymptomatic presentation, characteristic histopathological findings, and excellent prognosis. Clinicians may be successful in identifying patients with early bile duct cancers, if they have a high index of suspicion and knowledge regarding this disease entity.

Reference

1. Khan SA, Miras A, Pelling M, Taylor-Robinson SD. Cholangiocarcinoma and its management. Gut 2007;56:1755-1756.
2. Cha JM, Kim MH, Jang SJ. Early bile duct cancer. World J Gastroenterol 2007;13: 3409-3416.
3. Cha JM, Kim MH, Lee SK, et al. Clinicopathological review of 61 patients with early bile duct cancer. Clinical Oncology 2006;18:669-677.
4. Tsunoda T, Eto T, Koga M, et al. Early carcinoma of the extrahepatic bile duct. Jpn J Surg 1989;19:691-698.
5. Yamaguchi K. Early bile duct carcinoma. Aust N Z J Surg 1992;62:525-529.
6. Mizumoto R, Ogura Y, Kusuda T. Definition and diagnosis of early cancer of the biliary tract. Hepatogastroenterology 1993;40:69-77.
7. Bhuiya MR, Nimura Y, Kamiya J, Kondo S, Nagino M, Hayakawa N. Clinicopathologic factors influencing survival of patients with bile duct carcinoma: multivariate statistical analysis. World J Surg 1993;17:653-657.
8. Kurosaki I, Tsukada K, Watanabe H, Hatakeyama K. Prognostic determinants in extrahepatic bile duct cancer. Hepatogastroenterology 1998;45:905-909.
9. Tamada K, Tomiyama T, Wada S, et al. Cholangiographic findings of early-stage extrahepatic bile duct carcinoma. J Gastroenterol 2001;36:827-841.
10. Lim JH, Jang KT, Choi DI, Lee WJ, Lim HK. Early bile duct carcinoma: comparison of imaging features with pathologic findings. Radiology 2006;238:542-548.
11. Kim HJ, Bang SM, Park SW, et al. Assessement of the definition of early extrahepatic bile duct cancer through the prognosis analysis who had received curative resection. Korean J Gastroenterol 2007;50:101-107.
12. Okuda K, Nakanuma Y, Miyazaki M. Cholangiocarcinoma: recent progress. Part 1: epidemiology and etiology. J Gastroenterol Hepatol 2002;17:1049-1055.
13. Nakeeb A, Pitt HA, Sohn TA, et al. Cholangiocarcinoma: a spectrum of intrahepatic, perihilar, and distal tumors. Ann Surg 1996;224:463-475.
14. Crawford JM. Development of the intrahepatic biliary tree. Semin Liver Dis 2002;22: 213-226.

15. Nakanuma Y, Hoso M, Sanzen T, Sasaki M. Microstructure and development of the normal and pathologic biliary tract in humans, including blood supply. Microsc Res Tech 1997;38:552-570.

16. Hong SM, Kang GH, Lee HY, Ro JY. Smooth muscle distribution in the extrahepatic bile duct: histologic and immunohistochemical studies of 122 cases. Am J Surg Pathol 2000;24:660-667.

17. Hong SM, Presley AE, Stelow EB, Frierson HF Jr, Moskaluk CA. Reconsideration of the histologic definitions used in the pathologic staging of extrahepatic bile duct carcinoma. Am J Surg Pathol 2006;30:744-749.

18. Alpini GD. Biliary wound healing, ductular reactions, and IL-6/gp130 signaling in the development of liver disease. World J Gastroenterol 2006;12:3512-3522.

19. Hidaka E, Yanagisawa A, Makoto S, Takano K, Kato H. The opinions from the standpoint of pathology concerning "General Rules for surgical and pathological studies on cancer of the biliary tract, the 4th edition." Kan Tan Sui 2000;41:543-550 (In Japanese).

20. Huang JL, Biehl TR, Lee FL, Zimmer PW, Ryan JA Jr. Outcomes after resection of cholangiocarcinoma. Am J Surg 2004;187:612-617.

21. Okabayashi T, Yamamoto J, Kosuge T, et al. A new staging system for mass-forming intrahepatic cholangiocarcinoma: analysis of preoperative and postoperative variables. Cancer 2001;92:2374-2383.

22. Greene FL, Page DL, Fleming ID, et al. AJCC cancer staging manual, 6th ed. New York: Springer-Verlag, 2002.

23. Fleming ID, Cooper JS, Hensen DE, et al. AJCC cancer staging manual, 5th ed. Philadelphia. Lippincott Raven, 1998.

24. Hong SM, Kim MJ, Pi DY, et al. Analysis of extrahepatic bile duct carcinomas according to the new American joint committee on cancer staging system focused on tumor classification problems in 222 patients. Cancer 2005;104:802-810.

25. Lazaridis KN, Gores GJ. Cholangiocarcinoma. Gastroenterology 2005;128:1655-1667.

26. Olnes MJ, Erlich R. A review and update on cholangiocarcinoma. Oncology. 2004;66: 167-179.

27. De Groen PC, Gores GJ, LaRusso NF, Gunderson LL, Nagomey DM. Biliary Tract Cancers. N Engl J Med 1999;341:1368-1378.

28. Kim MH, Yasuda K. Percutaneous transhepatic cholangioscopic examination: a necessity for the biliary endoscopist. Gastrointest Endosc. 2001;53:695-697.

29. Khan SA, Thomas HC, Davidson BR, Taylor-Robinson SD. Cholangiocarcinoma. Lancet 2005;366:1303-1314.

30. Rosen CB, Nagorney DM, Wiesner RH, Coffey RJ Jr, LaRusso NF. Cholangiocarcinoma complicating primary sclerosing cholangitis. Ann Surg 1991;213:21-25.

31. Kim JY, Kim MH, Kim SD, et al. 28 cases of primary sclerosing cholangitis. Korean J Med 2004;66:127-134.

32. Takikawa H, Manabe T. Primary sclerosing cholangitis in Japan-analysis of 192 cases. J Gastroenterol 1997;32:134-137.

33. Lee SS, Kim MH, Lee SK, et al. Clinicopathologic review of 58 patients with biliary papillomatosis. Cancer 2004;100:783-793.

34. Lim JH. Park CK. Pathology of cholangiocarcinoma. Abdom Imaging 2004;29:540-547.

35. Rosai T. Rosai and Ackerman's surgical pathology. 9th ed. St Louis:Mosby, 2004: 1049-1050.

36. Kozuka S, Tsubone M, Hachisuka K. Evolution of carcinoma in the extrahepatic bile ducts. Cancer 1984;54:65-72.

37. Jeong S, Lee JI, Lee JW, et al. Papillary type of early common bile duct cancer. Gastrointest Endosc 2007;65:916-917.

38. Lim JH. Cholangiocarcinoma: recent advances in imaging and intervention. Abdom Imaging 2004;29:538-539.

39. Takehara Y. Preoperative assessment of extrahepatic cholangiocarcinoma with imaging. Abdom Imaging 2004;29:572-580.

40. Zandrino F, Curone P, Benzi L, Ferretti ML, Musante F. MR versus multislice CT cholangiography in evaluating patients with obstruction of the biliary tract. Abdom Imaging 2005;30:77-85.

41. Tischendorf JJW, Kruger M, Trautwein C, et al. Cholangioscopic characterization of dominant bile duct stenosis in patients with primary sclerosing cholangitis. Endoscopy 2006;38:665-669.

42. Hadjis NS, Collier NA, Blumgart LH. Malignant masquerade at the hilum of the liver. Brit J Surg 1985;72:659-661.

43. Albert MB, Steinberg W, Henry JP. Elevated serum levels of tumor marker CA19-9 in acute cholangitis. Dig Dis Sci 1988;33:1223-1225.

44. Tsuyuguchi T, Fukuda Y, Saisho H. Peroral cholangioscopy for the diagnosis and treatment of biliary diseases. J Hepatobiliary Pancreat Surg 2006;13:94-99.

45. Itoi T, Sofuni A, Itokawa F, et al. Peroral cholangioscopic diagnosis of biliary-tract diseases by using narrow-band imaging (with videos). Gastrointest Endosc 2007;66:730-736.

46. Toole DO, Palazzo L. Choledocholithiasis-a practical approach from the endosonographer. Endoscopy 2006;38 (S1):S23-S29.

47. DeWitt J, Misra VL, LeBlanc JK, McHenry L, Sherman S. EUS-guided FNA of proximal biliary strictures after negative ERCP brush cytology results. Gastrointest Endosc 2006;64:325-333.

48. Gores GJ. Early detection and treatment of cholangiocarcinoma. Liver Transpl 2000;6: S30-S34.

49. Kipp BR, Stadheim LM, Halling SA, et al. A comparison of routine cytology and fluorescence *in situ* hybridization for the detection of malignant bile duct strictures. Am J Gastroenterol 2004;99:1675-1681.

50. Rumalla A, Baron TH, Leontovich O, et al. Improved diagnostic yield of endoscopic biliary brush cytology by digital image analysis. Mayo Clin Proc 2001;76:29-33.

51. Kim JY, Kim MH, Lee TY, et al. Clinical role of 18F-FDG PET-CT in suspected and potentially operable cholangiocarcinoma: a prospective study compared with conventional imaging. Am J Gastroenterol 2008;103:1145-1151.

52. Khan SA, Davidson BR, Goldin R, et al. Guidelines for the diagnosis and treatment of cholangiocarcinoma: consensus document. Gut 2002;51:1-9.

53. Ouchi K, Matsuno S, Sato T. Long-term survival in carcinoma of the biliary tract. Arch Surg 1989;124:248-252.

Index